Screening in General Practice

Screening in General Practice

Edited by C. R. Hart

CHURCHILL LIVINGSTONE
Edinburgh London and New York 1975

Churchill Livingstone

Medical Division of Longman Group Limited

Distributed in the United States of America by
Longman Inc., New York and by associated
companies, branches and representatives throughout
the world.

First published 1975

ISBN 0 443 01208 3

Printed in Great Britain

Preface

Over the past two decades there has been a steadily mounting interest in the possibilities afforded by modern investigative techniques for the detection of disease processes at a very early stage in their development, with the hopeful objective of improving prognosis for both morbidity and mortality. Within the United Kingdom, the National Health Service presents a special opportunity for the conduct of such activities in a general practice setting.

The time has not yet arrived for the immediate introduction of a comprehensive nation-wide medical screening programme, and such a policy is not advocated in this book. All we have set out to do is to evaluate the present status of medical screening in general practice in this country, to discuss those procedures that are already established, and to indicate where possible the scope for future development. There is of course room for a wide range of opinions concerning the value and desirability of medical screening, and while there is a general consensus among the contributors, on specific issues each of us can accept responsibility solely for those views put forward in his or her individual chapter.

Screening as a discipline is still in its infancy, and it is important that its development should rest on a firm basis of established principles. But the situation is changing so rapidly under the impact of the new technology, that some of our contributors have accepted the dangerous task of peering into the future. In Chapter 6, Mr J.H. Evans and Dr A.M. Semmence discuss the application of computerisation to screening. The possibilities are limitless, the practical obstacles formidable. Looking still further ahead, in Chapter 2 Dr J. Tudor Hart propounds a novel concept of screening that is entirely his own. Whether or not his views gain general acceptance, only time will tell. In assessing the value of these contributions, account must be taken of the fact that the authors speak with more extensive first-hand experience of their subjects than most of us, and therefore with correspondingly greater authority.

We have tried to make the scope of this book as comprehensive as possible. It should serve as a textbook for medical students and health visitors, as a handbook for postgraduate seminars, and as a reference book for all members of the general practice team. It is to be hoped that it will not be overlooked by medical administrators. Some of the earlier chapters should prove of interest to our colleagues in the social sciences, and indeed to the lay public in general both at home and abroad, for medical screening raises wide-ranging issues of social policy.

On a more personal note, I am proud to have undertaken the editorship of these fundamental studies, which are evidence—if such were needed—of the strength and versatility of general practice in Britain today. I would like to offer my thanks to Dr Dennis Guttmann, Consultant Physician to Peterborough District Hospital, for reading through many of the chapters and for offering valuable suggestions for their improvement, and to my secretary Mrs Barbara Munton for her unfailing patience and efficiency with administration and typing.

Cyril Hart

Stilton, Peterborough. 1974

Contents

List of contributors

M.H.F. Coigley MB, BS, MRCGP
General Practitioner, Stratford on Avon, Warwickshire.

P.J. Constable MD, MRCGP, DObstRCOG
General Practitioner, Welwyn Garden City, Hertfordshire.

J.T. Cope MB, BS, MRCGP
General Practitioner, Swineshead, Lincolnshire.

D. Craddock MD, MRCGP, DObstRCOG
General Practitioner, South Croydon, Surrey.

R. Harvard Davis DM, FRCGP
Hon. Director, General Practice Unit,
Welsh National School of Medicine, Cardiff.

J.H. Evans BSc
Senior Systems Analyst, Oxford Regional Hospital Board.

Sheila Ganeri SRN, SCM, HV
Nursing Tutor, Leicester Royal Infirmary
Formerly Health Visitor, Telford, Shropshire.

George Gomcz MB, BS, MRCGP
General Practitioner, Wimbledon, London.
Clinical Assistant, Ear, Nose and Throat Department,
St. George's Hospital, London.

I. Gregg MA, BM, FRCGP
General Practitioner, Kingston upon Thames, Surrey.
Senior Lecturer and Director, Department of Clinical
Epidemiology in General Practice, Cardiothoracic Institute,
Brompton Hospital, London.

C.R. Hart MA, MB, MRCGP, FRHistS
General Practitioner, Yaxley, Peterborough.

J. Tudor Hart MB, DCH, FRCGP
General Practitioner, Glyncorrwg, Wales.

B.G. Harwin MB, MPhil, MRCPsych
Lecturer in Psychiatry, General Practice Research Unit,
Institute of Psychiatry, London.
Formerly General Practitioner, Orpington, Kent.

P.D. Hooper MB, ChB, MRCGP, DObstRCOG
General Practitioner, Newport, Isle of Wight.

G.H. Curtis Jenkins MA, MB, BChir, DObstRCOG
General Practitioner, Ashford, Middlesex.

I.F.W. Kerr MB, ChB, DObstRCOG
General Practitioner, Ashton under Lyne, Lancashire.

Gareth Lloyd MD, BSc, MRCOG, FRCGP
Senior Lecturer, Department of General Practice,
University of Manchester.

B.T.B. Manners MB, MRCP, MRCPath, MRCGP
Consultant Pathologist, St. Luke's Hospital, Guildford.
Formerly General Practitioner, Addlestone, Surrey.

R.M.A. Moore MB, BChir, MRCGP, DObstRCOG
General Practitioner, Shrewsbury, Shropshire.

J.R. Murray MB, BS, MRCGP, DObstRCOG
General Practitioner, Dereham, Norfolk.

L.A. Pike MB, FRCGP, DObstRCOG
General Practitioner, Birmingham.

R.J.F.H. Pinsent OBE, MA, MD, FRCGP, FRACGP
General Practitioner, Birmingham.
Research Adviser, General Practice Research Unit,
Royal College of General Practitioners.

I.H. Redhead MD, MRCGP
General Practitioner, Yaxley, Peterborough.

A.M. Semmence MSc, MD, FRCGP, DIH, DObstRCOG
General Practitioner, Abingdon, Berkshire.
Unit of Clinical Epidemiology, Oxford Regional Hospital Board.

R.G. Sinclair MB, ChB, MRCGP, DObstRCOG
General Practitioner, Falkirk, Scotland.

D.H. Smith MB, BS, MRCGP, DObstRCOG
   General Practitioner, Swineshead, Lincolnshire.

G. Teeling Smith BA, MPS
   Director, The Office of Health Economics, London.

M.K. Thompson MB, ChB, MRCGP, DObstRCOG
   General Practitioner, Croydon, Surrey.

E. Wilkes MBE, MA, MB, MRCP, FRCGP
   Professor of Community Care and General Practice,
   University of Sheffield.

B.E.P. Wookey MB, BS, MRCGP, DObstRCOG
   General Practitioner, Boston, Lincolnshire.

Definitions

Medical Screening. The detection of occult disease or defect by the application of tests, examinations, and other procedures which can be applied rapidly. Medical screening is not intended to be diagnostic; it sorts out apparently well persons who may have a disease from those who do not have the disease. (In Chapter 2, this established concept of medical screening is enlarged, to include the collection of medical information concerning patients that may have no immediate application, but is stored for future use in a data bank).

Health Check. Routine physical examination by a physician, directed to the uncovering of occult disease or defect. Usually the examination is preceded by history taking, and followed by other screening procedures; all the data are then gathered together for assessment by the physician.

Prescriptive Screening. This term is occasionally employed to describe screening undertaken with the deliberate objective of investigating, and where possible treating, abnormal conditions that are uncovered, as distinct from screening undertaken primarily for actuarial, statistical, or research purposes, or for storage of information in a data bank.

Mass Screening. The application of medical screening procedures economically to large unselected groups of apparently well persons. Mass screening is usually prescriptive. It can be monophasic or multiphasic.

Monophasic Screening. The application of one or more medical screening procedures to the detection of an individual disease or defect. Most monophasic screening is now selective in nature, investigation being confined to those people thought to be at special risk.

Multiphasic Screening. The combination into a battery of several medical screening procedures, aimed at the detection of a wide range of occult diseases or defects, performed wherever possible by technicians under medical direction, and applied to large groups of apparently well persons. By this definition, all multiphasic screening is mass screening.

Automated Multiphasic Screening (AMPS). The use of automated analytical machines to perform multiphasic screening tests. *Inter alia,* machines currently in use deal with blood chemistry, haematology, urinalysis, radiography, thermography, anthropometry, audiometry, retinoscopy, electrocardiography, spirometry, mapping of visual fields, and history taking. Increasingly, computers are being used to organise, record, analyse, and transmit data obtained from multiphasic screening. Ideally, screening of this degree of sophistication should always incorporate a health check.

Automated Multiphasic Health Testing (AMHT). This term is gradually replacing AMPS in American jargon, to indicate that screening procedures have been refined to secure more clearly diagnostic results from the programme.

Sensitivity and Specificity. Ideally, health tests should be sensitive enough to detect all those with the disease being sought for, and specific enough to detect only those with the disease. Mathematically, these values for a particular screening test may be defined as follows:-

$$\text{Sensitivity} = \frac{\text{number diagnosed by the particular test} \times 100}{\text{total number diagnosed}}$$

$$\text{Specificity} = \frac{\text{number non-diagnosed by the particular test} \times 100}{\text{total number non-diagnosed,}}$$

where 'non-diagnosed' refers to individuals in whom it is established that the disease or defect being sought for is not present.

I The Screening Programme

1 The History of Screening

Cyril Hart

'If preventable, why not prevented?'   King Edward VII.

The iceberg of disease

It is a truism that in medical science as in other departments of organised knowledge, the great wars of the past century have acted as catalysts for the development and application of fresh ideas. Just as the nursing profession was born from the horrors of the Crimea, so the very high rejection rate following medical examination of army volunteers during the Boer War led to the first realisation in this country of the extent of occult disease in the community. This experience was repeated during the two World Wars, not only in military medicine, but also in examination of the civilian population in connection with evacuation and rationing (Davidson *et al.*, 1943).

Whenever circumstances lead to the medical examination of a large number of people, no matter what the initial purpose, clinical interest rapidly develops in the detection of hitherto unrecognised disorders, and a screening situation exists. Routine examinations of school children, workers in industry, and applicants for insurances have been a feature of medical practice in this country since Victorian times, and to these have been added more recently ante-natal examinations, medical tests for drivers of lorries and public service vehicles, and the examination of immigrants. All these involve some form of screening. At the turn of the present century, Heiser commented on the prevalence of such conditions as deafness, valvular heart disease, hernia, tuberculosis, trachoma, and favus in immigrants at the port of Boston, USA (Wilson, 1966).

Many of these early examinations were hit or miss affairs, but in 1926 a survey was instituted at Peckham which enabled the health of a particular community to be monitored in an unhurried fashion over a period of years (Williamson and Pearse, 1938; Pearse and Crocker, 1943; Pearse, 1970). I well remember spending a day at the Peckham Health Centre as a raw medical student in the early post-war period. There we were introduced to the concept of the 'iceberg of disease'. This revelation of the staggering amount of undetected and untreated disease and defect in the population made such an impression on myself and my contemporaries, that it has motivated much of our activities since.

In 1963 J.M. Last of the Social Medicine Research Unit of the MRC attempted to quantify the iceberg by listing the unrecognised diseases in an average general practice; his estimates, extended slightly by R.F.L. Logan and the late C.L.E.H. Sharp, are reproduced in Table 1. As an indication of the size of the problem, the figures of this fundamental survey still have more than a purely historical value, for to a substantial extent they remain applicable to British general practice today.

Table 1. The iceberg of disease. Estimate of unrecognised diseases in an average general practice of 2,250 patients in England and Wales, 1962 (Last 1963; Logan 1964; Sharp 1968).

Disorder	Known to Practitioner	Total in Practice
Anaemia		
Males age 15-64	2	32 (Hb below 12 g%)
Males age 65+	1	24 (Hb below 12 g%)
Females age 15-64	19	132 (Hb below 11·5 g%)
Females age 65+	5	30 (Hb below 11·5 g%)
Cancer		
Cervix	½	3 invasive; 9 in situ
Breast	1	10 ('lumps')
Chronic bronchitis age 45-64		
Males	24	47
Females	19	24
Diabetes mellitus	14	31 (glycosuria + 'diabetic' GTT)
Epilepsy	8	14
Glaucoma age 45+	3	27 (early chronic)
Hypertensive disease age 45+		
Males	8	30 (diastolic ⟩ 100 mm Hg)
Females	24	131 (diastolic ⟩ 100 mm Hg)
Psychiatric disorders age 15+		
Males	32	91 ('conspicuous morbidity')
Females	72	144
Psychotic depression	12	125
Rheumatoid arthritis age 15+	11	25
Suicide attempts (annually)	3	6
Urinary infections age 15+		
Females	25	140 (bacilluria)

Early screening techniques and detection drives

It soon came to be realised that more was required than simple clinical examination to uncover the earliest stages of many of the commonest disorders, and progress in the past half century has been characterised by the development of a large number of screening techniques applicable to particular diseases. A few examples may be given. Mass radiography for TB, which started in this country soon after D'Abreu introduced the photofluorographic technique in 1939, has proved the most successful of all screening procedures. From infectious diseases, attention then switched to the early detection of malignant neoplasms, and in 1943 Papanicolau published his classical paper on the diagnosis of cervical cancer by exfoliative cytology (Papanicolau and Traut, 1943). A spatula for scraping the cervix to obtain specimens was developed a few years later, and it remains in general use today (Ayre, 1947). There was an immediate demand for laboratory facilities, and the first laboratory equipped for cervical cytology was opened in 1949 in British Columbia.

Interest in the early detection of metabolic disorders was stimulated by the publication in 1953 of a recommended diet for phenylketonuria, which offered hope for the first time for children born with this rare but dreaded error in the metabolism of phenylalanine (Bickel, Gerrard and Hickmans, 1953). As a result of this paper, the ferric chloride test on urine, first used by Fölling when he discovered the disease in 1934, began to be adopted more widely. A test using a paper strip impregnated with the solution, after the style of litmus paper, was developed ('Phenistix'), later to be superseded by the Guthrie test on a drop of blood obtained by pricking the baby's heel (Guthrie, 1966).

In another sphere, large-scale investigation of the early stages of chronic obstructive bronchitis has been made possible by the development of simple ventilatory function tests using the Wright Peak Flow Meter and the Vitalograph Spirometer, first marketed in 1959 and 1963 respectively. Technological advances of widespread application continue to be made at a remarkable rate. As recently as 1967, a dip-slide technique for culturing urinary pathogenic bacteria was first described by Guttmann and Naylor. Widespread use of the dip-slide from 1970 onwards has revolutionised the early detection of occult urinary infection (Arneil, 1972).

The spread of knowledge of these and other techniques was one of the most potent factors that led to the era of 'detection drives' for individual diseases, or mass monophasic screening, as some would call it today. The first diabetes survey in the USA was reported by Wilkerson and Krall in 1947, and a mass screening programme for glaucoma was described by Brav and Kirber in 1951. In 1955 it was decided to introduce a cervical cytology screening service based on the British Columbian laboratory that has been mentioned already (Kaiser *et al.*, 1960). A few years later, routine physical examination for asymptomatic breast cancer was first advocated, to be followed rapidly by mass soft-tissue X-ray detection of non-palpable breast tumours (Holleb *et al.*, 1960; Gershon-Cohen *et al.*, 1961).

The trend towards multiphasic screening

Until quite recently, health screening of a community has been regarded as something of a luxury, and it is not surprising that its early development has taken place largely in those countries where the standard of living is high—at least for some sections of the population. Specialised health checks on businessmen started in the USA in about 1947, and in 1951 the Kaiser Permanente organisation began to utilise screening methods as part of a periodic health examination. This was made available on a pre-payment basis to a large population on the western seaboard of the USA. As individual (monophasic) screening techniques were developed, they were incorporated piece-meal into the existing service, which was built up into a comprehensive multiphasic screening programme. By 1957 the Commission on Chronic Illnesses in the USA was able to list eight conditions for which it was considered that screening tests were applicable. The impact of multiphasic screening on periodic health examinations in the USA was reviewed by Breslow in 1959.

Meanwhile, in Sweden the brothers Gunner and Ingmar Jungner were experimenting with automatic mass analytical methods for quantitative estimation of the main constituents of blood serum. By 1961 they had developed a battery of ten chemical tests, and this was used straightway in a large scale multiphasic screening project mounted by the National Board of Health, to cover a population of 100,000 in the county of Värmland. The programme, completed in 1965, was highly successful, and vindicated the concept of auto-mated chemical health screening (Jungner, 1965; Engel, 1968). Later, the Swedes perfected a computerised 'Auto Chemist' giving reliable results for a wide range of tests, and capable of a very heavy workload (Jungner and Jungner, 1968).

The Americans were quick to see the revolutionary implications of this new development, and already by 1964 chemical screening had been integrated with the rest of the programme in two automated test laboratories run by the Permanente Organisation (Collen, 1965; 1968). By this time, the advantages of computerising the whole screening programme had come to be realised, and a year later the first textbook to deal with this new branch of medicine was published (Collen, Ruben and Davies, 1965). There resulted an explosion of activity throughout the USA, and computerised units for automated multiphasic screening (AMPS) were set up in many universities and hospitals. The early stages of this movement have been admirably described by Dr. Charles Hodes, a British general practitioner who spent six weeks studying these developments as a WHO Fellow in the autumn of 1968. The movement continues to spread at an astonishing pace, and it cannot be long before a network of screening clinics is established throughout the USA (Hsieh, Gilroy and Greberman, 1971; Gelman 1971; Branson and Constantine, 1972).

At the time of writing, several other developed countries are experiencing the birth pangs of similar programmes. In Western Germany, for example, the first commercially run screening clinic was set up in Wiesbaden in 1970, followed soon afterwards by others at Frankfurt and Munich. These have not proved viable propositions, but the trade unions have now moved into the field, with proposals for two more clinics based on hospitals in Hessen (Sault, 1973).

The first venture on these lines in Japan was the multiphasic health screening centre opened for employees of the Toshiba Electric Co. in May 1970. This progressive company has a commercial interest in developing automated screening techniques, and has pioneered in its own clinic the automation of respirometry, sphygmomanometry, and cervical smear testing (Yoshisuke Iwai, 1973). The pace of development in Japan has been such that AMPS is already said to be common there. (WMA Computer Panel, 1973).

In London, a health screening clinic was started by the Institute of Directors as early as 1964, and in 1970 a similar unit was set up by the British United Provident Association (Wright, 1971). On 1 January, 1972 the screening services of these two organisations were merged to form the Medical Centre at Webb House, 210 Pentonville Road, King's Cross. Here a fully computerised and automated unit, modelled on the latest American pattern, is currently carrying out health checks for subscribers at the rate of 15,000 examinations a year. Similar but smaller organisations have recently been started by Dr J.H. Briggs at the Cavendish Medical Centre, 99 New Cavendish St., London and by Dr David Thompson at the Medical Centre, Warwick House, 17-19 Warwick Rd., Old Trafford, Manchester. In 1973 an organisation known as Health Care commenced to offer a private biochemical screening service, using multichannel auto-analysers capable of determining 12 blood constituents, plus haematological and lipid analyses. This is available in Britain to industrial firms wishing their employees to be screened, the blood being collected within the factory. As yet, there is no sign of similar

facilities being developed within the framework of the National
Health Service.

Early screening in Britain

'One very important advantage that the medical care organisation
in this country has over the United States, is the concept of general
practice as a clear-cut mandate, as a responsibility for the health of
families. . .
The organisation of your services, subject as it is to improvement, at
least provides for physicians who have responsibility for populations
and for people whom they know, and with whom they can
deal, . . . and in relation to whom they can initiate action.'

C.G. Sheps, 1966.

The words are those of an American professor of preventive
medicine, when attending a symposium on screening in general
practice held at Edinburgh in 1964. It is interesting that he graduated
in medicine at Manchester. For better or for worse, the creation of
the National Health Service in 1948 has prevented the proliferation
over here of the subscriber-orientated hospital based multiphasic
screening clinics that are now so characteristic a feature of the North
American scene.

Because of the priority rightly given since the inception of the
NHS to the development and coordination of therapeutic medicine,
early screening activities in this country have proceeded on a very
patchy *ad hoc* basis, being regarded for the most part as a luxurious
optional extra rather than a basic necessity, and as something
supplemental to existing preventive measures, rather than integral
with them.

Initially, experiments in screening within the NHS were conducted
as often by medical personnel of hospital and public health
departments as by general practitioners. A classic early example was
the survey by Dr Arthur Exton-Smith, a consultant geriatrician, on
215 elderly patients whom he visited in their own homes in the
borough of St. Pancras in 1952. In the same year, a more ambitious
but differently organised geriatric programme was initiated at
Rutherglen Consultative Health Centre in Scotland. Here the Local
Health Authority and the Departments of Psychology and of
Geriatric Medicine at Glasgow University combined to offer a
comprehensive health screen to older people who, while feeling well,
desired a medical assessment, or who, because of illness, were
referred to the centre by their general practitioner. To date, some
2,000 people aged 60 and over have been screened (Andrews, Cowan

and Anderson, 1971; Cowan, 1972). It should be noted, however, that the Rutherglen programme is essentially a research project, and the screen is offered only on a selective basis.

Interest in geriatric screening on the part of hospital consultants has continued to date, but more often than not this is now carried out in conjunction with general practitioners. The trend was set in a survey mounted in Dr Roger Meyrick's practice at Hither Green in 1962, when patients were seen at a hospital clinic after a home visit by the general practitioner (Meyrick, 1962). Occasionally consultants in specialities other than geriatrics have worked jointly on a programme with the public health authorities, notably in the screening of phenylketonuria and diabetes (Guthrie Test Report, 1968; Sharp, 1964). On the whole, however, the number of hospital based screening surveys of any kind on the general population of this country has not been large.

Public health screening

The past decade has witnessed the build-up of a tradition of public health participation in screening in other spheres than preventive geriatrics. The pioneering work of Dr J.L. Burns, the Medical Officer of Health for Salford, has been inadequately reported; in 1960–2 he organised a unique multiphasic clinic in the town (Ferrer, 1968). Better known are the Bedford surveys into diabetes and glaucoma, held in 1962–6 (Sharp, 1964; Wright, 1966). Further screening in Bedford was brought to an end by Dr Sharp's untimely death. Meanwhile, interest had spread to Teeside, where after some preliminary experiments the MOH, Dr R.J. Donaldson, conducted a nine day multiphasic screen at Rotherham in 1966, attended by 5,500 people (Rotherham Report, 1969).

The results from Rotherham were valuable for statistical purposes and are often quoted, but perhaps of greater interest for our present review is the following description of the administrative arrangements, which were evidently run on a shoe-string. They appear decidedly primitive by modern standards, and illustrate vividly the drawbacks of short-term detection drives:

'We think the "open door" clinic with no appointments gives us a better representation of the population than if we had appointment clinics . . . we stress to them the limitations of the service. . . . The clinic itself is held in a large dance hall, and nine of the 11 test stations are around the hall. The other two, for breast cancer and cervical cytology, are in side rooms. The people coming in, after having registered, more or less chose their own test. . . . The staff are mainly from our own department, and work with a tremendous amount of energy and enthusiasm, and find it an exhausting but exhilarating experience. After the clinic is closed comes the tedious sentence of hard labour in getting the data ready for processing and despatch to the general practitioner.' (Donaldson, 1968; *see also* Donaldson and Howell, 1965).

Based on these and similar activities (developmental assessment of infants, for example) a case has been argued that 'screening procedures are the special prerogative of the Medical Officer of Health', but it has received little support (Ferrer, 1968). Valuable though these early public health surveys have been, they can hardly be thought of as satisfactory models for a nationwide screening programme. The trend of modern thinking in the public health departments is perhaps epitomised by a suggestion of Dr I.A. MacDougal, the County MOH for Hampshire, that local authority doctors might conduct screening clinics from health centres (MacDougal, 1970). It is difficult to predict what effect the current administrative reorganisation within the NHS will have upon public health screening, but doubtless the Community Physician will have a major role to play.

Screening in British general practice

The inception of the National Health Service in 1948 had a profound effect on the organisation of general practice in this country. In the early years of the service, general practitioners were too busy accustoming themselves to working in the new regime to wish to take on extra responsibilities in preventive medicine, and it was not until 1954 that the foundation of Darbishire House Health Centre as a teaching unit of the Manchester Medical School enabled some experimental work to be undertaken. Dr H.W. Ashworth, the first general practitioner appointed there, began to investigate the incidence of anaemia among his patients as soon as the health centre opened (Ashworth, 1963). In 1958 routine multiphasic health testing of the 45—54 age group was undertaken in the practice. At this date many of the more useful screening techniques had still to be developed, and Dr Ashworth was sceptical as to the value of his investigations (Ashworth, 1959; 1964).

In the same year, 1958, Dr I.H. Redhead carried out a diabetes detection drive on 2,000 patients in his Newcastle practice—the first practice-based survey of the incidence of diabetes in this country (Redhead, 1960). The following decade witnessed many such drives, mostly for the detection of diabetes and carcinoma of the cervix, within the framework of general practice. Between 1962 and 1965 Dr I. Gregg carried out screening tests using the Wright Peak Flow

Meter to detect symptomless airways obstruction in early chronic bronchitics in his practice at Kingston upon Thames (Gregg, 1966). Multiphasic detection drives were held in rural practices in Lincolnshire and Derbyshire (Cope and Smith, 1967; 1972; Evans, Wilkes and Dalrymple-Smith, 1969). The description of the arrangements for the Derbyshire survey deserves to go on record here, both for comparison with the Rotherham survey and also as a classic contribution to the literature of screening in general practice.

'The screening clinic was held in our surgery headquarters on two half days only, and coincided with a visit from the Mobile Mass X-ray Unit a few hundred yards away. The only publicity was a circular letter which we sent to each household registered with the practice under the National Health Service. Patients under 15 years of age were not permitted to attend, and the elderly were gently discouraged from doing so.

With much help from varied sources it was possible to provide a wide range of tests. We crowded into our waiting room, registration, tests for anaemia and glycosuria, the measurement of weight, blood pressure, and Wright Peak Flow Meter reading, a history of cough and sputum and smoking, and a personality adjustment rating. The small examination room housed the electro-cardiograph and its technicians. One consulting room had observers examining for goitre (endemic in Derbyshire, Ed.) and technicians taking venous blood for biochemical estimations. Another separate consulting room was used for breast examination and cervical cytology. Working conditions were noisy, tiring and very crowded.

In the two half-days 791 patients were screened—about a quarter of those eligible. The total was made up of 355 males and 436 females. The average age of men attending was 47, of women 48 years. In the same two days, the Mobile Mass X-ray Unit took over 1,000 chest X-rays.

The enthusiasm of the patients was indeed obvious. We attempted to spread the load by asking patients to attend in an alphabetical sequence, but we offered them only a queue in the open air. Despite a staff of about 25 people, this queue was usually 10 or 20 yards long, and on one of our two days it was raining. The patients had replied on a tear-off strip telling us how many were intending to come. We catered for about 800 on the basis of their replies. We could not have coped with more.'

Short-term detection drives of this nature, or 'health fairs' as they are picturesquely described in the USA, served to alert general practitioners to the usefulness of multiphasic screening, and during the past decade there has been a quiet but steady development of practice-based experiments. Many of these pioneering studies have remained unrecorded in the literature, and the present writer was surprised and impressed by the number of practices found to be undertaking screening, and the extent of their commitment, during his preliminary enquiries leading up to the preparation of this book.

A substantial proportion of ordinary run-of-the-mill practices—not just those that happen to be research orientated—are now involved with screening at infant welfare, antenatal, and cervical cytology clinics held in the practice premises, and there is a growing movement towards geriatric screening. Undoubtedly the creation of a health team and the possession of an age-sex register leads naturally to an increase of screening activity within a practice, and the trend is all away from detection drives, towards a continuous and comprehensive cover for all the practice population at risk.

The move towards a planned screening programme

On July 7, 1965, a colloquium was held at Magdalen College, Oxford under the auspices of the Office of Health Economics, to discuss surveillance and early diagnosis in general practice. It was attended by members of the faculties of medicine of various British universities, by medical officers of health, representatives of the Medical Research Council and of the Ministry of Health, by a number of leading members of the College of General Practitioners, and by distinguished visitors from Sweden and the USA (Wilson, 1966).

The contrast between the proceedings of this august assembly and the hectic activities of the detection drives currently being held in Rotherham and Derbyshire could not have been more marked. Nevertheless, the colloquium proved just as decisive an event as the detection drives in the history of medical screening in this country. The discussion centred around such topics as: Who should be screened? Who should do it? Why will they do it? How is it to be organised? What procedures should be used? What are the long-term benefits? What is the cost? Can any list of priorities be given (a) for individual clinical practice and (b) for social policy?

One of the many valuable contributions to the colloquium was that of Dr J.M.G. Wilson, then a Senior Medical Officer of the Ministry of Health, who listed the following principles of case finding:

Wilson's criteria

1 The condition sought should be an important problem.
2 There should be an accepted treatment for patients with recognised disease.
3 Facilities for diagnosis and treatment should be available.

4 There should be a recognised latent or early symptomatic stage.

5 There should be a suitable test or examination.

6 The test or examination should be acceptable to the population.

7 The natural history of the condition, including its development from latent to declared disease, should be adequately understood.

8 There should be an agreed policy on whom to treat as patients.

9 The cost of case-finding (including diagnosis and subsequent treatment of patients) should be economically balanced in relation to the possible expenditure on medical care as a whole.

10 Case-finding should be a continuing process and not a 'once for all' project.

Dr Wilson's criteria were difficult to meet then, and remain so today. Editorials appeared in the Lancet and BMJ counselling caution, and recommending that carefully designed research studies should evaluate programmes of prescriptive screening before their general introduction as a branch of preventive medicine. A number of long-term screening investigations were put in hand in the departments of general practice of universities in the national capitals of Cardiff (Winter et al., 1972), Belfast (Irwin and Neill, 1970), and Edinburgh (Scott and Robertson, 1968; Illingworth, 1970; Percy-Robb et al., 1971).

The most ambitious of these was the South East London Screening Survey, in which long-term multiphasic screening was offered to the middle aged patients of two group practices, the sessions being conducted of an evening in Local Health Authority clinics. This study, by far the most elaborate of its kind, was organised by the Department of Clinical Epidemiology and Social Medicine at St Thomas's Medical School, under the direction of Professor W.W. Holland and with support from the (then) Ministry of Health. Designed as a five-year longitudinal survey, it was commenced in November, 1967. As yet it has only been reported on as to methodology (Trevellyan, 1973), and the full results of the survey are unlikely to be published before the end of 1974.

There is no doubt that the results of this valuable investigation, when available, will have a big impact on the planning of screening programmes in this country. However, the considerable time interval between initiating and reporting a longitudinal survey of this kind poses a dilemma for those who advocate full evaluation of prescriptive screening before its general introduction. While the survey has been in progress, epoch-making administrative changes have occurred within the NHS, and clinical medicine has not stood still. What was possible in 1967, before the era of dip-slides and health visitor attachment, has only limited relevance to what is both possible and desirable today. Because of such considerations as these, a number of general practices have started modest screening programmes of their own, before awaiting the results of such long-term investigations. Moreover, practices are beginning to realise the inherent value of building up a data bank concerning patients at risk for various disease processes. Screening is not longer solely a research activity. There are, of course, dangers, and it is to be hoped that the information offered in this book will help practitioners to minimise them.

Few can have foreseen at the time the opportunity to develop preventive medicine in a general practice setting that the advent of the NHS brought with it. It has taken a long while for the seed to germinate, and even now it is not yet in full flower. Only when the radical administrative changes initiated in the past decade are completed, and general practice is fully organised on a team basis in proper premises, with attachment of ancillary staff (to use an obsolescent term) the rule rather than the exception, with its record system fully developed, and with the integration of its services with those of hospital and public health medicine a reality; only when all this is achieved, will the introduction of a national screening programme become a practical proposition. The argument then will not be whether it is desirable, but whether we can afford it.

REFERENCES

Andrews, G. R., Cowan, N. R., & Anderson, W. F. (1971). The practice of geriatric medicine in the community. In *Problems and Progress in Medical Care.* Edited by Gordon MacLachlan. Nuffield Provincial Hospitals Trust.
Arneil, G. C. (1972). Urinary tract infection in children. *Update,* 1115.
Ashworth, H. W. (1959). Routine medical examination. *Medical World,* p. 90.
Ashworth, H. W. (1963). An experiment in presymptomatic diagnosis. *Journal of the College of General Practitioners,* 6, 71.
Ashworth, H. W. (1964). Presymptomatic diagnosis of carcinoma of the cervix. *Medical World,* p. 153.
Ayre, J. E. (1947). *American Journal of Obstetrics and Gynaecology,* 53, 609.
Bickel, H., Gerrard, J., & Hickmans, E. M. (1953). *Lancet,* 2, 812.
Branson, M. H., & Constantine H. P. (1972). Designing multiphasic screening. *Hospitals* 46/9, 47.
Brav, S. S., & Kirber, H. P. (1951). Mass screening for glaucoma. *Journal of the American Medical Association,* 147, 1127.
Breslow, L. (1959). Periodic health examinations and multiple screening. *American Journal of Public Health,* 49, 1151.
Collen, M. F. (1965). A multiphasic screening programme. In *Surveillance and Early Diagnosis in General Practice.* Edited by G. Teeling-Smith. Office of Health Economics.
Collen, M. F. (1968). Automated multiphasic screening. In *Presymptomatic Detection and Early Diagnosis,* chap. 2. Edited by C.L.E.H. Sharp and H. Keen. London: Pitman.

Collen, M. F., Rubin, L., & Davis, L. (1965). Computers in multiphasic screening. In *Computers in Biomedical Research.* Edited by R.W. Stacey and B.D. Waxman. Vols 1 and 11, New York: Academic Press. 1, 339.

Commission on Chronic Illness (1957). *Chronic Illness in the United States of America,* vol. 1, *The Prevention of Chronic Illness.* Harvard University Press. Cambridge, Massachusetts.

Cope, J. T., & Smith, D. H. (1967). A health week in rural general practice. *British Medical Journal,* 2, 756.

Cope, J. T. & Smith, D. H. (1972). A second multiple screening clinic in a rural general practice. *Journal of the Royal College of General Practitioners,* 22, 113.

Cowan, N. R. (1972). The early recognition of disease in older people. In *Symposia on Geriatric Medicine,* 1, 41—49. West Midland Institute of Geriatric Medicine and Gerontology.

Davidson, L. S. P., Donaldson, G. M. M., Lindsay, S. T., & McSorley, J. G. (1943). Nutritional iron deficiency anaemia in wartime. *British Medical Journal,* 2, 95.

Donaldson, R. J. (1968). Screening procedures and the local authority. *Journal of the Royal College of General Practitioners,* 16, supplement no. 2, 37—41.

Donaldson, R. J., & Howell, J. M. (1965). Rotherham multiple screening clinic. *British Medical Journal,* 2, 1034.

Engel, A. (1968). Mass screening for asymptomatic disease as a public health measure. In *Perspectives in Health Planning,* chap. 3. University of London: Athlone Press.

Evans, S. M., Wilkes, E., & Dalrymple-Smith, D. (1969). Presymptomatic diagnosis. *Journal of the Royal College of General Practitioners,* 17, 237—240.

Exton-Smith, A. N. (1952). An investigation of the aged sick in their homes. *British Medical Journal,* 2, 182—186.

Ferrer, H. P. (1968). *Screening for Health.* London: Butterworths.

Gelman, A. C. (1971). *Multiphasic Health Testing Systems: Reviews and Annotations.* U.S. Department of Health, Education and Welfare. Rochville.

Gershon-Cohen, J., Hermel, M. B., & Berger, S. M. (1961). Detection of breast cancer by periodic X-ray examination. *Journal of the American Medical Association,* 176, 1114—1116.

Gregg, I. (1966). The recognition of early chronic bronchitis. *Journal of the College of General Practitioners,* 11, Supplement no. 2.

Guthrie, R. (1966). *Procedings of the International Conference on Inborn Errors of Metabolism,* 20. U.S. Department of Health, Education, and Welfare. Washington D.C.

Guthrie Test Report (1968). Population screening by the Guthrie Test for phenylketonuria in South-East Scotland. Report by the consultant paediatricians and medical officers of health of the South-East Scotland Hospital Region. *British Medical Journal,* 1, 674—676.

Guttmann, D., & Naylor, G. R. E. (1967). Dip-slide: an aid to quantitative urine culture in general practice. *British Medical Journal,* 3, 343.

Hodes, C. (1969). *A Report of a Visit to the United States of America as WHO Fellow to Study Multiphasic Screening.* BMA Library (Cyclostyled copy).

Holleb, A. I., Venet, L., Day, E., & Hayt, S. (1960). Breast cancer detection by routine physical examinations. *New York Journal of Medicine,* 60, 823—827.

Hsieh, R. K. C., Gilroy, F. D., & Greberman, M. (1971). *Automated Multiphasic Health Testing: A Health Services R & D. Laboratory.* U.S. Department of Health, Education, and Welfare. Washington D.C.

Illingworth, D. G. (1970). *The Health Check in Practice.* Hemel Hempstead: Educare.

Irwin, W. G., & Neill, D. W. (1970). Biochemical screening in general practice. *British Medical Journal,* 4, 56.

Jungner, G. (1965). Chemical health screening. In *Surveillance and Early Diagnosis in General Practice.* Edited by G. Teeling-Smith. Office of Health Economics.

Jungner, G., & Jungner, I. (1968). Chemical Health Screening. In *Presymptomatic Detection and Early Diagnosis,* pp. 67-108. Edited by C.L.H.E. Sharp and H. Keen. London: Pitmans.

Kaiser, R. F., et al (1960). *Journal of the National Cancer Institute,* 25, 863.

Last, J. M. (1963). The clinical iceberg in England and Wales. *Lancet,* 2, 28—31.

Logan, R. F. L. (1964). Control of chronic disease in general practice and industry. *Journal of the College of General Practitioners,* 11, supplement no. 1. 94—100.

Mac Dougall, I. A. (1970). *Health Trends,* 2, 70.

Meyrick, R. (1962). A geriatric survey in general practice. *Lancet,* 1, 393—395.

Papanicolau, G. N., & Traut, H. F. (1943). *Diagnosis of Uterine Cancer by Vaginal Smear.* New York: Commonwealth Fund.

Pearse, I. H. (1970). Periodic overhaul of the uncomplaining. *Journal of the Royal College of General Practitioners,* **20,** 146–152.

Pearse, I. H., & Crocker, L. (1943). *The Peckham Experiment.* London: Allen & Unwin.

Percy-Robb, I. W., Cruikshank, D., Lamont, L., & Whitby, L. G. (1971). Biochemical screening programme in general practice; a clinical follow-up. *British Medical Journal,* **1,** 596–599.

Redhead, I. H. (1960). The incidence of glycosuria and diabetes mellitus in general practice. *British Medical Journal,* **1,** 695.

Rotherham Report (1969). *A Multiple Health Screening Clinic, Rotherham 1966: a Social and Economic Assessment.* Report prepared by the Social Science Research Unit, London. HMSO.

Sault, J. (1973). Diagnoscreen in West Germany. In *Doctor,* **3,** no. 2.

Scott, R., and Robertson, P. D. (1968). Multiple screening in general practice. *British Medical Journal,* **2,** 643–647.

Sharp, C. L. E. H. (1964). Diabetes survey in Bedford. *Proceedings of the Royal Society of Medicine,* **57,** 193–196.

Sharp, C. L. E. H. (1968). Opportunities and problems presented by screening procedures. In *Presymptomatic Detection and Early Diagnosis,* chap. 1. Edited by C. L. E. H. Sharp and H. Keen. London: Pitmans.

Sheps, C. G. (1966). *Journal of the College of General Practitioners,* **11,** supplement no. 1, 105–106.

Trevelyan, H. (1973). Study to evaluate the effects of multiphasic screening within general practice in Britain: design and method. *Preventive Medicine,* **1,** 278–294.

Wilkerson, H. L. C., & Krall, L. P. (1947). Diabetes in a New England town. *Journal of the American Medical Association,* **135,** 209–216.

Williamson, G. S., & Pearse, I. H. (1938). *Biologists in Search of Material.* London: Faber & Faber.

Wilson, J. M. G. (1966). Some principles of early diagnosis and detection. In *Surveillance and Early Diagnosis in General Practice.* Edited by G. Teeling-Smith. London: Office of Health Economics.

Winter, C. J., Clay, S., & Davis, R. H. (1972). School medical examination in an integrated group practice. *Journal of the Royal College of General Practitioners,* **2,** 327.

WMA Computer Panel (1973). Report on computers and community health in Japan, by Dr Masakazu Kurata. *British Medical Journal,* **4,** 292.

Wright, H. B. (1971). The implications of automated health screening for the delivery of medical care. *Community Health,* **3,** 71–80.

Wright, J. E. (1966). The Bedford glaucoma survey. In *Glaucoma.* Edited by L. B. Hunt. London: Livingstone.

Yoshisuke, I. (1973). Recent data and their analysis from the Toshiba multiphasic health screening centre. *Medical and Biological Engineering,* **11,** 15–26.

2 Screening in Primary Care *Julian Tudor Hart*

'Doctors are just like other Englishmen: most of them have no honour and no conscience: what they commonly mistake for these is sentimentality, and an intense dread of doing anything that everybody else does not do, or omitting to do anything that everyone else does.'

George Bernard Shaw. *The doctor's dilemma*, 1906.

Screening, anywhere, is a planned procedure, and any plan must derive from an ideal, abstracted description of the reality in which it will operate. Most of the failures and disappointments of screening, and they are many, arise from errors of theory, and need never have occurred. Because it is so important that general practice in this country should move rationally toward a greater congruity with the problems it is meant to solve, we cannot afford early defeats that may discredit and impede this work. A sophisticated theory of screening has already been elaborated by epidemiologists and public health administrators (Wilson and Jungner, 1968), largely on the basis of experience in these two fields. For reasons which I shall explain, this theory is not fully applicable or adequate for our purpose in primary care, and attempts to apply it directly to our quite different situation can only result in discouragement and waste. We have got to elaborate our own theory, suited to screening that is both effective and feasible in the normal conditions in which British general practitioners work.

The application of simple sorting procedures to whole defined populations has a long and rather unsatisfactory history. The idea that early detection of disease must make its treatment easier and more effective is attractive, but seldom fully realised; even the idea that it must at least do no harm, even if it does no good, has not always proved true. Until its abolition in 1886, the Contagious Diseases Act provided that in garrison towns and naval stations any

17

girl seen consorting with a soldier or sailor, or anonymously reported to have done so, was liable to compulsory pelvic examination for the presence of venereal disease; for which, of course, no reliable diagnostic test existed at that time (Petrie, 1971). Its effect, and perhaps part of its purpose, was simply to humiliate. The greatest number of lives ever saved by any screening procedure must surely have been during the 1914—18 war, when almost any loud systolic murmur was diagnosed as valvular disease of the heart, and disqualified a man for the trenches. The main benefit of systematic screening of schoolchildren and recruits for the grosser kinds of disease and unfitness before 1948 was the evidence it gave for campaigns for the prevention of such disease by adequate wages, housing and nutrition, since very little effective treatment was available. The only really effective screening procedures were elaborated by the Local Authority clinics for infants and expectant mothers; these were the basis for an anticipatory care that has now replaced the treatment of gross disease in both these fields, and their experience is highly relevant to any theory of screening in primary care.

The renewed interest in screening of the past 10 years derives little from these sources, and depends much more on two new factors. The first of these is the new technology that permits rapid, cheap and accurate measurement of many variables in blood and urine, the mechanical recording of aspects of heart and lung function, and computer-assisted storage and retrieval of huge volumes of data. The second is the experience of epidemiologists in using and evaluating these techniques in large population surveys. The initial and still largely dominant conception of screening resulting from these was an episodic, once-for-all campaign of intensive case-finding, aiming at a rapid throughput using special staff and equipment, and without responsibility for continued care and follow-up. A later modification has been the more or less independent but permanent screening unit, sometimes attached to a hospital. Such influence as there has been from primary care has come chiefly from the experience of 'health checks' in the USA, notably the Kaiser Permanente scheme (OHE, 1966). These are essentially a marketed commodity, developed without regard to feasibility if applied to the whole population; their counterpart in this country is the Institute of Directors scheme. Such schemes are not economically viable on a universal basis, and it is not possible to derive valid conclusions from their experience because of their biassed and unmeasured social selection. Claims for their effectiveness in reducing mortality—for instance, that regularly screened business executives have a 28 percent lower mortality than that in white males in the USA generally (Thorner and Crumpacker, 1961)—are not well substantiated.

There is no doubt that epidemiology has added new dimensions to the theory of screening, particularly in imposing a more critical approach. One of the worst features of military and local authority clinic screening was the way in which routine examinations degenerated into rituals, unrelated to the ideas and enthusiasm that often set them up. So long as clinical diagnosis by physical signs was regarded as more or less infallible, this was bound to happen; the delineation of lung cavities by percussion ceased, and was perceived to be fallible, when routine chest X-rays became accessible to junior hospital staff, but not a moment before. Epidemiologists, notably A.L. Cochrane, showed real courage in exposing the limitations of all clinical, laboratory, and radiological measurements and descriptive definitions, the large margins of difference between observers, and inconsistency within observers, as well as the great variability of things measured in relation to time, eating, activity, and so on. For instance, seven skilled observers interpreting 600 chest X-rays found active tuberculosis in from five to 20 subjects, a fourfold difference (Cochrane, 1950); four experienced observers reading ECG's found from four to 20 percent compatible with coronary disease (Higgins, Cochrane and Thomas, 1963). Similar results apply to virtually every diagnostic procedure taken in isolation, but the painful conclusions from this evidence have yet to be fully accepted.

Epidemiologists have also emphasised the importance of high response rates, and the often unpredictable qualities of reluctant respondents and non-respondents. Cochrane (1950) divided 600 men co-operating after various degrees of persuasion in a mass chest X-ray survey for coalworkers' pneumoconiosis and pulmonary tuberculosis into three groups of 200 each, by order of coming up. He found over-representation of pneumoconiosis in the first group (most wanting screening), and over-representation of tuberculosis in the last group (most resistant to screening). Obviously in most clinical situations non-consulters are healthier than consulters, but the process of recognising and accepting symptoms as illness, and then of acting appropriately to the adoption of the sick role, is exceedingly complex (Robinson, 1971). This process differs between symptoms, between localities, and between social groups; but a small group of sick people who deny illness by avoiding its recognition exists for most diseases, notably cancer of the breast (Aitken-Swan and Paterson, 1955), and probably of the bladder and rectum. Paradoxically, such people may welcome diagnosis made on the doctor's initiative, for it is just the decision to consult, or to consult overtly and effectively, which they may fear to take. If their doctor takes it for them, he is more likely to get a welcome than a rebuff. Screening procedures that cover only 30 or 40 percent of a population, or even the 70 percent attained by the Värmland scheme in Sweden (OHE, 1966), are almost certainly not reaching those who seldom or never consult a general practitioner, and may yield misleading conclusions on both the costs and the benefits of complete (95 per cent-plus) coverage.

Epidemiologists have also undermined traditional simplistic views of the definition of disease entities. The difference between a severe insulin-dependent diabetic and a healthy man is a qualitative one, not merely a matter of degree; but it is not of the same nature as the difference between a camel and a horse. The WHO definition of diabetes is arbitrary and wholly quantitative; it is based simply on blood levels of glucose at a standard time after ingestion of a standard load, and even then has to introduce a 'doubtful' range between 121 and 140 mg per cent. The same is true of high blood pressure, ischaemic heart disease, stroke (the standard epidemiological definition requires a neurological deficit clinically demonstrable for more than 24 hours), peripheral arterial disease, many cancers (of the cervix *in situ*, histological cancer of the prostate, transitional cancers of the bladder, variants of Hodgkin's disease), nearly all mental illness—in fact, nearly all the common killers and disablers of industrialised mankind. The classical presentations of these diseases at a more or less terminal or irreversible stage present no difficulty, but these are not the cases we find by screening; in general it may be said that every important qualitative diagnostic entity, however sharply defined when viewed in isolation or from afar, disintegrates into quantity if we examine it closely enough, especially around the edges.

No, the real difference between what is currently regarded as diabetes, and what is not, lies in the collective eyes of the beholders; it lies in the decision to include one within the field of medical care, and to discard the other. Such an operational definition will now include the fat first-degree relatives of diabetics, with borderline glucose tolerance, for advice on diet and exercise and perhaps for annual follow-up; it would not have done so 20 years ago. Any condition causally related to disability or mortality, in which treatment is shown (or, more frequently, is supposed) to alter the outcome favourably, will be defined as disease; so that definitions will depend upon available remedies and avoiding actions. Pickering is almost certainly right in regarding 'hypertension' as one end of a continuous distribution, but clinically it will continue to be defined as 'that level of blood pressure at which I consider the initiation of treatment or continued supervision'; and with certain provisos, that is a good definition, so long as the 'I' becomes 'we'. The definition of all diseases is to an important extent a strategic one, which depends not only on what is 'absolutely' going on in the patient, but also 'relatively' on our means of perceiving and interfering with what is going on, and the balance of risks and advantages in doing so; these will change with time, and so will our working definitions.

This implies that clinical definitions should often differ from epidemiological research definitions, and that clinical definitions at primary care level for the diagnosis of self-selecting symptomatic patients may differ from those for the screening of asymptomatic patients. The significance of bacteriuria with a colony count less than 10^5 is quite different in a miserable child who does not eat, from the same finding in a well child; the first must be repeated several times before we accept a negative. More important, screening may require a revision of traditional clinical definitions in all situations. Elwood's investigation of iron-deficiency anaemia led him to doubt whether the disease existed at all (Elwood, Waters, Green and Wood, 1967). This was because he failed to find any correlation between symptoms and haemoglobin level in the range eight to 14 grams per cent, and also found that more severe anaemia than this occurred in less than one per cent of non-pregnant women. This suggests that hypochromic microcytic anaemia as a sole finding may be of small significance in itself unless it is severe, and that the symptoms associated with it by tradition may be fortuitous—a situation exactly similar to that found in hypertension. However, it fails to take account of valuable experience from general practice, which should modify this generally debunking approach. A new doctor taking over a high-morbidity industrial practice from an exhausted predecessor will detect over the first five years (if he looks for them) perhaps eight to 12 severe microcytic anaemias (less than eight grams) in middle-aged women, perhaps one or two of these with dysphagia, and new cases will subsequently present at a rate of perhaps one a year. Their detection and treatment not only relieves the dyspnoea and exhaustion to which these women have gradually accommodated, but may also prevent the later onset of pharyngeal cancer; and Fry (1966) has shown that without very careful follow-up these anaemias usually recur, even after prolonged and apparently adequate treatment. The point is, of course, that the one per cent prevalence of severe anaemias, both microcytic and macrocytic, is well worth looking for. It is chastening to recall that more than 40 years after Minott and Murphy there are still about 400 certified deaths annually from pernicious anaemia (Minott and Murphy, 1926). Nearly all of these occur in the aged, but usually these old men and women are otherwise well, and deaths should not and need not occur from this cause. If we are serious about eliminating preventable deaths, we must adjust our minds to small returns.

Does the unpresented case actually wish to be found, and if doctors take the initiative in this search does this in itself create more problems than it solves? The doctor who encourages patients to think that annual physical examination prevents serious illness is (on present evidence) fooling the patient and perhaps himself also; but the rapid 'complete' physical examination we were taught was not designed to do this job, whereas a screening programme is, and we have good reasons to think it may be effective in some directions. Providing we do not encourage naïve expectations by making inflated claims for it, our ethical position is secure. General practitioners are quite familiar with the problems of patients who more or less conceal illness, and screening creates a less novel situation for them than for doctors with a hospital or research background. We do not regard the routine recording of blood pressure or body weight as an intrusion on privacy, merely because the patient attended with a complaint to which these measurements are irrelevant; we are carrying out normal routine measures of health surveillance, and screening is only an extension of this, if it is done within primary care.

However, the attitude of most epidemiologists to screening is now sceptical, and there is a general feeling that it has been oversold— particularly those programmes operating outside the normal machinery of the health service (intervention screening). This attitude is shared by many thoughtful and experienced general practitioners. Van den Dool, in the Netherlands, a little-recognised pioneer of screening in primary care, applied intensive multiphasic screening to a stable rural population of 4,000 three times over a period of 10 years (Van den Dool, 1970 a and b). His team included workers from a university department. He achieved response rates of 80, 85, and 90 per cent successively. He concluded that this style of case finding was inappropriate to primary care, wasteful, and failed to make use of the natural advantages of the primary care setting. Instead, he proposed the development of a style of 'anticipatory care', in which the primary doctor uses all his contacts with his population to build up a comprehensive profile of those variables relevant to the early diagnosis of reversible disease.

The same view was taken by Keith Hodgkin and John Fry in 1965 (OHE, 1966), who claimed that good British GPs were already carrying out an effective screening function by their attention to continuity of care, combined with high rates of contact with their populations. They see between 70 and 75 per cent of their patients in any one year (85 to 90 per cent of those aged 65 and over), and 95 per cent of them over five years. As Dr Fry said, 'we do not have to have mass community surveys because we are seeing them all the time.' The British general practitioner is paid to care for a defined population, not only on demand at times of self-reported illness, but all the time. This may not be an interpretation of the terms of service that most GPs would now accept, but at least they *can* make such an interpretation, and put it into practice, within the present frame, in a way that is not possible where patients move about from one doctor to another on a fee-paying basis, and where direct access to specialist advice displaces an unknown proportion of primary consultations. The British GP in the National Health Service is as accessible as he chooses to be, without serious financial barriers to his patients.

This opportunity exists, and perhaps some doctors are able to make full use of it to maintain a full profile of essential data on all their patients, without creating any special procedures or investigations to accomplish this. However, when I looked at carefully maintained records accumulated over six years in a stable industrial practice with very high consultation rates, I found I had recorded blood pressure readings in only about half of my adult patients (Hart, 1970). Without a system for recording data essential to anticipatory care, but irrelevant to current symptoms, such data are recorded incompletely or not at all. The traditions of industrial primary care do not progress to such anticipatory care without effort; we inherit stubborn traditions of 'perfunctory care by perfunctory men' (Hart, 1972), in which possibility and reality are usually widely separate. There are no grounds at present to expect any rapid improvement in this position, and doctors working in hospitals know quite well the relative infrequency of continuous personal anticipatory care, particularly in urban industrial areas.

However, for exactly the reasons given by Hodgkin and Fry, screening should be developed within our present framework of primary care, and not by intervening agencies. The development of the school medical service and of local authority infant and antenatal screening services were originally a social necessity, because in the first quarter of the 20th century no substantial number of general practitioners was able or willing to provide these services. The situation now is quite different: probably at least 25 per cent of British GPs would accept—in work, not words—continuing responsibility for the anticipatory care of their defined populations, unrelated to expressed patient demand, if (and only if) they were convinced of its usefulness, and were given the staff, buildings and equipment needed to carry it out. This would be a sufficient basis for a realistic perspective of extending the responsibilities of primary care from exclusive concern with individually presented symptoms, to include an active concern for the whole community served; a substantial advance on these lines would be possible within one generation. Such a perspective is essential; for however unsure we may be of the present effectiveness of presymptomatic diagnosis in affecting the outcome of disease, we may be quite certain that medical science is now moving rapidly in this direction. If new scientific knowledge is to be applied, we must have an appropriate social structure of primary care, and doctors' shops dealing out hastily conceived remedies to symptomatic customers will not do.

Already we have a situation in which most strokes could be prevented by control of high blood pressure, and in which about 80 per cent of those with high blood pressure could be controlled by relatively simple treatment. The doctor who is called to his patient with irreversible brain damage, and who has no record of the pre-ictal blood pressure, is not delivering medical science effectively to his patients; yet we know this is a common situation, and will remain so until some form of screening for blood pressure becomes a normal feature of good primary care. The theory and technique of doing this need not differ very much from those that will be required for the anticipation of other diseases, as they also become treatable at a presymptomatic stage.

To sum up, there appear to be five questions that must be answered, in general and in each local circumstance, for planning screening programmes in primary care:

1 What information do we need about the whole population for whose continuing care we are responsible, to sort it into its component risk groups?

2 What additional information do we need about each of these risk groups, both for casefinding and as baseline data?

3 How is the information to be obtained, initially and for subsequent updating?

4 How is the information to be recorded, retrieved, and linked or integrated with the clinical record?

5 How can such a semicontinuous screening system be developed from existing positions in primary care?

The detailed answers to these questions depend on current knowledge and technique, but we should be able to elaborate a system that can accommodate new methods as they become available. The area covered differs from Wilson and Jungner's definition of prescriptive screening, because in effect it includes the whole of the *data base* (Weed, 1969) required for anticipatory continuing care, not only that required for current case finding.

What information do we need?

For the whole population we must have personal identification data permitting the segregation of risk groups. This *identification data base* would include names, maiden names, and dates of birth, occupational data including current place of work and previous contact with serious industrial hazards (for example, asbestos and rubber processing), data on immigrants, addresses and kinship data to permit the segregation of families and households, data on serious functional and social disabilities (living alone, bedfastness, long-term unemployment, single-parent families, presence of handicapped child, sensory impairments and so on). All this data could be obtained by a self-administered questionnaire, to which could be added blood group and other genetic constants that cannot be self-reported.

From this data, various risk groups can be identified, requiring different screening data; at least, we need separate groups for infancy, pre-school children, primary schoolchildren, secondary schoolchildren, adults 16–34 and 35–64, and the elderly, each divided by sex. The data needed for the anticipatory care of each of these is different, each has a different clinical *risk-group data base*.

Some of this information will be of the sort classically associated with prescriptive screening, variables relevant to the finding of current latent or unpresented disease; examination for dislocation of the hip, absent or reduced femoral pulses, sensory defects in infancy and old age, and so on. But much more of it will be relevant less to a search for current asymptomatic disease than as a baseline measurement permitting rapid and accurate diagnosis of illness occurring later on. For instance, the routine measurement of serum cholesterol in middle-age may be of some value in selecting high-risk groups for coronary disease, who can then be offered dietary and perhaps other advice; but it also means that a woman of 53 with a baseline cholesterol of 153 mg per cent in 1971, seen with minimal symptoms and signs of hypothyroidism in 1973 and a serum cholesterol of 630 mg per cent, is diagnosed more quickly and efficiently than she might have been. Electrocardiography as a routine screening procedure is of doubtful value, since it leads very seldom to any effective clinical decision; but if the tracings are stored so that they are quickly available in the event of later sternal pain, and can be compared with a new ECG, diagnosis can be far more rapid and efficient, particularly in the prodromal period of infarction. So with a great many other variables—serum creatinine and urea, proteinuria, haemoglobin level, chest X-rays, neonatal head circumference, bodyweight and skinfold thickness, peak expiratory flow rate and spirometry: all are more often useful as baselines for the rapid recognition of significant change in continuing anticipatory care, than for current case-finding.

This aspect of screening has been neglected by intervention-screeners, because they have no means of using their information for the future care of the patient. In primary care nothing need be wasted, and all of this information can be used to reduce the primitive, episodic aspect of primary care, and to raise it to a level of continuous health supervision.

How do we get it?

If we accept that there is a minimum data base appropriate to the anticipatory care of various age/sex groups and perhaps a few social and occupational sub-groups, how is this to be obtained? Certainly intensive surveys with rapid recruitment are not the only means of doing this, in fact for us they are the most difficult and least efficient way, since they do not make use of the unstructured and incomplete screening function that already exists in the British style of primary care; they can throw an impossible burden on referral and follow-up services for cases found, and they make thorough investigation of those cases very difficult.

If there is a place at all for intensive screening, it is in the initial collection of base data, to shift a population rapidly onto a fully screened basis, or at least to do this for its most vulnerable risk groups. The most urgent and rewarding of these is probably the geriatric group, but even for this extra help may be needed to complete screening within one year.

Most of the data can be collected by natural recruitment: standardised examination and recording in infancy as new babies are born, and of entrants to the other age-groups as they reach qualifying birth dates. Some of these are socially nodal points—puberty, school-leaving, running up to retirement, and so on, each presenting problems that may be usefully discussed without the usual obligation to have a symptom; advice on contraception and sterilisation is an obvious example. Within one five-year span it should be possible to pass all groups of a practice population through an appropriate screening procedure, bearing in mind that a great deal of the most useful material will be obtained by self-administered questionnaire (Hall, 1972).

How is it to be recorded and retrieved?

The present 18 x 12 cm general practice record card and envelope will have to be replaced sometime during the next five years, because it cannot accommodate more than 15 years' recording for high-morbidity cases, on any system. It has survived so long only because serious record-keeping was seldom attempted in panel practice before the NHS. It is sure to be replaced by the A4 international size folder, broadly similar to present hospital notes.

The techniques exist for recording, storage, updating and rapid retrieval of vast numbers of simple items of information, providing these can be coded or quantified (Gruer, 1972). Satisfactory software has not yet been fully evolved for anticipatory primary care, but we now have enough general practitioners accustomed to diagnosis on agreed criteria using standardised terms (which could avoid a lot of coding) to develop this on a fairly small pilot basis, and to have a national system available within five years. The limiting factor is not mainly economic, as often supposed, but the proportion of doctors prepared to accept the discipline of precise recording in a common language; a great many still seem to equate clinical freedom with the right to use private languages which defy all criticism.

The technical means for storage and retrieval of almost unlimited quantities of data is already available, but we have got to make up our minds how we are going to use them. It is almost certainly not useful to attempt continuous total morbidity recording, as in the national morbidity surveys of 1955-6 (Logan and Cushion, 1958) and 1970-73; what and how we record should depend on the purposes likely to be served by retrieval. The informal day-to-day clinical record will remain, because much of it cannot be reduced to quantified or codeable items without losing valuable information, but certain key items must be routinely transferred to computerised data storage. All intermittent screening data should enter computer storage, and be available as a continuously updated profile of clinical and social variables relevant to anticipatory care, and a cumulative history of major events and measurements of lasting significance.

A signalling system will be necessary to alert secretarial staff that the data base for a consulting patient is incomplete, so that it can be updated at that consultation, or arrangements can be made for updating after recovery if the patient has an acute illness. All the records will have to be searched for outstanding signals of incomplete data from time to time, so that non-consulters reaching a five year span can be contacted by ancillary staff.

How can screening be developed from existing primary care?

This important question has been insufficiently discussed. The pilot stage of comprehensive screening is likely to occur for the most part in university departments of community care (Holland, 1973).

In the past, at least, these departments have not always shown effective concern that their techniques should be reproducible in the setting of urban industrial practice; because this is the biggest, sickest, and most technically backward area of primary care, it is the test of all really effective innovation.

In the first place, and above all in industrial practice, people tend to consult frequently and rather superficially, rather than occasionally and in depth; though not in itself desirable, this frequent contact can be used for updating of data, as already discussed. Secondly, the dissatisfaction of both patients and doctors with existing traditions of practice can be an incentive to change. For those doctors in industrial practice who have not accepted defeat, its most frustrating aspect is the lack of congruity between needs and resources. This depends partly on the overall social setting within which we work (Hart, 1971), and partly on a grossly excessive load of detailed tactical decision-making on individual sickness episodes coupled with an almost total absence of strategic decisions and forward planning. The possession of an accessible and complete data base for his population gives the industrial GP the means to plan rational changes in the style and content of his work, away from expensive, wasteful, often irrational and sometimes dangerous treatment of symptoms (often in fairly minor and self-limiting illness), towards rational anticipatory care, and a treatment style that does not use steam-hammers to crack peanuts. For the new generation of GPs in particular, this is a most important incentive.

In non-industrial practice the introduction of screening should be easier, and for those already running their own infant, antenatal and geriatric clinics, the extension to other groups should be simple.

Finally, the screening idea involves the practice population as a whole, in some cases even as a community. There are important and as yet untapped resources in this fact. Collectively, people want anticipatory care. Cartwright (1967) found that 64 per cent of people would like regular check-ups on their health, and two-thirds of these wanted this to be done by their own doctor; more young people were in favour than old people. It is true that she found about one-third opposed or indifferent, but many of their reasons related to their actual experience with general practitioners who were not oriented to prevention. In my own practice, in which screening procedures have been applied to from 94 to 100 per cent of the population several times, less than two per cent expressed opposition or reservations when their opinion was asked. The goodwill and co-operation aroused by serious attempts to organise for a more preventive style of care spill over into every other kind of clinical and social contact.

The accumulation and maintenance of a complete data base for a whole population is laborious, and evidence of real concern; properly planned, it can make that concern effective, move us further away from slipshod illusion, towards a more critical and rational anticipatory care, yet with a human face.

REFERENCES

Aitken-Swan, J., & Paterson, R. (1955). The cancer patient: delay in seeking advice. *British Medical Journal,* 1, 623.

Cartwright, A. (1967). *Patients and their doctors: a study of general practice.* London: Routledge & Kegan Paul.

Cochrane, A. L. (1950). contribution to discussion in *The application of scientific methods to industrial and service medicine: proceedings of a conference March 29–31, 1950.* London: HMSO.

Elwood, P. C., Waters, W. E., Green, W. J., & Wood, M. M. (1967). Evaluation of a screening survey for anaemia in adult non-pregnant women. *British Medical Journal,* 4, 714.

Fry, J. (1966). *Profiles of disease.* Edinburgh: Livingstone.

Gruer, K. T. (1972). Livingston new town—using a computer for general practice records. *Journal of the Royal College of General Practitioners,* 22, 100.

Hall, G. H. (1972). Experience with outpatient medical questionnaires.

Hart, J. T. (1970). Semicontinuous screening of a whole community for hypertension. *Lancet,* 2, 223.

Hart, J. T. (1971). The inverse care law. *Lancet,* 1, 405.

Hart, J. T. (1972). Primary care in the industrial areas of Britain; evolution and current problems. *International Journal of Health Services,* 2, 349.

Higgins, I. T. T., Cochrane, A. L., & Thomas, A. J. (1963). Epidemiological studies of coronary disease. *British Journal of Preventive and Social Medicine,* 17, 153.

Holland, W. (1973). Contribution in *Portfolio for Health 2: The developing programme of the DHSS in health services research.* ed. D. McLachlan. Oxford University Press.

Logan, W. P. D., & Cushion, A. A. (1958). *Morbidity statistics from general practice,* volume 1 (general). General Register Office, Studies on medical and population subjects no. 14. London: HMSO.

Minot, G. R. & Murphy, W. D. (1926). Observations of patients with pernicious anaemia partaking of a special diet. In *Classic Descriptions of Disease* by Major, R. H. Charles C. Thomas: Springfield, Illinois. 1945.

OHE (Office of Health Economics) (1966). *Surveillance and early diagnosis in general practice: report of a symposium.* London: OHE.

Petrie, G. (1971). *A singular iniquity: the campaigns of Josephine Butler.* London: Macmillan.

Robinson, D. (1971). *The process of becoming ill.* London: Routledge & Kegan Paul.

Thorner, R. M., & Crumpacker, E. L. (1961). *Archives of Environmental Health,* 3, 523, quoted in *Lancet* 1969, 2, 833.

Van Den Dool, C. W. A. (1970a) *Huisarts en Wetenschap,* 13, 3.

Van Den Dool, C. W. A. (1970b). *Huisarts en Wetenschap,* 13, 59.

Weed, L. (1969). *Medical records, medical education and patient care.* Cleveland: Case University Press.

Wilson, J. M. G., & Jungner, G., (1968). *Principles and practice of screening for disease.* Public Health Papers no. 34, Geneva: WHO.

3 The Economics of Screening

G. Teeling-Smith

De omnibus dubitandum.

It is an interesting observation that the development of screening programmes and presymptomatic treatment was probably more responsible than any other single factor for the introduction of rational economic principles into the assessment of medical care. With traditional clinical medicine, it had usually been assumed that the more treatment one could afford, the better the prognosis would be. It was only with the introduction of screening programmes during the early 1960's that the question came seriously to be asked 'Is this diagnosis and treatment worthwhile in relation to its cost and the benefit it will yield?' During the last decade we have started to ask the same question of the treatment of symptomatic disease also. However, in the first place it arose in relation to screening, and probably it arose because it was obvious to anyone who considered the matter that if screening were uncritically introduced, the potential workload and cost would be infinite. If every apparently healthy person could be regarded as a potential presymptomatic victim of every disease, the scope for clinical, radiographic and biochemical investigation would be unlimited. Indeed it has been said that the healthy patient would be one who had not been properly investigated.

Hence during the 1960's Wilson (1966) and others started to expound certain criteria which needed to be satisfied if any screening programme were to be justified. The first and most obvious was that there must be available an effective treatment which could be shown to improve the prognosis once a positive result has been obtained from a screening test. There is very little benefit for the patient in diagnosing a disease—at whatever stage—if no effective treatment for it exists. Second, the treatment must also be acceptable to the patient, in some cases for the rest of their lives. Third, the diagnostic test must be reasonably accurate. One which was so unselective that it yielded a large proportion of false positives or which was so insensitive that it yielded a large proportion of false negatives could be dangerously misleading. Fourth, the condition to be screened for must be sufficiently common among the particular population being screened. What would represent 'sufficiently' in this sense, of course, must depend to some extent on the seriousness of the disease, and also the extent to which earlier detection would significantly improve its prognosis. The value of presymptomatic detection is reduced considerably if equally effective therapy can be instituted when symptoms are first reported. Indeed, it could be argued that the existence of the National Health Service, which allows patients easy and inexpensive access to medical care at an early symptomatic stage in their illness, renders the introduction of a national screening programme less urgent in this country than in most other parts of the world. Tuberculosis, for example, can in general now safely be left to the symptomatic stage before treatment is begun, and hence Mass Miniature Radiography is being withdrawn (Cochrane, 1972). The rarity of cases in the population as a whole (as opposed to immigrants) meant that largely 'unnecessary' presymptomatic detection was, even by 1966, costing over £600 per case detected (Cochrane and Fletcher, 1968).

Fifth, as a corollary, the cost of contacting the population and of carrying out the tests must be reasonable. Again, what would be 'reasonable' in a particular case will depend on the seriousness of the condition. Detection of a treatable cancer would justify much larger expenditure than the detection of a trivial orthopoedic abnormality. Obviously, too, the cost per case detected will depend on the prevalence of the condition being sought and also its rate of progression through the latent or presymptomatic stages. With lung cancer, for example, which progresses fairly quickly to a symptomatic stage, it has been estimated that radiological screening would need to be repeated at least at six monthly intervals to be effective (Wilson, 1966). This would not only be uneconomic but could well cause more harm than good. On the other hand, screening once during pregnancy for asymptomatic bacteriuria will effectively pick up most cases, so that this is fully justified in economic as well as medical terms, especially now that dip-slides are available (Asscher, 1970). In particular, and of special relevance to screening in general practice, the cost of a screening programme will depend on the circumstances under which the patient is contacted. A patient screened a long distance from his home in purpose-built premises by specially trained staff involves a very different cost from his being given a specific diagnostic test in the course of a routine visit to his general practitioner.

Finally, it is important that as large a proportion as possible of the whole population at risk should be included in the screening programme, and that those not at risk should be excluded from it. Hence the haphazard 'open door health weeks' are now economically indefensible, involving widespread waste of resources.

It was relatively easy, in the 1960's, to state these general principles which should be taken into account in deciding whether a particular screening programme could be justified on economic grounds or not. As an aside, it should perhaps be explained that 'being justified on economic grounds' does not mean that 'it will pay off in financial terms'. Practically no medical care does that, despite frequent contrary assertions*. An 'economic' justification for a particular treatment implies that the benefit to the population from having it available is greater than if the treatment were abandoned and the resources so released were used to provide alternative forms of medical care. That is, if a treatment (or screening programme) is extremely costly and brings little or no benefit, it would be better to discontinue it and to use the resources instead to meet some of the present unmet needs in diseases where the effectiveness of treatment is beyond doubt.

However, having stated those principles and explained the overall economic objective, it is immediately clear that it is exceedingly hard to decide in particular cases whether a screening programme is economically justified or not. This is because, just as the economic principles in the evaluation of medical care had not been generally applied until the introduction of screening, there had previously been no systematic attempt to assess the effectiveness of medical care using the principle of the randomised controlled trial. Although the assessment of individual pharmaceutical preparations in double blind randomised trials had been accepted as routine in Britain by the 1950's, application of the same principle to whole systems of medical care did not become widespread until the late 1960's. As already stated, it was usually assumed that 'more was better'. An extra diagnostic investigation, a few extra days in bed, or surgery rather than non-surgery were all generally believed to bring benefit. Hence systematic scientific evidence on what benefit one could expect from treatment following early diagnosis was generally absent. Yet it was no longer possible to assume automatically that treatment would be of benefit, when the numbers of new treatments

*The control of tuberculosis, and the conquest of childhood infections are two of the few examples where medical progress has paid off in financial terms.

which might be started as a result of screening programmes would be so great.

The extent of the problem was highlighted by what Last (1963) described as the 'clinical iceberg'. Table 1 (p. 4) shows his estimates of the numbers of new cases for treatment which could have been expected to be revealed by national screening programmes. If all these cases were indeed to be detected and treated, there needed to be some proof, rather than merely a 'clinical impression', that they would in fact benefit from the treatment.

This general difficulty was made greater during the 1960's by the realisation of the full extent of the 'borderline' problem in defining the presence or absence of a disease state. This other aggravating factor is illustrated in Figure I, which shows the particular difficulty arising in cases where the 'normal' and 'diseased' distribution curves for the population overlap. For people falling in the shaded area, it is impossible to tell from the biochemical (or physical) measurement whether they are in the upper 'tail' of the distribution curve for the healthy population or in the lower part of the distribution of the disease group. As the diagram also shows, taking any reasonable measurements to define healthy normals and 'obviously' diseased groups respectively, it is likely that these definitions will nevertheless include a small proportion of 'false negatives' and 'false positives'. The inset on the diagram shows the only distribution pattern in which the diseased population could be unequivocally distinguised

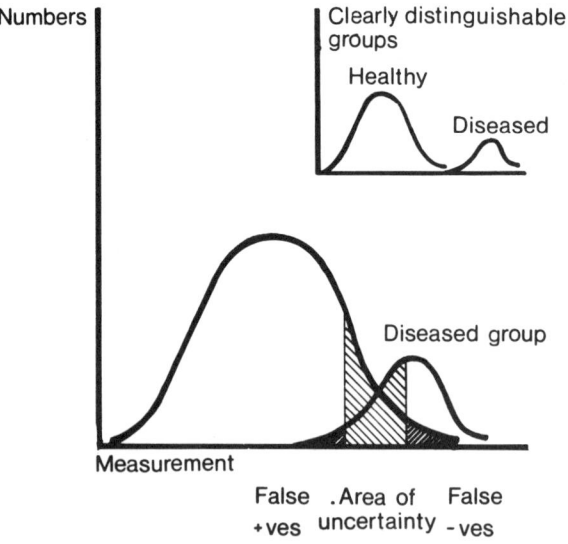

Figure 1. The borderline between health and disease.

from the healthy, and certainly that pattern does not apply, for example, in the case of body weight, blood pressure, blood cholesterol, or haemoglobin measurements.

Hence, on very rational grounds, instead of indiscriminately introducing screening programmes on a national basis (except in the case of cervical cytology) it was decided instead to undertake randomised controlled trials to evaluate the cost and benefit of screening for different diseases. Typical of these studies were the diabetes screening trial in Bedford and the multi-centre trial of blood cholesterol screening under the auspices of the World Health Organisation (Keen, 1971; Heady, 1973). Their objective was to answer for the particular disease as many as possible of the questions which were relevant in making a rational decision on whether screening was worthwhile, and in deciding what criteria should determine whether particular biochemical or other measurements indicated the need for treatment or not. In most cases, these trials needed to run for ten years or more before statistically significant answers could be obtained. This is, of course, because of the chronic progressive nature of the diseases both in their presymptomatic and symptomatic phases. The complications of diabetes, for example, often develop only many years after a raised blood sugar level has been measurable. An acute coronary episode may not occur until decades after a raised cholesterol level has been detectable. Hence, prevention of complications by lowering the blood sugar levels or blood cholesterol levels may only become significant after correspondingly long periods.

The result is that in general it is still not possible to state categorically which conditions are worth screening for in terms of benefits in relation to cost. Nor in many cases—for example in the case of high blood pressure—can one state specifically which findings justify treatment and which do not. Nevertheless, although one cannot set out precise conclusions or rules, it is possible to give some better economic guidance than was available when the problem first became apparent in the 1960's.

First, there is now no doubt that if it is practicable for a particular screening programme to be undertaken in general practice rather than elsewhere, this is an ideal location. Such programmes do not necessarily imply very great reorganisation of the practice, but can be a logical extension of good general practice as it has already developed. Indeed in many cases such development has already occurred. The principal advantage is that the population at risk is clearly defined, and in addition if age-sex registers are maintained the population can be subdivided conveniently into different risk groups for different diseases; for example, middle-aged males for hypertension and middle-aged females for cancer of the cervix. In some practices the patient's place of residence may in addition indicate social class and this, for example, would be relevant in defining the population most at risk for the latter disease. Moreover, about two-thirds of those on the list of an average National Health Service general practice will contact their practitioner routinely each year. Thus, if one is planning a screening programme over, say, an eighteen-month period, only a third or less of patients would need to be specially contacted. When a test for high blood pressure or obesity is undertaken during a regular surgery visit the economic cost is negligible.

If the practice records are maintained to indicate family relationships, this too will help to identify particular risk groups. And of course if a small high risk sub-group within the practice can be identified, the economic justification for screening them becomes much more obvious than if the whole practice has to be screened simply to pick up those in the high risk group. This is the case, for example, with relatives of patients having glaucoma. The picking out of immigrants for screening for tuberculosis is another illustration, although here the screening itself will normally have to be done by referral to an X-ray unit.

The question of special remuneration for screening in general practice has arisen already in the case of cervical cytology. It would, however, perhaps be unfortunate if special incentive payments had to be given for each new screening procedure which became accepted as a logical part of general practice. It would imply a shift away from the capitation basis of remuneration towards a fee for item of service basis. It is outside the scope of this book to discuss the implications, but they certainly should not be forgotten if there were to be further discussions on remuneration for screening procedures. A more helpful way of spending government money on screening services based on general practice might well be to subsidise the employment of additional ancillary staff specifically for screening. In many cases such staff could shoulder the main screening workload, leaving to the general practitioner a much less time consuming (and therefore more economic) supervisory role.

If general practitioners will accept screening as a rational addition to their other responsibilities, what economic considerations should they take into account in deciding which groups of patients to screen in respect of which diseases? There seems at present no justification in this country for what the Americans call multiphasic screening; that is, the indiscriminate application of an extensive battery of tests to large groups of individuals. Economic logic argues for a much more selective approach, which, as already indicated, can probably be largely meshed into the routine general practice activity.

The age-specific epidemiology and the natural history of the different diseases must be the starting point for a rational policy. High blood pressure in middle-aged males has been quoted as an excellent example (Holland, 1967; Coope, 1974). It is a relatively common condition with a long presymptomatic phase, where there has for sometime been strong statistical evidence that raised pressure causes early mortality (Metropolitan Life Insurance Company, 1961). It is interesting, however, that although early detection is almost certainly worthwhile in terms of patient survival (and reduction of morbidity) it represents no economic saving to the nation. Because most deaths due to high blood pressure occur during retirement, their prevention adds to the economic burden rather than reducing it. This, however, is no argument against such a screening programme.

Another example of a prevalent and generally treatable disease is obesity. Here detection is even simpler than with hypertension, although in both cases the major stumbling block is patient acceptance of the treatment which is available—in this case, in the long-term, strict dieting. However, the inclusion of obesity exemplifies that many of the conditions for which there is the best economic justification for screening are the relatively simple and unglamorous ones. This is particularly the case with the elderly and the very elderly. With them it is often, for example, trouble with their feet or just progressive lack of interest in life which eventually precipitates their need for institutionalisation.

Regular observation for deterioration of this sort involves very little cost, particularly if health visitors or other ancillary staff can be effectively used, as Williamson (1966) has shown in an experiment in Edinburgh. By contrast with the economic arguments in favour of such 'bread and butter' screening, there is little evidence at present to support, for example, routine electrocardiography or similar technologically glamorous procedures. This again is one of the arguments in favour of general practice as the most appropriate location for present screening programmes. It also means that there is little to be said at present in favour of several practices combining to provide routine screening facilities, except perhaps in the sphere of computerisation.

Another consideration favouring the introduction of particular screening programmes is if the particular group at risk will be in routine contact with the medical services anyway. Two examples of this, although probably not directly affecting general practice, are bacteriuria in pregnancy and phenylketonuria in infancy. Screening for the latter, in particular, would be difficult to justify in economic terms—because of its extremely low incidence—if the test were not so simple and if the health visitor who undertakes it were not in any case visiting the house.

At the other extreme, in contrast to the common conditions when prognosis can be favourably affected if they are detected at the presymptomatic stage, are the very rare conditions where the danger is often not so much that diagnosis is left too late as that it is never made at all, even when symptoms appear. Here there is little or no economic justification for a screening programme, and in medical terms the need is often for a greater awareness of the possibility of the unexpected at the clinical stage. An example here would be porphyria. It is far too rare, and the diagnostic tests too inconvenient, ever to consider a screening programme—although such would be potentially lifesaving in a handful of cases. However, because of its very rarity, there is always a danger that the symptoms it causes may be misinterpreted when they occur.

Finally, to put the whole question of the economics of screening into perspective, it is necessary to return to the statement at the beginning of this chapter, that it was the prospect of presymptomatic diagnosis which hastened the application of rational economic principles to medical care planning. It still remains true that there is a serious imbalance between the amount of economic assessment attempted in preventive medicine (and especially screening) as compared with that applied to conventional therapeutic medicine.

This chapter has described some principles which can be used in helping to decide whether the expense of a particular screening programme is justified for a particular sector of the population. It has also described many of the reasons why such programmes can often be more economically undertaken in general practice than in special centres or clinics. However, what is sometimes overlooked is that very similar principles and arguments apply also to much of conventional therapeutic medicine. The same critical assessment of whether different therapeutic regimes are worthwhile for different types of symptomatic illness is necessary, but is too rarely undertaken (Glass, 1973). Corresponding arguments about bringing as much conventional medical care as possible into the normal scope of general practice are just as applicable, but they are less frequently voiced.

This is not just an academic observation. It has very serious practical consequences. Because diagnostic and therapeutic procedures for symptomatic illnesses are still accepted uncritically, without systematic assessment of their benefit in relation to cost, there is little pressure to discontinue ineffective or inefficient practices, especially in hospital. By contrast, presymptomatic diagnosis can only be introduced routinely under the National Health Service once rigorous economic proof of efficacy has been obtained, and the difficulty in obtaining such proof within a reasonable time span has been described. The result of this is that health care planning still leans much too heavily towards conventional therapeutic medicine rather than a presymptomatic or preventive approach.

This is not to argue that screening should have been allowed to be introduced with the same economically uncritical attitude as has conventionally applied in the case of therapeutic medicine. Rather it is to be urged that the sound economic principles which have emerged as a result of critical assessment of screening programmes should be applied to health service activities as a whole. It is perhaps in general practice more than anywhere else that this attitude could be developed. The central position of general practitioners under the Health Service system could then enable them to disseminate this philosophy both to patients and to hospitals. The economic principles developed in relation to screening could as a result have a much more far-reaching influence in health care than in the relatively narrow field in which they originated.

REFERENCES

Asscher, A. W. (1970). *The Early Diagnosis of Urinary Tract Infection.* London: Office of Health Economics.

Cochrane, A. L. (1972). *Effectiveness and Efficiency; Random Reflections on Health Services.* Oxford: Nuffield Provincial Hospitals Trust.

Cochrane, A. L. & Fletcher, C. M. (1968). *The Early Diagnosis of Some Diseases of the Lung.* London: Office of Health Economics.

Coope, J. (1974). A screening clinic for hypertension in general practice. *Journal of the Royal College of General Practitioners,* 24, 161.

Glass, N. J. (1973). Cost-benefit analysis and health services. *Health Trends,* 5, 51—56.

Heady, J. A. (1973). Primary prevention of ischaemic heart disease; cooperative trial using clofibrate; methods and progress. *Bulletin of the World Health Organisation,* 48, 243—256.

Holland, W. W. (1967). *The Early Diagnosis of Raised Arterial Blood Pressure.* London: Office of Health Economics.

Keen, H. (1971). Factors influencing the progress of atherosclerosis in the diabetic. *Acta Diabetologica Latina,* Vol. III, Supplement I.

Last, J. M. (1963). The clinical iceberg in England and Wales. *Lancet,* 2, 28—31.

Metropolitan Life Insurance Company (1961). *Blood Pressure; Insurance Experience and its Implication.* New York.

Williamson, J. (1966). 'Detecting disease in clinical geriatrics', In: *Surveillance and Early Diagnosis in General Practice,* Edited by G. Teeling-Smith. London: Office of Health Economics.

Wilson, J. M. G. (1966). 'Some principles of early diagnosis and detection', In: *ibid.*

4 The Organisation of Screening

Cyril Hart

'The present organisation of general practice as regards orientation of doctors, professional time available, records, premises, and laboratory facilities, is all against surveillance and early detection in that environment.'

J.M.G. Wilson (1965).

'The group practice or health centre, which can bring together in a well-equipped locus the family doctor, public health medical staff, nurses, and health visitors, together with secretarial help, well-organised records and accessible laboratory and other diagnostic facilities, gives promise of providing the ideal *milieu* for well-considered population screening.'

J.M.G. Wilson (1968).

These two statements by a distinguished senior medical officer of the (then) Ministry of Health epitomise the possibilities opened up by the revolutionary change in the organisation of general practice that we have witnessed in the past decade. Indeed, it can be argued that for the most part the ideal *milieu* is now within our reach; what is needed is a fresh orientation of the practice team, so that the potentialities of this new framework can be fully exploited. If we are to apply to the general population lessons learned from the pioneering surveys of recent years, we are faced with a long hard slog to establish medical screening as a valued part of the normal activity of the average general practice in this country.

Some of the organisational advantages of screening within a general practice setting will now be recounted. Here are preserved the personal medical records of the population. The practice premises are accessible to those under investigation, and in these premises the great bulk of screening information can be collected and processed. Only a few techniques, such as radiology and thermal mammography, may still require on the part of those being screened a visit to a specialised centre; and even in these cases, the administration of the screen is handled most conveniently by the general practice team (Davis, 1968).

A high percentage response can be expected when the screening team is the practice team, already known to the population under investigation, and trusted by them. The same team is responsible for recording abnormalities that the screen uncovers, and for explaining their significance and implications to those affected. Perhaps most important of all, the team responsible for detection is also responsible for continuing surveillance; they manage the investigation and treatment of diseases and defects uncovered by the screen, and when necessary they arrange periodic recall for further screening of those in whom no fresh pathology has been found. Experience has shown that effective follow-up is less likely with screens conducted outside the general practice framework (Hart, 1962; Butterfield, 1964; Cochrane, 1965; Bloor and Gill, 1972).

Another great advantage of general practice-orientated screening is that the programme can be varied according to local needs and local resources, both for detection and for follow-up. The introduction of a screening programme calls for a searching preliminary assessment as to its desirability and practicability, followed by much careful preparation for its implementation. The greater the effort devoted to this planning stage, the easier it will be to work the programme and the more effective will be its result.

Planning the programme

The idea of a screen may come from some outside agency, or it may originate with the practice health visitor, but perhaps it is most likely that one of the medical members of the team will be the prime mover. Setting aside for a moment the situation within single-handed practices, it is probable that the idea will first be discussed informally between the doctors within the group. Enthusiasm may vary from partner to partner. Individual attitudes are influenced by a wide variety of factors, both tangible and intangible. What proportion of the practice commitment should be devoted to preventive medicine, and how should this be allocated between health education, screening, inoculations, and epidemiology? How much effort, both mental and physical, will be required to adjust one's existing pattern of practice to this new-fangled slant on medical care? Will the work load of the practice bear any substantial increase? Would the introduction of screening alter the distribution of the work load between the partners? How much in terms of remuneration does each partner stand to lose, due to increase in overheads? Has not experience taught that the more facilities we offer to our patients, the more is expected of us?

Human nature being what it is, the introduction of a screening programme within a general practice is likely to depend as much on such considerations as these, as on any assessment of its possible benefit to the practice population. Nevertheless, in spite of all such problems, medical screening is already well on the way to becoming an established feature of British general practice; its use is increasing, and one can predict with confidence that it will continue to increase.

Suppose, then, that a measure of agreement is reached in principle within the partnership. The next step is to widen the discussion by taking in the non-medical members of the practice team. A preliminary meeting of the whole team should be called, at which the project is outlined by one of the partners. Some indication must be given as to the extent of the programme envisaged, but at this stage its scope should be regarded as tentative, and subject to modification as planning proceeds. Usually it will be best to keep the project within very modest bounds at the outset, allowing for the possibility of expansion by degrees, spread out over a period of years.

Possible repercussions on the work of each member of the practice team must then be explored. Both the health visitor and the practice nurse are likely to be much more heavily involved than the doctors in running the screening programme, and their whole-hearted support is essential to its success. Careful assessment is also needed of the effect of the programme on the receptionist, the secretary, and (if the group has one) the practice manager.

The health visitor's part in the programme is discussed in a later chapter. She is particularly valuable in the initial stage, selling the whole idea to the general public. Those being screened are entitled to a full explanation of what is sought of them, and why. An introductory leaflet may suffice, but a personal visit from the health visitor is a far more satisfactory arrangement, if time can be found. Failing this, she could invite selected groups of patients to a talk at the practice premises; those who attend are bound to discuss the idea with others.

Within the practice premises, most screening procedures can be delegated to the practice nurse, who may herself superintend the activities of one or more subordinates. A fundamental principle of the screening process is to employ at each stage staff with the minimum necessary qualifications (Wilson, 1968). Thus, collection of blood samples must be the nurse's own direct responsibility, but most of the other routine procedures such as weighing and measuring, the use of questionnaires, collection of urine samples, blood pressure recording, spirometry, and even electrocardiography, could be delegated to suitable personnel, trained within the practice for these specific tasks. Additional secretarial and receptionist staff may also be needed, and some arrangement may have to be worked out for the transport of specimens to the hospital laboratory.

In the summer months, students may be specially employed for carrying out, under supervision, particular aspects of the screening programme. It should be possible to secure from the Area Health Authority 70 per cent reimbursement of their salaries. Alternatively, it has been suggested that help should be sought from local voluntary organisations such as the RWVS and the Royal Red Cross (Hodes, 1969). All temporary helpers, whether paid or voluntary, must be carefully instructed in the precise details of the tasks allotted to them, and all must be made fully aware of the confidential nature of the data they are collecting. Circumstances may require that they sign a statement pledging secrecy concerning information coming to their knowledge as a result of their work; and temporary staff should not, of course be allowed free access to the practice files.

While these staffing arrangements are being planned, one of the partners should undertake to gather information and experience gleaned from previous screening surveys. This investigation might commence profitably with a review of the relevant literature. A general bibliography will be found at the end of this book, and it can be extended from the lists of references at the end of individual chapters. More detailed bibliographies on special topics can be obtained from the librarian of the Royal College of General Practitioners, and for members and associates of the College there is a free photo-copying service. The librarian at the local postgraduate centre may also be able to help. Most local Faculty Boards of the Royal College have research and practice organisation committees whose expertise can be sought; alternatively, an approach can be made to the central committees of the College. Deplorably, there are at present no postgraduate courses devoted to screening in general practice, nor is the subject catered for sufficiently in the training of health visitors.

In the early stages of planning, one must approach also those agencies outside the practice team who may be affected by the screen. Plans should be discussed with those consultants at the local District Hospital whose departments may be involved both in detection and in after-care. In particular, cooperation should be sought from the local radiologist, haematologist, and biochemist. Important sections of the screen may require modification in cases where local hospital facilities are insufficient to carry the additional load. The Regional and Area Health Authorities may be able to help here; the latter will also need to be put in the picture in case of administrative repercussions with the staff attached to the practice. In most cases, the best person to contact will be the Community Physician. It may be that the Area Health Authority can offer the use of computer facilities, or at least help with the age and sex register.

A further meeting of the practice team is desirable at this stage, so that information gathered by individuals can be pooled, snags identified, and a more detailed assessment of the possibilities be made. It should now be possible to decide on the extent of the programme, and to suggest a date for its introduction. There is still much to do in the way of detailed planning however, before the programme can be put into operation.

Much depends on the amount of floor space available, and on the convenience of its arrangement for screening purposes. Can a room be sound-proofed for audiometry, and blacked out for vision testing? Is there space for a spirometer, and a small quiet room with a couch, free from electrical interference, for the ECG? Are dressing rooms available, and what are the facilities for collecting blood samples? Listed thus, the problems may appear insuperable, but in practice one finds that very often a modest expenditure on modernising the layout of one's premises results in substantial benefit in terms of improved operational efficiency. In cases where empty accommodation is not available, it may be found that the existing use of rooms can be improved upon.

The larger the practice, the greater the potentiality for adaptation, and the easier to finance the purchase of specialised equipment. Even in a single-handed practice, it is surprising how much can be done by improvisation; moreover, it can be a distinct advantage not to have to debate every step with a number of partners. With a continuous screening programme, the number of patients screened in any one week can be quite small, particularly after the initial coverage of the whole practice has been completed, and only repeat screening is required. Nevertheless, accommodation can be a problem. Every practice contemplating a change of premises should bear in mind the need for screening facilities when planning the new building.

The timetable for screening depends to a large extent on the present use of practice accommodation. In many cases the practice nurse will work in a treatment room. If this is not fully in use each morning and afternoon, it may be possible to fit in one or more screening sessions during normal working hours. Alternatively, one evening during the week, or Saturday morning, can be devoted to screening. One great advantage of screening timetables lies in their non-urgent nature, which allows of considerable flexibility. The number of screening sessions can be reduced during periods when the ordinary workload of the practice is high, and the sessions can be cut out altogether when essential members of the practice team are on holiday or sick leave.

Each programme will require special documentation, and usually this will entail printing coloured record sheets; much time and thought has to be given to these, for upon them the success of the screen depends. Necessary details of identity are entered on these forms by the practice receptionist or filing clerk before the patient attends for the screening appointment. After the findings of the various tests have been entered on the record sheets, they are processed for statistical purposes, then (in most cases) filed in the normal record envelope. The integration of screening records with the rest of the practice filing system calls for care (Acheson, 1968). Unfortunately, recording methods are at present in the melting pot, due to the impending introduction of A4 filing, and the possibility of future computerisation. As general practice screening develops, standardised methods of documentation and record linkage with the hospitals will doubtless be worked out.

Questionnaires filled in by the patients have an important part to play in general practice screening. These require to be planned carefully for different age groups. Details of family history, of occupations, and of exposure to different types of risk, are of major significance. The whole subject of questionnaires receives special treatment in chapter 25.

Finally, every programme must be assessed, before its introduction, for its subsequent effect upon the work load of the practice. It must be remembered that the value of a screen rests largely on the follow-up. The significance of all freshly discovered abnormalities must be assessed. Most will need further investigation; some require monitoring and treatment spread over many years. Special appointment sessions may well become necessary for the routine control of cases of obesity, diabetes, and hypertension thrown up by the screen (Coope, 1974). Moreover, provision must be made for repeat screens at suitable intervals. Practitioners will be aware of this problem in the case of cervical cytology screening (Husain 1968). As the programme developes, its effectiveness needs auditing from time to time. Unproductive tests must be withdrawn and fresh procedures introduced, as soon as practicable, after their value becomes established. This ruthless pruning and grafting is essential to the health of the screening programme.

The programme in operation

As an example of planning and logistics, we may instance the introduction of a continuous screen for the total geriatric population of a two-partner practice having 6,500 patients. It was found from the age and sex register that approximately 10 per cent of the total list consisted of patients aged 65 and over; this is a little lower than the national average. Two forms were designed, each of a distinctive colour, and of a size and thickness similar to those of the standard continuation card (form EC7) at present in use with NHS record envelopes (form EC6).

The first card was used by the health visitor for a medico-social investigation which she completed during a visit to the patient's home. Each week she would select four names from the age and sex register. Her visit commenced with an explanation of the scope and purpose of the screen, and an invitation to the selected patient to take part in it. No pressure was brought to bear on the few who refused. After completing her survey and recording it on her card, she gave to each patient an appointment to attend at the practice surgery for the next stage of the screen. Each home visit took approximately half an hour.

The surgery appointments were usually for Wednesday mornings, when the partner responsible for the screen had some free time. Patients were booked at half-hourly intervals from 8.30 a.m. to 10 a.m. Sometimes, when the partner wanted Wednesday morning free, the arrangements were varied—e.g. two were seen on Tuesday morning and two more on Thursday morning, before the routine practice appointment session. When the doctor was ill or on holiday, or extra busy due to his partner's absence, screening sessions were suspended.

Each patient brought a urine specimen (bottle left by the health visitor). On arrival, height, weight, blood pressure and urinalysis were recorded by the practice nurse. Meanwhile, during the week before the patient's arrival, the receptionist had prepared all the necessary documentation, and the doctor had entered a précis of major items from the patient's case notes on to the second special record card printed for the screen. This preliminary review proved an invaluable pointer to items to be concentrated upon during the ensuing medical examination. The health check was comprehensive, commencing with a history of present symptoms taken directly from the patient (with hindsight, it has been realised that much of the foregoing information could have been obtained by means of a questionnaire completed by the patient, assisted where necessary by the receptionist. This would have saved much valuable professional time). Special attention was paid to such items as nutrition of the feet, size of the prostate, lens translucency, and other conditions in which degenerative changes were to be expected. Care was taken to keep the room warm.

Upon completion of the medical examination, the patient was presented with letters (prepared previously by the receptionist) for a chest film, blood test, and dipslide culture, all of which were undertaken during a single visit, without appointment, to the District General Hospital. Finally, when all the relevant information had been gathered together, arrangements were made for any necessary surveillance or treatment. Those in whom no fresh pathology was found, were so informed.

In this practice, it was estimated that if one partner saw four patients weekly for forty weeks each year, the whole geriatric population would be screened within approximately four years. This estimate rested on the assumptions that the response would be 100 per cent, and that all the patients were mobile enough to attend the surgery. Neither assumption, of course, is valid. Between 10 and 20 per cent of the geriatric population is housebound; but only a proportion of the housebound are suitable for inclusion within the screen anyway. The remainder, most of them very aged, are already under routine surveillance for severely disabling conditions. Screening has little relevance in this situation.

The prediction of a four-year screening cycle is therefore about right. It follows that initially, a total geriatric screen in a high list general practice can be expected to involve an average commitment of one hour per week per partner, for forty weeks in each of the first four years. Subsequently, the medical commitment would fall considerably, for repeat screens could be more selective; they would concentrate on the more worthwhile diseases and those most likely to occur in the particular patient, reserving the full screening process for those patients freshly attaining the age of 65, and for older patients moving into the area and coming on to the practice list.

Anyone who has worked such a programme will soon conclude that the time and effort is well worthwhile. The pay-off in terms of fresh treatable pathology is substantial, but the advantages do not end here. The practitioner is encouraged to interest himself in geriatric medicine, the health visitor's geriatric work is more purposeful and effective, the practice team learns to work as a unit, the comprehensive nature of the survey ensures that no old person is left neglected, and the patients themselves—some of whom have not seen a doctor for decades—are extraordinarily grateful for the interest taken in their welfare. Far from screening leading to impersonal, bureaucratic medicine, each individual is made to feel that he or she is still valued by society.

Considerable space has been devoted to this particular survey because it illustrates so many fundamental principles of organisation. Not all practices will be ready as yet to mount such a programme;

but it is suggested that as screening activities are extended within a practice, the geriatric population should be given a fair degree of priority.

Not all screening within a practice will be confined to patients grouped by age, nor is a fully comprehensive set of investigations necessary for every patient. Much effective work can be done on small groups of patients subject to particular risks, once these groups can be identified by questionnaires, and once special practice 'at risk' registers have been compiled. Screening of close relatives of patients having chronic glaucoma forms a case in point. Such a selective screen can be expected to throw up a high incidence of new cases, giving a maximum return for a minimum of effort.

By far the greater part of the effort goes into planning and establishing the initial stages of a screen; once the routine has been established, and the primary survey of the practice population completed, maintenance of a continuous screen is much less costly in time, effort, and materials than might be expected. As yet, this important principle of screening has hardly been appreciated. It is all too easy to be put off by the problem of overcoming the initial inertia, and to overlook this substantial reduction of screening commitment in the long term. All screening in general practice should be continuous.

Comprehensive screening

The time has not yet arrived for a national screening programme applicable to all National Health Service practices, with standardised procedures and recording of data. There is indeed no ideal programme for the perfect practice, for the possible range of screening activity is limitless. Limits are in fact set as much by operational efficiency, by the orientation of the practice team, and by the extent of other practice commitments, as by straightforward economic considerations. Before long, one of the most sensitive indications of the quality of a particular general practice will be the extent and efficiency of its screening programme.

For those idealists in search of a fully comprehensive programme for their own practice, suggestions for its content will be found in later chapters in this book. It is necessary to build up screening activities gradually; nothing should be undertaken that cannot be properly digested by the practice team. The worst possible propaganda for screening occurs when an elaborate programme is introduced with a fanfare, only to be hastily abandoned when the full implications of the commitment are brought home to the horrified practitioners.

REFERENCES

Acheson, E. D. (1968). Records and file organisation for population screening procedures. In *Presymptomatic Detection and Early Diagnosis,* chap. 4. Edited by C. Sharp and H. Keen, London: Pitman.

Bloor, M. J. & Gill, D. G. (1972). Screening of the well child: a discussion of some of the problems involved. *Community Medicine,* 135.

Butterfield, W. J. H. (1964). Summary of results of the Bedford diabetes survey. *Proceedings of the Royal Society of Medicine,* 57, 196–200.

Cochrane, A. L. (1965). In *Surveillance and Early Diagnosis in General Practice,* 24. Edited by G. Teeling-Smith. Office of Health Economics 1966.

Coope, J. (1974). A screening clinic for hypertension in general practice. *Journal of the Royal College of General Practitioners,* 24, 161.

Davis, R. H. (1968). Presymptomatic Screening from the viewpoint of general practice. *Journal of the Royal College of General Practitioners,* 16, supplement no. 2, 42–47.

Hart, C. J. R. (1962). Urine tests at pre-employment examinations in industry. *Practitioner,* 188, 797–9.

Hodes, C. (1969). *Report of a Visit to the U.S.A. in 1968 to study Multiphasic Screening,* 31, (Cyclostyle copy in B.M.A. library).

Husain, O. A. N. (1968). *The Early Diagnosis of Cancer of the Cervix.* London: Office of Health Economics. Early Diagnosis Paper No. 3.

Wilson, J. M. G. (1965). In *Surveillance and Early Diagnosis in General Practice.* Edited by G. Teeling-Smith, Office of Health Economics, 1966.

Wilson, J. M. G. (1968). In *Presymptomatic Detection and Early Diagnosis.* Edited by C. Sharp and H. Keen, London: Pitman.

5 The Age-Sex Register   R.J.F.H. Pinsent

'Take ye the sum of all the Congregation of the
Children of Israel, after their families, by
the house of their fathers, with the number
of their names . . . . ,'

Numbers, Chapter I, verse 2.

The idea that a general practice is a population with characteristics
which can be described and defined in considerable detail, and with
fair accuracy, is a fairly recent one. Before the Second World War the
circumstances of private medical care led each practitioner to collect
information of those who consulted him. These were the traditional
clinical records kept by the doctors about sick people and as essential
for purposes of accountancy as for medical care. In a sense the
contents of these personal files constituted a medical list, though
there was no way in which the doctor could know if the patient had
transferred his allegiance elsewhere—except perhaps by the return of
bills unpaid.

The doctor could not at any time have any idea whom he might be
called upon to see. He might suppose that if he had looked after
three members of a household of five, he would be called to the two
healthy members when their turn came to be sick. This did not
necessarily follow unless the whole family had made a special point
of discussing the future with their doctor. The doctor could know
neither the upper total of those for whom he was at risk nor the
lower, of those for whom he was likely to continue care.

Whatever else the National Health Service may or may not have
done, it made the construction of a 'practice list' quite easy. The
decision by the paymasters to remunerate doctors on a capitation
basis made it essential that the doctor knows exactly for whom he

51

was at risk and precisely for whom he would be paid. Actuarial need is a great stimulus to exact documentation. Thus it came about that individual doctors had personal lists of National Health Service patients, and as partnership practice replaced solo these lists merged to become the practice lists which we know today. These are, correctly, lists of persons who may or may not be patients and there can be very few people in the country who are not listed with a general practitioner.

With the establishment of lists the provision of a national documentation system became a practical proposition. The idea of a medical record envelope was not new, these had come in for limited sections of the population with the first National Insurance Acts. Naturally each doctor or practice received a medical record envelope for every person. Here in fact, was the practice population. Following tradition practitioners filed the envelopes in cabinet drawers, in alphabetic order, just as their predecessors had filed their clinical notes. To preserve the proprieties male and female medical record envelopes were filed separately.

The information on the basic medical record was quite comprehensive; sex and date of birth were (or should have been) included and a start could be made on defining the demography of the practice, for an age-sex register is no more than a demographic portrayal of a population, the population for whom the doctor and the practice are at risk.

The early age-sex registers were ledgers (Records and Statistics Unit, 1963). They were made up by doctors who wished to compare the rates of incidence and prevalence of illnessses in their practices with those in the practices of others. They served this purpose better to begin with, within a short time of their construction from the primary records, but as the patients left the list, or were newly added, erasures and additions spoilt the original alphabetic arrangement and the ledgers became difficult to handle. Two facing ledger pages held names and addresses of all those born in a given year. Loose leaf ledger carcasses were used to allow expansion where it was necessary, but few ledgers lasted more than five years before becoming unworkable.

The first large screening programme to be carried out was based on ledger indexes. This was the Birmingham Diabetes Survey which was carried out in a group of Midland practices in 1960 (British Medical Journal, 1962). It was, in fact, the existence of age-sex registers that led to the concept of the survey and special registers were compiled for those practices taking part which did not already have them. In this survey every person on the list was contacted, either directly when they attended to consult, or by post, or by visits made by the doctors or others working with them. A urine specimen from each member of each household was tested using an enzyme strip; the strip was placed in a specially designed container with an attached identification label, and then returned to the practice.

The age-sex registers were used to identify the people, and as their completed urine tests were interpreted the names were marked off. It was very simple, quite primitive, but it turned out to be an accurate and effective method. Those patients whose urine tests showed glycosuria were listed separately, and were later recalled for glucose tolerance tests to be done. The same ledgers were used, in this study, to provide controls whose urine tests were normal, matched to the glycosurics by age and sex. It was a feature of this particular screening exercise that both the patients with glycosuria and their controls were to be followed up and reviewed at five year intervals to discover changes in the glucose tolerance test results and see which patients subsequently developed florid diabetes.

The ledger method of maintaining an age-sex register (Evolving Age-Sex Register, 1968) was superseded by the card index. This had the very real advantage that it could be kept up to date as soon as entries to or departures from the practice took place. Cards for those temporarily absent could be extracted and placed in a temporary file pending their return. A running audit could be kept using a marker card for each age group, enabling a quick count of the whole practice to be made, or a count of individuals in a selected age group.

Any card index can be used but many practices have adopted the size of card recommended by the Research Unit of the Royal College of General Practitioners. These cards measure 5in x 3in (12·7 cm x 7·6 cm), the sexes being distinguished by colour, females pink and males blue. The cards may be blank and made up by hand or typescript. One way to make a number of cards up quickly is to use adhesive labels prepared in an endless roll for insertion into the typewriter. The completed labels are torn along a perforated line and stuck to the standard card.

Because the card is of standard size metal filing cabinets of the right dimensions are easy to get and not expensive. They are of modular design and can be added to as the list increases and the years go by. Cards are filed by year of birth, by sex, alphabetically within each year group. The groups are separated one from another by a marked signal card placed behind each 'block' of cards. These cards can themselves be used for the running audit if it is desired to maintain this.

Blank cards, made up according to the idea of the practice, form the basic age-sex register. The Royal College of General Practitioners has, however, developed a form of structured card which encourages users to record more than the minimum of information and some aspects of their design make the undertaking of practice screening programmes just a little easier. From properly completed cards it is possible to tell almost at a glance who has been screened for what, and possibly, even, when.

The Birmingham Diabetes Survey exemplified the use of an age-sex register in studying the whole population on the medical lists of the practices which took part. There are not many conditions for which such an extensive survey is required unless the definition of 'screening' is extended to include morbidity surveys. Technically a morbidity survey is almost an exercise in screening, but not quite. Morbidity surveys of the kind carried out by the Royal College of General Practitioners and the Office of Population Censuses and Surveys are concerned with illness that leads the person on the practice list to consult, and takes no count of those who do not do so. A true screening programme is one in which the doctor seeks to contact every person in the sample with which he is concerned.

It will be clear that an accurate age-sex register is an ideal source of samples. The doctor has only to decide on the pattern of his screening programme and then go to his card index to find details of the people whom he will wish to approach. Suppose he wishes to undertake a cervical smear programme, he will go to the pink cards and list those women in the age group with which he is concerned. He may wish to apply a battery of tests to all men, or all women over a given age. By counting up the numbers he can at once make an estimate of the work that is likely to be involved. In addition to identifying populations to be screened, the register has a contribution to make to the practical design of many screening programmes. Many an over-ambitious plan has been brought down to reasonable proportions simply by finding out how many people in the practice are going to have to be looked at.

The plan of a screening exercise may be based on the card index itself or on a list or series of lists made up from it. If the activities concerned require a sequence of activities it may be better to make up separate working ledgers. Supposing every member of an age group is to be invited to attend for examination, an alphabetically arranged nominal roll is prepared for a start. Vertical columns are added for insertion of dates on which action was taken, and for its results. The first date is that of the first communication sent, then a column for the response. Supposing the first approach is ignored an entry is made for the date of the second, and a note of plans to visit if necessary. Suppose acceptance, a column is used for the date of the appointment, and further columns for the results of whatever the tests may be. An elaborate study can be set out stage by stage either in ledgers or on a kind of latin square using suitable graph paper. A 'remarks' column is usually worthwhile, as well as horizontal and vertical column total spaces.

Simpler studies can be monitored from the cards themselves and it is a convenience to use a colour tagging system. Colour tags are used in age-sex registers for a number of purposes, including the identification of at risk groups and patients with certain chronic illnesses which may easily be overlooked. There is a standard colour code for this purpose, introduced by the Royal College of General Practitioners, and the use of these colours should be avoided. Tags may be of metal or plastic. Metal tags can be obtained which clip on to the top edge of the age-sex card and if these are not too large they do not interfere with the opening and shutting of the drawer. In use, however, they exert leverage forces on the edge of the card because they are rigid and increase the wear and tear on the card.

Plastic adhesive tape can be used, and if short lengths are folded upon themselves they can be applied to the upper edge of the cards with about an eighth of an inch projecting. This can readily be seen. In planning the study both colour and position of the tag can be used. In principle a tag is applied to the card when something has been done, and not until then. A red tag at the leftmost edge may indicate a first letter, a black beside it a negative reply, and so across the upper edge. The tag on the right serves to indicate the point that the patient has reached in the sequence of events required by the screening exercise. A schedule of colour tags is, of course, prepared in advance for reference, but the progress of each patient can be assessed at a glance by one familiar with the set up of the study.

A colour code can be devised for findings, and for action taken. after some abnormality has been found. There are, however, limits to the use of tags where the number of alternative courses of action is large. There comes a point beyond which colour and pattern must give place to numerically recorded information, with mechanical analysis in mind. Using blank cards, of course, information derived from a screening study may be entered in clear on the reverse of the card. This may take up most of the space there is, and leave little room for another screening programme in which the patient may be involved later. An alternative, therefore, is to make out a special card, in some neutral colour, containing the basic information about both patient and study, and file this immediately behind the age-sex register card. This 'doppelganger' can carry all the tags and entries required for the programme and all the cards relating to the particular study can subsequently be removed from the main file, for storage elsewhere.

Where numbers of people to be screened are large, and where the number of variations to be examined is also large, the observer may be faced with an analysis problem. This may be overcome by the use of some mechanical means of analysis of data recorded on the age-sex register card, and to make this possible the Research Unit of the College has introduced cards of special design. These are standardised in content and layout and entries are coded at the time of entry. The cards were designed with the 80 column counter-sorter in mind, and information from the age-sex cards themselves can be punched either on to analysis cards or computer input tape.

Figure 2. Royal College of General Practitioners Research Unit. Age-Sex Register Card.

A.S.R.2a COLLEGE OF GENERAL PRACTITIONERS RECORDS and STATISTICS UNIT

Card	Dr. Code							Surname of Patient				Forename		Date of Birth			Sex	MS	SS
1	2	3	4	5	6	7	8	9	10	11		12		13-14	15-16	17-18	19	20	21

Addresses	N.H.S. No.			E.C.
1.	Date (Entry)	22-23	24-25	26-27
2.	Date (Removal)	28-29	30-31	32-33
3.	Reason			34 35
Occupation	Card to E.C. / /19			

A	B	C	D	E	F	G	H	I	J	K	L	M	N	O	P	Q	R	S	T	U	V	W	X	Y	Z
36	37	38	39	40	41	42	43	44	45	46	47	48	49	50	51	52	53	54	55	56	57	58	59	60	61

Along the bottom edge of the card there is a row of alphabetically designated boxes, each representing a çolumn on the 'Hollerith' analysis card. These can be used to carry information relevant to the study in hand. Though seldom needed, up to nine alternatives may be accepted by each column. These cards were designed to have a greater capability to accommodate information than is likely to be required in any routine study. At the same time the non-specific designation of the columns allows flexibility. The alphabet of columns can be used in a different way, also, for it serves as a series of signal stations right across the card, each of which can be marked off as an action is completed. Unlike colour tagging—for which signal stations are set out on the top of the card—each card must be separately withdrawn for inspection.

Insofar as the object of a screening programme is to reveal the prevalence of a phenomenon in a population, with the calculation of a rate for its occurrence comparable with that from other populations, an age-sex register is an absolute necessity. Where no register exists one has to be made for the purpose of each study as it is decided upon. To be sure that all subjects in the required sub-population are included, every medical record envelope must be examined and while this task is in progress it is surely logical to make out a whole practice card index register that can be kept up to date and used for any new programmes the practice may decide on later.

The accuracy of a register compiled from medical record envelopes may not be absolute, and when an age-sex register is being set up with an eye to the future it is best to have the register checked against the master list held by the Executive Council* of the National Health Service in the name of the doctor or the practice. Clerks to Executive Councils have sometimes been most helpful in arranging for physical checks, card against card, in newly established registers and some practitioners have, by arrangements with their Executive Council, had their registers made up for them direct from the EC files. This is the best situation of all for sometimes additional information, say precise date of birth, is entered on the EC file but omitted from the Medical Record Envelope. The accuracy of a survey or a study is that of its weakest element and when a register has been prepared to a high standard of accuracy the incentive to keep it so is that much greater.

Age-sex registers are not, however, simply screening devices. They complement other methods of data elicitation and recording wherever the twin needs of incidence and prevalence require to be met. They are an essential component of Morbidity Surveys such as that carried out by the Royal College of General Practitioners with the Office of Population Censuses and Surveys, and the Department of Health and Social Security in 1971/72. At the time of writing only the methodology of this survey has been published (Morbidity Statistics from General Practice, 1973) but standardised registers were made to work in over 50 practices. The register's two companions are the Diagnostic Index and the Summary Card, each of which is an instrument which enables the user to find out more about what is happening to the patients who form the population which is his practice.

The Diagnostic Index, its evolution from the 'E Book' and its use in relating practice morbidity patterns to time and persons, have been described elsewhere (The Diagnostic Index, 1971). Like an

*With the recent NHS reorganisation, the Executive Councils have now been replaced by the Family Practitioner Committees of the Area Health Authorities. These new Committees have the same function as their predecessors regarding NHS records.

age-sex register it is multifunctional, serving not only as a visual index to the illnesses met with in the practice but also as a source of data on the occurrence of illness. The College's Summary Cards enable consecutive illnesses affecting one individual to be brought together and examined both visually and by modern methods of mechanical data processing (The analysis of summarised data using 'S' cards, 1972). Both are used with a classification of disease adapted to the circumstances of general practice rather than hospital work. This short list of rubrics relatable to those in the International Classification of Diseases and Causes of Death is itself being further developed to increase its value in international studies.

These are research tools, the use of which may not be screening in the strictest sense. A new research device introduced by the Research Unit, the 'package programme', introduces the principle of screening into the dimension of practice activities. The practices themselves become the objects of scrutiny, and various aspects of their work and performance are examined. What is the referral pattern of a practice by specialty? How many patients use an appointments system correctly? What is the practices' rate of prescribing of tranquillizers or diuretics? This kind of screening is evidence of the maturing of the National Health Service and of the wish of the doctors who take part in it to measure their performance to show where they can do better. It is screening in the context of operational research, just as much as the quest for glycosuria in a population is legitimate epidemiology. It is a growing point in general practice.

There are now numerous sources of advice and help to be called on by doctors who wish to carry out screening programmes, and early discussion is always wise. This should be local, including the Community Physician who may be able to help considerably. Now, in a number of regions, there are medical schools with Departments of General Practice. In these reside not only the skills and experience necessary but also, sometimes, access to mechanical analytical facilities not otherwise readily available. Doctors in Scotland have available to them the Scottish General Practice Research Support Unit based on the Medical School in Dundee, and those elsewhere can approach the Research Unit of the Royal College of General Practitioners in Birmingham, for advice and help. This Unit can supply standardised cards and other materials at reasonable cost.

Long before computers were dreamt of it was clear that if man was to survive he would have to become a numerate as well as a literate animal. The twin concepts of incidence and prevalence bring the need for numeracy into general practice, and the age-sex register can be seen as the fulfillment of that need.

REFERENCES

The Records and Statistics Unit (1963). *Journal of the College of General Practitioners*, **6**, 196.
British Medical Journal (1962). i, pp 1497–1503.
The Evolving Age-Sex Register (1968). *Journal of the Royal College of General Practitioners*, **16**, 127.
Morbidity Statistics from General Practice, Second National Study, Preliminary Report Method, March 1973.
The Diagnostic Index (1971). *Journal of the Royal College of General Practitioners*, **21**, 609.
The analysis of summarised data using 'S' cards (1972). *Journal of the Royal College of General Practitioners*, **22**, 377.

6 *The Computer* *J.H. Evans and A.M. Semmence*

> 'Swift as a shadow, short as any dream,
> brief as the lightning in the collied
> night . . . .
> the jaws of darkness do
> devour it up,
> so quick bright things
> come to confusion.'
>
> Shakespeare: *A Midsummer Night's Dream*
> Act 1, Scene 1.

A basic requirement for screening in general practice in the United Kingdom is an age-sex register, which has already been described by Dr Pinsent. With the refinements he has outlined it is possible to screen for particular diseases as well as particular age groups. However, the duplication of recording involved in keeping registers up to date can be laborious.

It is useful, for example, for a health visitor making a geriatric survey to have a list of all patients living in a particular district or a particular village. To produce such lists manually is time consuming, and so is the effort of addressing envelopes if postal surveys are undertaken.

A computer makes it possible to maintain age, sex and address registers with a minimum of effort, and 'at risk' registers can readily be derived from them. The technique of automated data handling in screening has been detailed by Wilson and Jungner (1968).

The construction of a computer-held basic practice file may be rather more time consuming from the secretary's point of view than an age and sex register because of the amount of data about each patient which is usually recorded in it. However, amending and using the register are very much easier. Many different methods have been used to construct the basic file, and a number of them have been reviewed by Dinwoodie (1970).

The ease with which it can be done is exemplified by the method used in one practice in the Oxford Community Health Project (OCHP), which is concerned with the development of computer-based facilities in general practice.

Experience has shown that patients' NHS record envelopes are unsuitable as source documents for preparation of a computer input. They cannot be taken out of the practice for several days, which may be necessary if a punching bureau is being used, and punch operators unfamiliar with the practice make many mistakes in copying the data. Area Health Authority indexes of patients, particularly of their addresses, may not be up to date.

A register of the patients was therefore prepared by the secretarial staff of the practice. To the data appearing on the front of the patient's record envelope—surname, forenames, sex, general practitioner (GP) code, date of registration, date of birth, National Health Service number, home address, distance in miles from practice headquarters, and dispensing code—were added the GP code of the doctor usually seen by the patient, a geographical zone code and a unique serial number and check character, the whole constituting the patient's basic record. By allocating nine zones to the practice, each village in it can be identified by a combination of the zone and the mileage.

The method of input is an OCR typewriter, the use of which does not require special training. Its typescript (Fig. 3) can be converted directly to magnetic tape using the optical character reader (OCR).

Only new or changed items of information, together with the person number and attached check character (records prefaced by 'X' in Fig. 3) need be presented, so that updating is easy. The typewritten sheets are sent by post to an OCR bureau and the magnetic tape subsequently produced is sent to the main computer used by the Project.

Collection of the minimum information necessary to be certain that data refer to a particular patient and to no other can be a time-consuming process. Usually surname, forename and date of birth are required. A personal number allocated serially is an easier method of identification. However, mistakes may occur, for example, in transposing the digits. The addition of a computer-generated check character (Smythe, 1968) which detects all transposition and transcription errors, together with a high proportion of random errors, overcomes this problem. If the figures in number 33243 had been transposed and written say, 32343, the arithmetical process used by the computer would produce a remainder of 20

PAGE 195 CH 5/FEB/71 42 JG

A T32563* SN STEVENS* FN JOHN* SX M* GP 2* DM 14/09/63*
DB 21/10/22* NH QUBJ 213* HA 7 PARSONS/WOOTTON/NR ABINGDON/BERKS*
UD 2* AZ 5* ML 3* DS 1*

A C32564* SN STEVENS* FN MARY* SX F* GP 2* DM 14/09/63*
DB 15*02/33* NH DUA 237867* HA 7 PARSONS RD/WOOTTON/NR ABINGDON/BERKS*
UD 2* AZ 5* NL 3* DS 1*

X T32563* HA 7 PARSONS ROAD/WOOTTON/NR ABINGDON/BERKS*

A L32565* SN STEVENS* FN MARGARET* SX F* GP 2* DM 14/04/58*
DB 28/03/58* NH PONQ 618* HA 7 PARSONS ROAD/WOOTTON/NR ABINGDON/BERKS*
UD 2* AZ 5* ML 3* DS 1*

A U32566* SN STONE* FN PEGGY* SX F* GP 2* DM 15/04/58*
DB 22/03/58* NH PONR 823* HA 28 HONEY LANE/SUTTON COURTENAY/BERKS*
UD 2* AZ 8* ML 3* DS 1*

A D32567* SN STONE* FN RUTH* SX F* GP 2* DM 17/10/49*
DB 06/12/37* NH DUAA 674* HA 28 HONEY LANE/SUTTON COURTENAY/BERKS*
UD 2* AZ 8* ML 3* DS 1*

A X32463* SN STUART* FN ALBERT* SX M* GP 2* DM 03/11/58*
DB 17/05/03* NH DTA 4317211* HA 90 FRAMES ROAD/ABINGDON/BERKS*
UD 2* AZ 8* ML -* DS 2*

X X32463* HA 6 MILTON LANE/SUTTON COURTENAY/BERKS* AZ 4* ML 4* DS 1*

AZ = ADDRESS ZONE. ML = MILEAGE. UD = USUAL DOCTOR
DS = DISPENSING CODE.

Figure 3. Specimen OCR input sheet. (fictitious records).

Table 2. Use of check character in patient number 33243.

Weights

3 x 19 =	57	Modulus 23	
3 x 7 =	21		
2 x 4 =	8		
4 x 9 =	36		
3 x 15 =	45		
		Multiple of modulus next above	
	167	167 is 8 x 23 = 184	

184 minus 167 = 17, corresponding to T in alphabet
Check Character is T

Weights of 19, 7, 4, 9 and 15 are allocated to the 5 digits of the number. Each digit is then multiplied by its corresponding weight and the results totalled (167). A modulus of 23 (the number of letters of the alphabet less I, 0 and Z) has been selected in our system. The multiple of the modulus next above the total (8 x 23 = 184) is selected and the total (167) subtracted.

ALPHA LISTING OF WOMEN REACHING 35 YEARS BETWEEN JULY 1970 AND JUNE 1971 INC

PERSON NUMBER	SURNAME	FORENAME	DATE OF BIRTH	S X	A Z	M L	G P	U D	D S	ADDRESS
X30219	AINSLEY	ROSEMARY OLI	06 03 36	F	6	03	2	2	1	2 DARK LANE/ABINGDON/BERKS
U30070	BARNARD	JANET ELIZAB	20 02 36	F	8	01	2	2	2	20 LUCCA DRIVE/ABINGDON/BERKS
S31258	BUCKELL	LYNDA	28 06 36	F	1		2	2	2	0 FARINGDON ROAD/ABINGDON/BERKS
X35709	DOOEY	LINDA	11 11 35	F	7	02	3	3	1	0 WHITES LANE/RADLEY/ABINGDON/BERKS
R33723	GEE	AVRILE	17 07 35	F	8	01	3	3	2	1 OVERMEAD/ABINGDON/BERKS
E34150	HARRIS	LINDA CAROL	03 05 36	F	2	01	3	3	2	97 WORDSWORTH ROAD/ABINGDON/BERKS
X30523	JARVIS	HILDA M	15 12 35	F	5	02	2	2	1	324 WHITE CROSS/ABINGDON/BERKS
V32508	PATERSON	DOROTHEA IRE	27 09 35	F	1		2	2	2	3 LARKHILL ROAD/ABINGDON/BERKS
Q33262	WORTH	JANET	30 10 35	F	2	02	2	2	1	55 ABINGDON ROAD/DRAYTON/BERKS

9 RECORDS ACCEPTED FROM 1183 ON THE FILE

Fig. 4. Computer produced listings (fictitious records).

(check character W), and the piece of information about the patient whose serial number was T33243 would be rejected (Table 2).

In the Community Health Project each participating practice is allocated a unique block of numbers approximately equal to the current practice list size. These numbers are produced by computer with an attached check character and are allocated to patients, the number then being the means of identification of the individual.

The computer can produce lists of patients sorted alphabetically by address zone, by age, or by any of the other variables listed in the basic record (Fig. 4).

The cost of constructing registers for the practices in the OCHP has varied with local methods and circumstances (Evans, 1972). In the practice described the time taken by the secretaries in 1970/1971 to complete a current practice register for 3,247 patients amounted to 147 hours. At 35p per hour this cost £51, of which £36 were recoverable from the Executive Council; OCR bureau costs were £65 and computer processing £83. Costs per 1000 records worked out at £61, of which £11 were recoverable from the Executive Council. Thus, the cost to the practice was 5p per record. Keeping the record up to date is relatively inexpensive and, depending on the turnover in the practice, costs between £2 and £3 per month for each 1000 patients on file.

Though there may still be some debate about the value of unselected screening for cervical cancer, a question Dr Gareth Lloyd discusses in chapter 31, the value of the computer in any screening campaign is exemplified by the call and recall 'package' scheme for cervical cytology being designed for practices in the OCHP. This scheme selects patients by age, marital status and high risk factors. Optionally it selects patients due for recall, either because the interval since the last smear (specified by the general practitioner) has elapsed, or (if no interval is stated) the last smear was more than six years before. Adhesive name and address labels and a list of patients may be produced. Depending on the response to the first call or recall, up to two further approaches may be made. The general practitioner specifies the 'lapse time' before a further approach. If no response is forthcoming from the patient within this time, the computer prints a list and an adhesive label as required for each non-responder.

Results of smears can be stored in the computer held file, whether in response to the computer call or recall 'package', or because the patient has requested one, or because the smear has been done by another agency such as a Family Planning Clinic. The prior recording of the results of smears previously carried out on patients in the practice prevents these patients being selected for a first call.

PRACTICE	AGE GROUP	HAD HYSTERECTOMY		ALREADY HAD SMEAR		NEVER HAD SMEAR		TOTAL
		No.	%	No.	%	No.	%	
A	20 — 34	—	—	215	72·4	82	27·6	297
A	35 — 49	8	2·8	208	73·8	66	23·4	282
B	35 — 49	4	1·8	51	23·4	163	74·8	218
C	35 — 49	71	8·0	280	31·5	539	60·5	890
A	50 and over	43	9·3	130	28·0	291	62·7	464
A	All ages	51	4·9	553	53·0	439	42·1	1043
D	All ages	93	2·8	938	28·1	2306	69·1	3337

Table 3. Women at risk in 4 practices.

Reasons for not doing a smear, because the patient refused or failed to respond to all approaches, or is pregnant, or has had a hysterectomy, or because of some other reason, can be included in the file. Doing so will exclude them from selection for call or recall. Identification of patients with known high risk factors such as low social class or high parity ensures early selection by the computer.

The package will include a statistical analysis of performance showing the proportion of the 'at risk' population which has been screened for cervical cancer, the response rates to call or recall, and results of smears analysed by various factors.

The user controls the total number of patients selected each time the program is run, whether recalls are included or not, how many approaches are made and when (for example, two letters followed by one visit), and the characteristics of the population to be selected for first call.

The practice must decide how many patients to select each month or quarter. Analysis of 11 OCHP practices shows that women aged between 20 and 65 years form approximately 25 to 30 per cent of the practice lists. The percentages of women at risk in selected populations are shown in Table 3. There are wide variations, due largely to differing practice attitudes to cervical cytology, but the figures suggest that between half and three quarters of women at risk have never had smears.

The expected response rate also affects the number of patients selected. If, on average, only half of the patients selected attend for a smear, then the user can select twice as many as can be accommodated in the time available. Expected response rates are difficult to predict since they depend so much on the approach taken by the practice. The package therefore allows for the number of patients to be specified each time the program is run, thus allowing the user to find the optimum number by trial and error.

All these functions can of course be quite adequately carried out manually, probably more cheaply than by computer if the cost of setting up the basic file is included. It is probably true that an expensive computing facility used solely as an aid to screening procedure does not make economic sense, especially for the relatively small populations involved. However, in considering the wider applications of computers in primary medical care, where the establishment of a basic record for all patients is indispensable, the additional facilities required for a screening programme are relatively easy to provide, especially since many of the items of information required for a screening programme may be relevant to other applications. The use of computers in screening should, therefore, be viewed in the wider context of the applications of computers in primary care.

Confidentiality

Once clinical data e.g. the results of cervical smears or the reasons for categorising 'high risk' patients are linked with the basic record, then problems of confidentiality arise.

It would obviously be possible to withhold from the computer all personal identification data such as name and address, since the computer requires only a number to identify an individual. However, if the user wants the computer to produce an adhesive label containing the patient's name and address to attach to the envelope of a letter inviting a woman to attend for a smear, then obviously these items must be included in the computer file. The alternative is for the practice staff to translate the numbers listed by the computer into names and addresses, but some of the advantages of using the computer are thereby lost.

Accepting therefore that there are sound operational reasons for storing personal identifiable clinical and social information in a computer then the general practitioner must satisfy himself that all reasonable precautions are taken to safeguard that information from unauthorised use and that he remains the sole arbiter of the uses to which the information is put. For their part, the custodians of the computer system must take all possible measures to secure the information (comparisons between security of computer records and paper records are irrelevant). These will be both political and technical. At the technical level, use of passwords, scrambling of information on compute: files, the use of selective keys allowing any enquirer access to only authorised items of information are all well established procedures and go a long way towards ensuring the security of computer held information.

At present the sheer labour of linking manually records from banks, tax authorities, the police, credit agencies and Health and Social Security Departments would be a major deterrent to creating a centralised data bank. Once all these records are computerised the technical difficulties of doing so would be much smaller. That it should not be allowed to happen is a political matter which depends on the decisions of the electorate and the integrity and ethical standards of the professions involved.

Future trends

Though item of service payments may not always constitute a large part of general practitioner incomes in the future, and the items for which payment is made may change, now that there is a financial incentive in knowing which women over 35 in a practice have not had a cervical smear, which patients have not been immunised against rubella or tetanus, and, if current negotiations are successful, which fit babies have not been screened, a growing demand for computer facilities in general practice can be expected, quite apart from the question of possible improvement in the quality of medical care.

Probably the next stage in the development of computers in general practice will be the extension of the 'basic practice file' facilities offered by organisations such as the OCHP. This 'batch mode' process with its relatively slow turnround (lists of patients sorted by various criteria according to the instructions of the general practitioner and returned to him in the post within say a week) is easy and economical to arrange. If such demand exists (and experience in the Oxford area suggests that it does) and resources were provided to meet it, facilities could be organised on a large scale relatively quickly.

The stage beyond this could be a computer held medical summary (by a 'batch mode' process) for each patient. A problem orientated medical record (POMR) in which emphysema appeared on the problem list would as a by-product produce a listing, at the appropriate time, containing the patient's name for influenza vaccination. A record in which a husband's occupation (coded according to the Registrar General's Classification) was Class IV or V and which contained details of a large number of pregnancies would generate, as a by-product, a listing in which the patient concerned was given priority for cervical cytology. The enormous labour in converting and updating the present record system (even after its conversion to A4 and POMR records) suggests that this development on a wide scale may be a decade away.

The association of the most recently prescribed industrial disease, nasal cancer, with woodworking in the furniture industry was demonstrated by a system of medical record linkage (Acheson, Cowdell, Hadfield and Macbeth, 1968). Similar rises in morbidity can point to hazards in the environment whether natural, social or occupational but imply the patient collection of data of potential hazards, some of them perhaps not of immediate relevance, over a number of years. The general practitioner in the United Kingdom is in a unique position to make this collection and to screen groups at high risk from whatever cause. To do so without the aid of computers with their enormous capacity for storage, linkage and analysis of data, would be unthinkable.

So far the GP has not been involved with the paraphernalia of the computing industry. Developments in replacing the conventional paper record with, for example, visual display units (television screen and typewriter keyboards) are at present very expensive and hence not widely applicable. They will, however, become cheaper and more widespread in the future and will involve the medical profession in some fundamental changes in its attitude to the provision of health care.

REFERENCES

Acheson, E. D., Cowdell, R. H., Hadfield, E., Macbeth, R. G. (1968). *British Medical Journal,* 2, 587.

Dinwoodie, H. P. (1970). Simple computer facilities in general practice—a study of the problems involved. *Journal of the Royal College of General Practitioners,* 19, 269.

Evans, J. H. (1972). *Symposium on Community Health Information Systems,* Oxford. September 5th—8th 1972. Department of the Regius Professor of Medicine, University of Oxford.

Smythe, M. (1968). in *Record Linkage in Medicine,* p. 179 ed. E. D. Acheson, Edinburgh: E. & S. Livingstone.

Wilson, J. M. G., & Jungner, G. (1968). *Principles and Practice of Screening for Disease.* Public Health Paper No. 34. Geneva: World Health Organisation.

7 The Health Visitor
Sheila Ganeri

> 'O, Sir, you are old;
> Nature in you stands on the very verge
> Of her confine: your should be rul'd and led
> By some discretion, that discerns your state
> Better than you yourself.'
>
> Shakespeare: *King Lear*, Act II, Scene IV.

His family cast him out into the storm, which he defies, and he fights impotently against the elements. It is a matter of choice whether we think of his madness as coming from the degenerative processes of old age in which his behaviour becomes troublesome, or whether we think of him as justly rebelling against, and being driven mad by, the ingratitude of his daughters.

None of the problems of old age—personal, family or communal— are new. What is new is the fact that more people live to a greater age and, therefore, any problems which exist are multiplied. The economic aspects have to be faced, and it may become more important than ever to find value in the capacity and competence that old people still have in family, social and occupational life.

The role of the Health Visitor

In this context, it is relevant ·to explain the role of the health visitor and the part she plays in the screening programme. It has been said that no other worker at present has a range of knowledge and skills comparable with those of the health visitor. The service the health visitor offers is essential if medico-social problems are to be contained within manageable proportions in relation to available resources in money and personnel, quite apart from the promotion of the health of the community in its widest sense.

71

Many general practitioners do not appreciate, nor do they understand, the role of the health visitor. This has to change, and will do so as more health visitors become attached to general practice teams, and general practitioners become aware of what they can contribute to patient care. Bearing in mind that soon after reorganisation of the National Health Service in April, 1974 all health visitors will be attached to general practitioners, it is essential that good relationships should be developed at an early stage. If the health visitor, as many do, condemns the general practitioner for his lack of interest in her work, then she must take the initiative and show that she can be a valuable member of the practice team, and in this way the patient will be the beneficiary. Many general practitioners still need educating as to her role, which will now be described.

The international definition states that public health nursing is a special field which combines the skills of nursing, public health and some phases of social assistance. It functions as part of the total health programme for the promotion of health, the improvement of conditions in the social and physical environment, rehabilitation, and the prevention of illness and disability. The health visitor is a nurse with post-registration qualifications who provides a continuing service to families and individuals in the community. Her work has five main aspects:

1 The prevention of mental, physical and emotional ill health and its consequences.
2 Early detection of ill health and the surveillance of high risk groups.
3 Recognition and identification of need, and mobilisation of appropriate resources where necessary.
4 Health teaching.
5 Provision of care; this will include support during periods of stress, and advice and guidance in cases of illness as well as in the care and management of children. The health visitor is not, however, actively engaged in technical nursing procedures.

She is a practitioner in her own right, detecting cases of need on her own initiative as well as acting upon referrals. She has skills and knowledge particular to her work, and these are drawn from her nursing background and from the additional preparation in her health visitor course. She brings to her work in the community:

1 Observational skills.
2 Skills in developing inter-personal relationships.
3 Skills in teaching individuals and groups.
4 Skills in organisation and planning in her own sphere.

The knowledge she brings to her service is obtained:

1 From her nursing background.
   (a) Human biology.
   (b) Principles of bacteriology.
   (c) Disease processes.
   (d) Therapeutic methods.
2 From her midwifery training.
   (a) Pre-natal development.
   (b) Factors influencing the subsequent health of the child.
   (c) Care of the mother and baby following delivery.
   (d) Emotional factors associated with pregnancy and childbirth.
3 From her health visiting course.
   (a) The development of the individual at all stages in the life cycle; 'from the cradle to the grave'.
   (b) The development of the individual in relation to his social and cultural group.
   (c) The development of social policy.
   (d) The changing pattern of health and disease and the methods used to determine priorities in the Services.
   (e) The principles and practice of health visiting.

The health visitor acts as a go-between for the Area Health Authority, the practice team, and the patients. She is the practice expert in preventive medicine, which in addition to screening includes health education, epidemiology and immunisation.

Screening

In smaller practices where there is no manager, the health visitor may well be in charge of the organisation of the whole screening programme. As part of her health education work, she introduces the patients to the concept of screening, its advantages, and its limitations. She must always explain the details of the programme. She may also need to educate the general practitioners to the value of screening. She should orientate the practice towards preventive medicine. She should also tactfully co-ordinate screening by area health authority staff—e.g. school clinics—with that of the practice within which she works. She should ensure there is no duplication of effort, and see to it that screens performed outside the practice, e.g. at hospital, or by area health staff, are reported to the practice, and assimilated into the patients' notes.

To some extent the quality of health visiting is affected by the philosophy of the employing authority, some hindering development and others encouraging professional growth. Since, however, the skills and knowledge we have outlined are basic, it follows that they are applicable to any situation in which the health visitor operates, and to any combination of duties. The Royal College of Nursing believes there is an ever-increasing need for health visitors to work alongside general practitioners in a team approach to the health of the community.

Unfortunately, as yet there is certainly not enough attention given to screening in the health visitor training syllabus. This is a tragic drawback since her role is based almost solely on preventive medicine. It is to be hoped that the Council for the training and education of health visitors will be made aware of this in the future.

The particular activities of the practice health visitor in relation to screening might include:

(a) Follow-up of the neonate after the midwife has left.
(b) Developmental paediatrics: a well baby clinic should be established in all practices.
(c) Routine screening for phenylketonuria.
(d) Organisation of cervical cytology.
(e) Administration of screening questionnaires.
(f) Special clinics e.g. obesity, anti-smoking.
(g) Assistance with geriatric screening.
(h) Immunisations.

The screening of patients could be endless; unfortunately time, manpower and money does bring its limitations; in present circumstances, each practice has to decide how much is to be done for its patients as a whole.

The health visitor monitors the whole screening programme; she identifies and tries to overcome any difficulties. She should encourage and persuade patients to take part in the screening programme, always bearing in mind that they cannot be forced; it is a free country, but surely prevention is better than cure. The health visitor should then assist in the follow up of freshly identified conditions arising from the screen. She should also keep up to date with screening literature in professional journals, and bring new ideas to the notice of the general practitioner. The health visitor must also keep careful records of her own participation in the screening programme, so that these may be passed to her successor at any time, should she be away from the practice. The health visitor should not initiate any screening procedure within the practice without the prior agreement of the general practitioner. In return, she should be entitled to be consulted by the general practitioner at every stage in the introduction of a screening programme; this would, of course, apply only to health visitors attached to a practice. The health visitor is more concerned with the general organisation and smooth running of the screening programme, than with carrying out individual screening procedures herself; usually these procedures can be delegated to other less-trained personnel.

Developmental assessment

With regard to the important subject of developmental assessment of the under-fives, it is becoming increasingly realised that this should be the function of the general practice team. Weighing and measuring and routine urine testing can perfectly well be undertaken by a receptionist or by similar ancillary staff, but there is need for a more careful delineation than hitherto realised between the parts to be played by the health visitor and by the general practitioner. Aspects of the programme that should lie well within the competence of the health visitor, when properly trained, include simple tests of sight and hearing, recording of milestones, and (with the aid of a questionnaire) the taking of case histories from the mothers, with special reference to behavioural anomalies and symptoms suggestive of backwardness, incoordination, and weakness or spasticity of particular muscle groups. Such essentially medical surveillance as routine neurological and cardiac examination falls, of course, within the province of the medically qualified doctor—ideally the child's own general practitioner. But the whole programme calls for more integration than it receives at present, and the health visitor has an important part to play in securing its efficient coordination and recording.

Geriatric screening

When asked to take part in a screening programme of the elderly, I experienced a sense of great joy that someone had at last recognised the need to screen the elderly in our society. I thought of an eighteenth century writer who said: 'Old age is such a charming condition. What a pity it lasts such a short time.' Perhaps there was something personal in the feeling. One remembers that George Bernard Shaw, on reaching his ninetieth birthday, was very concerned at the idea of mortality, and felt that at least for a few selected people there should be some lengthening of the ordinary span of life.

It then became my role to gain the full co-operation and acceptance of the patient and to allay any anxiety about health raised in the patients' minds by the screening programme. Each week certain patients were selected from the age/sex register and visited by me at their own homes. This visit was quite informal and it was stressed to the patient that this was a purely voluntary scheme, part of the preventive medicine programme of the practice, and that it was being carried out solely for their benefit and future health and happiness. During my visits only one patient declined the offer of screening; fortunately his medical condition was already well known to the practice.

On my visits I took with me a printed card in the form of a questionnaire, in order to assess the medical and social needs of the patients; this assisted the general practitioner with his part of the medical screen, which came later. An assessment could be made regarding housing, finance, family help, general health of the patient (e.g. diet, vision, hearing, bowel and micturition function, and so on), and whether or not the patient was receiving any help he might need from other agencies. The patient was asked to take a specimen of urine to the surgery and given an appointment for a health check there. I found the patients delighted to feel that an interest was being taken in them; many had not seen a doctor for several years. Many expressed anxieties which were easily dealt with, but which would never have been known had the screening programme not been carried out. I was given full access to the patients' records and told about their medical and social history beforehand. This greatly helped in my general approach to the patients, most of whom I had not seen before. This initial visit took away any fears on the part of the patients; they were made to feel that they had complete freedom of choice regarding the screen, and that no pressures would be brought to bear upon them.

I was able to explain to the patient the psychological and physiological processes of ageing. Old age is frequently discussed not as a stage of life but as a problem of residential accommodation, social amenities and medical attention. It is still appropriate to deal with the life of old people in the different aspects, physical, intellectual, emotional and social. The physical changes were explained to the patient, the wear and tear on various tissues. There are changes which are to be expected and which are normal. The rate of metabolism is reduced, some tissues may shrink, and many old people find they need to eat less, and so become thinner. Ageing people often accommodate themselves very well to the metabolic change by slowing down many of their activities, while yet finding themselves able to preserve some interest in restricted fields. Changes take place in the central nervous system, and the total amount of mental activity is reduced. The deterioration seems less marked in those of high intelligence, and it is one of the unfair aspects of nature that those who have more, often have it longer. Many patients expressed fears of loss of memory. Sometimes the difficulty of conversation with an old person is that particular topics of long ago become repeated time and again, and interest is lost in their conversation. Old people sometimes become separated from members of their family on this account—their lack of capacity to enter into the day-to-day life of the home. Important events occur in a household, and the old person has no foreknowledge of them; this can lead to a feeling of confusion, of uncertainty, and to the expression of a belief that he is no longer valued by the family. Physical, intellectual and emotional characteristics thus become linked with one another in the changing nature of behaviour which results from degenerative processes. There are social implications too, with regard to the various aspects of any care and treatment. My visits gave me an opportunity to talk to the patients generally and specifically about their anxieties and fears of growing old.

In place of all the tales of woe so often related to me about the National Health Service, I found it rewarding to see the surprise in the faces of the patients visited, when they realised that something was being offered them, without them having to do the asking. Not only did this help the screening programme, but it helped me as a health visitor to identify medico-social needs. I learned much about the worries of the elderly expressed about the younger members of the family, especially the grandchildren, and occasionally this led to my detection that something was indeed wrong with the child, and help was offered. All kinds of problems were brought to light during my visits, and had it not been for my involvement in the screening programme, families in need, children 'at risk', and so on may have slipped through the net. From the health visitor's point of view one of the advantages of a screening programme is that it can act as a foundation upon which other domiciliary work can be built up. Certainly it led to an improved image of general practice in the eyes of the family, which resulted in turn in an improved relationship between the family and the whole general practice team; and for me as a health visitor, it became a way into the family as a whole. One wishes that more general practitioners could be motivated into taking part in screening programmes of their choice, thus taking away from the patients the general feeling that the doctor is far too busy to care.

Continuity of care

There is a final point to be made. To develop a substantial range of screening activities within a particular practice, requires on the part of all concerned a very considerable amount of time and effort. The health visitor has a major role to play in all this, and it would be all too easy for the whole structure to break down should she leave the practice without an immediate replacement. In such an eventuality, someone must accept the responsibility of ensuring that continuity of screening is preserved within the practice. When Health Service reorganisation is complete, this responsibility could well fall upon the shoulders of the Community Physician. A practice cannot gear itself to working with a health visitor as a member of the practice team, then suddenly ungear itself. The present shortage of health visitors does occasionally lead to this deplorable situation. It is a problem that calls for more recognition and consideration than it receives at present from the powers that be.

If screening is to be developed to its full potential in British general practice, a major increase in the number of health visitors, and a radical improvement in the quality of their training, will undoubtedly be needed.

> 'What we have done
> Will not be lost to all eternity.
> Everything ripens at its time
> And becomes fruit at its hour.'

II Screening by Groups

8 The Newborn

'The rewards of prevention in childhood are unique because the benefits may last a whole lifetime.'

M.C. Joseph and R.C. MacKeith, 1966.

'Is my baby normal, doctor?' is the question, often unspoken, on the lips of every new mother—especially for the first time. As a result of work done in the past 15 years, we are now in a position to answer that question far more accurately than ever before. Ten years ago it was considered sufficient when examining a new baby (if it was done at all) to listen to the heart and lungs, palpate the abdomen and examine the perineum. We now have, in addition to the ordinary clinical examination, a battery of tests available to assess the neurological equipment of a new baby which is, after all, the most vulnerable body system, especially in the perinatal period, as well as a multitude of biochemical tests for the detection of metabolic disease. In fact, from a screening point of view it is a matter of some difficulty to select those tests which will provide the best returns out of the plethora available.

History

Arnold Gesell in America was the first to make any attempt at a scientific study of the growth and development of infants; he was followed in this country by such people as Professor R.S. Illingworth (1971), Dr Mary Sheridan (1960) and Dr R.C. MacKeith (1969). In France André Thomas and Mme. Saint Anne Dargassie, and in Holland Heinz Prechtl and David Beintema (1964) studied the central nervous system, while in Italy the pioneer work of Ortolani

(DHSS, 1969) on congenital dislocation of the hip should be mentioned.

The awareness in this country of certain pre- and perinatal factors liable to increase the incidence of abnormality resulted in the concept of the 'At Risk' register, but it has since been shown that screening of infants on the 'At Risk' register will uncover only about half of the abnormalities (Rogers, 1968; Hooper, 1971). There is thus a move for the periodic screening of all infants and there is at the time of writing a sub-committee of the Royal College of General Practitioners working on a suitable screening programme for use in general practice for children under school age.

What is one looking for in a neonatal screening examination? Primarily the search is for structural abnormalities in all systems and these can frequently be discovered by careful routine examination. The incidence of some of the more common ones is:

Down's syndrome	2 per 1,000
Hydrocephalus	1 per 2,000 live births
Congenital disease of heart	6 per 1,000 live births
Congenital dislocation of hip	1 per 1,500 live births
Undescended testes	30 per 1,000 of full term infants

But beyond this are disorders of funtion, and here one is concerned principally with the nervous system and its derivatives—the eyes and ears. Here one must be careful and Professor Illingworth has rightly stressed the importance of knowing what each test is intended to demonstrate. So one is looking for deficiency of sight or hearing responses, abnormal tone and defective responses indicating cerebral dysfunction and disordered function of the spinal cord reflexes and tracts. Finally there are the tests for metabolic disorders which involve the aid of the laboratory.

One or two further aspects of the neonatal examination must be stressed. Firstly, the importance of an accurate and careful antenatal history cannot be overestimated; in general practice this presents no problem as the doctor has usually been at least partly concerned in the antenatal care of the mother. Secondly, the neonatal examination must be seen not as an end, but a beginning. It is the base line from which all future observations of a child must be made. Thirdly it opens the door for the mother to discuss her otherwise unspoken anxieties about the baby, and for the doctor to assess the effect of the new arrival on the home. For the mother, and frequently the father, to witness this careful examination of their new baby which ends with the triumphant demonstration of the placing and walking response does more to inspire confidence and instil unity of care than all the talk and tablets in the armamentarium.

Is it worth it?

It is frequently argued against screening that the effort is not worth the return in terms of abnormalities discovered, that nothing can be done when they are discovered, that one merely induces unnecessary anxiety in the parents, and that the general practitioner sees so few abnormalities that he will not recognise one when he sees it. The truth is that repeated observation of the normal child is in itself a rewarding experience and gives a growing realisation of the range of normality, so that after a time the abnormal child 'sticks up like a sore thumb'—one cannot help but recognise it. With each examination taking about 10 minutes, one possibly abnormal child discovered and treated early each year makes the effort worth it. What can be done when an abnormality is discovered? The explosive advances of the past decade in cardiac and neurosurgery have made mandatory the early and accurate delineation of deformity of the cardio-vascular and central nervous systems. The benefit of a low phenylalanine diet in phenylketonuric infants has been amply demonstrated. Who is to say that advances will not be made in other areas? And when they come we must be prepared for them. As for inducing unnecessary parental anxiety, the experience of the writer is the exact opposite; many parents will harbour unspoken worries about their child for months for fear of being thought foolish by their doctor. To have the fear laid to rest, or, if valid, the realisation that the doctor knows and cares and will do his best to help and to get treatment started early, is a far more common and relevant experience.

How accurate is the examination?

Of course we can always go on perfecting our technique, but the examination about to be described has been used by the author for nearly ten years, and has so far proved to be reliable (Hooper, 1971). We investigated the 151 children born into the practice in 1967 and followed them carefully till the age of 18 months; and at the age of four-and-a-half years we re-examined 87 of them. At the neonatal examination 18 cases showed some abnormality (see Table 4). Six infants showed some deficiency in the neurological tests (see Table 5); in each case the findings were isolated, but required careful observation and by the age of 18 months they were all developing normally. Thus, Elaine had no walking response at birth; she was late in smiling at nine weeks; at six months she could not bear weight on her legs, did not reach for a rattle nor show recognition of her mother. Yet by 18 months she was normal and at four-and-a-half

D

Table 4. Abnormalities found at neonatal examination of 151 infants.

Abnormality	Number found
Erb's Palsy	1
Sterno-mastoid Tumour	1
Umbilical hernia	3
Talipes Equinovarus	2
Hydrocoele	1
Multiple skeletal abnormalities	1
Congenital Dislocation of Hip	1
? Ventricular Septal Defect	1
Persistent Jaundice	3

Table 5. Developmental deficiencies found at neonatal examination of 151 infants.

Deficiency	Number found
Moro response absent or difficult to elicit	3
Grasp response absent	1
Placing and walking response absent or difficult to obtain	4

years performed all her tests readily and appeared quite bright. It might be inferred from this that our efforts have been wasted, but our contention is that it is only in this way that we shall make an early diagnosis, as in the case of Peter who was noted at the neonatal examination to have an unusually active Moro response and who at the age of three months was showing definite signs of spasticity with tightly clenched fists (which is unusual at three months) and increased muscle tone in the limbs; by the age of six months it was possible to make a fairly confident diagnosis of spastic cerebral palsy which after being fully confirmed, led on to suitable treatment, which when started early probably gives much better results.

Of the 143 infants who appeared neurologically normal at the neonatal examination 83 were traced and re-examined at the age of four-and-a-half years. In none was there any neurological abnormality which should have been detected in the early months of life. Six cases (seven per cent) showed evidence of some intellectual delay, but these could probably be attributed to hereditary or environmental factors.

Prechtl (1965) investigated newborn children born after obstetrical complications. Of 102 infants without neurological signs 86 per cent were normal two to four years later, while of 150 infants with neurological signs 40 per cent were normal two to four years later.

These figures, we think, support our general impression over the past ten years, that a properly conducted neonatal examination will almost certainly reveal those children who are likely to show abnormalities or delay later, and fully justify the few 'false positives' which later become normal.

Who should do the neonatal examination?

The neonatal examination is performed once and never repeated; if the chance is missed it can never return, and the valuable information it affords is lost forever. As it is essentially a clinical examination it should surely be done by a doctor, whether he be a general practitioner or a member of the medical staff of a maternity unit. The only part that may justifiably be delegated to a nurse or health visitor would be the taking of the blood sample for the phenylketonuria test.

When does the neonatal examination take place?

The child is examined briefly at birth to exclude major abnormalities such as imperforate anus, oesophageal atresia or cyanotic congenital heart disorder which demand immediate specialist care. But it is best to delay a complete examination for three or four days to allow extra-uterine life to be established, and the examination is best done before 21 days.

The history

The list of factors which can influence the future growth of the foetus and infant is almost endless and comprehensive lists are available in many text books. Here only the commoner ones are listed.

Pre-natal. Virus infections in the first trimester—notably rubella, but other infections, e.g. syphilis, toxoplasmosis, cytomegalic inclusion disease. Maternal illness, e.g. diabetes, thyrotoxicosis treated medically. Drugs taken by mother, e.g. streptomycin, steroids, anti-epileptic drugs, irradiation. Complications of pregnancy, e.g. pre-eclamptic toxaemia, ante-partum haemorrhage, Rhesus immunisation, hydramnios.

Intra-natal. Short gestation and low birth weight, light for dates. Foetal anoxia (Apgar score).

Post-natal. Convulsions and cyanotic spells, hyperbilirubinaemia (kernicterus and later athetoid cerebral palsy and deafness), hyper-excitability or apathy.

The examination

The sequence in which the examination is conducted is not important; in examining the new baby one has to be guided by the state of the child; for instance it is best to examine the heart and feel the femoral pulses early on in case the baby should start crying and make auscultation difficult. So that while it may be said that it is simplest to 'Start at the top and work down', it is better to postpone those tests which are most likely to upset the baby. In the experience of the author this applies especially to examination of the palate and the hip test.

The infant is fully undressed and placed on the mother's bed or a suitable table lying on a nappy (with another nappy readily available in case of need). He is observed for skin condition, jaundice, spontaneous movements and obvious abnormalities, such as syndactyly or talipes. The muscle tone of the limbs is assessed by gently flexing and extending the arms and legs. The head circumference is then measured and in doing so the fontanelles and skull surface palpated. The eyes, if open, are examined for cataract and squint. The external ears are inspected (abnormal and low-set ears are sometimes associated with renal abnormality—Potter's facies). If the baby is crying the palate is examined for cleft palate. The auditory response may be tested now by ringing a bell or rattling a rattle above the baby's head (so that he cannot see it). In a positive response the baby will quieten, or open its eyes or become momentarily still. Next the front of the chest is percussed, followed by auscultation of the heart and lungs. It must be ascertained that the lungs are fully aerated. Crepitations may suggest the presence of fibro-cystic disease of the lungs. A heart murmur will suggest the possibility of a congenital heart lesion.

The child is then turned over and supported on the palm of one hand in the position of *ventral suspension*. In this position several features can be examined. The examination of the lungs posteriorly is completed. The spine is examined; spinal anomalies may be suggested by the presence of a tuft of dark hair over the lower lumbar spine, or a dermal sinus leading to the spinal meninges—not to be confused with the much more common post-anal dimple, the bottom of which can usually be easily identified. Lateral flexion of the spine is tested by laying the child on its side across the palm, first one side and then the other, and may reveal a congenital scoliosis. Finally the position of ventral suspension itself is most important. In this position the normal child will show evidence of extension (elevation) of the head and legs, maintained perhaps only momentarily, perhaps the head only. It is a test of general muscle tone. With the hypotonic child the head and legs will hang down limply as in a short gestation baby, or perhaps be our first indication that the child suffers from brain damage, e.g. the flaccid stage of cerebral palsy.

The child is then laid on the bed in the prone position. Here the normal full-term child will turn its head to one side to enable it to breathe, and show the primitive crawling response, with elevation of the buttock. In a short gestation infant the buttocks are not lifted from the bed. The movements should by symmetrical. The abdomen is best palpated in this position, with the hand passing round from behind on each side. In the right upper quadrant one palpates for enlarged liver, in the left for enlarged spleen, and in both lower quadrants for enlarged (polycystic) kidneys.

The child is then turned over and picked up to do the *Moro response*. This is a most important response; Mitchell (1960) concludes 'it seems most probable that the Moro reflex results from summation of a number of different reflexes originating in the neck muscles and labyrinths', but it tests also the integrity of the neural connections involving vestibule, medulla and the cervical cord; it also demonstrates hyper- or hypo-tonicity of the arms, and their mobility (e.g. absence of injury). The response may be symmetrical or asymmetrical; it may occur spontaneously or to the minutest of stimuli (low threshold), or be difficult to obtain (high threshold). Total absence of the response in the neonatal period is suggestive of higher brain damage, e.g. mental subnormality or cerebral palsy. By three months the response has totally disappeared in 56 per cent (Hooper, 1971); it has disappeared in the great majority by four to five months and persistence beyond this time is suggestive of cerebral dysfunction and spasticity. The response is best obtained by sudden extension of the neck, and this can be achieved in one of two ways. With the child lying supine the head is supported in the hand an inch or so above the bed. The hand is then suddenly removed, allowing the head to fall back on to the bed; or the child is supported lying on its back along one arm of the examiner, while the head is supported in the other hand which is then rapidly lowered an inch or so. The response consists of the rapid abduction of the arms at the shoulder, with the elbows, wrists and fingers extended though commonly the index finger is flexed. This is followed by adduction at the shoulders and flexion of the elbows and wrists.

Next, one attempts to elicit the *grasp reflex*. This tests the integrity of the spinal reflexes of the cervical cord, and sensory and motor functions of the hand, and is presumably a remnant from the time when we were monkeys and hung from trees or grasped the hair of the maternal bosom prior to sucking. Without touching the dorsum of the hand, a pencil or a finger is passed across the palm from the ulnar side. This produces flexion of the fingers around the finger or pencil. This can be followed by the *traction response*. When the fingers are firmly grasping the pencil it is drawn gently upwards, when the grip will be intensified and there will be flexion at the elbow and shoulder so that the infant can be suspended by its own grip. The symmetry or otherwise is noted; the response may be modified by hyper- or hypo-tonicity of the arm from any cause.

The child is then laid supine and the inguinal region inspected for hernia, the scrotum for the position of the testes and the penis for hypospadias; in the female the vulva and introitus are inspected. The femoral triangles are palpated for pulsation of the femoral artery on each side.

The child is now picked up to do the *placing and walking responses*. These responses test the integrity of the sensory and motor nerves of the legs, of the spinal reflexes, of the lumbar enlargement, and probably of the long tracts of the spinal cord. Total absence of the response suggests major brain damage. The responses are noted for symmetry and may be modified by hyper- or hypo-tonicity from any cause. The child is held upright from behind, with one hand round each side of the chest under the axilla. The dorsal surface of the foot is then brought into gentle contact with the overlapping edge of a table and the response is flexion of the hip and knee so that the foot is lifted and placed on the table. The test is repeated for the other side. This is the placing response. The feet are then rested on the table with the child still in the upright position and stepping movements will occur; the aftercoming foot may catch on the forward leg and have to be disengaged. This is the walking response.

This is followed by testing the *light response*. The child is taken to a source of diffuse light—usually a window—and held as for the start of the Moro response with the crown of the head pointing towards the light. The examiner then rotates slowly through 90° so that the light falls on one side of the child's face, and he will turn his head towards the light. It is, of course, important to ascertain that rotation of the head is mechanically possible, e.g. no sternomastoid tumour. The examiner then turns toward the light again, and when the child's head has assumed the mid-position the test is repeated for the other side. The advantage of testing in this way is that it can be done with the eyes closed. If it has been impossible to inspect the eyes previously the child is then held up high in the prone position facing the light when he will almost certainly open his eyes, allowing them to be inspected for cataract, etc. The child is then returned to the bed and if the palate has not been inspected this is done now, using a spatula or the handle of a spoon if necessary.

Finally comes the test for congenital dislocation of the hip. The thighs are flexed to a right angle and then grasped with the thumb on the medial side of the thigh and the fingers over the great trochanter, while the knee rests in the palm of the hand. Downward pressure is exerted on the femur by the hand in an attempt to dislocate the femoral head in a backward direction out of the acetabulum. The thighs are then abducted to a right angle, and in the process, the fingers push the great trochanter forward to force the femoral head back into the acetabulum. If this movement is associated with a click (audible or palpable) then the hip is dislocated, or at least unstable. This completes the clinical examination.

Screening for metabolic disease

There is a vast array of metabolic disorders, mostly genetically determined, and very rare, which may cause mental retardation (Council of Europe Report, 1973). Because of their rarity it is not economical to screen for all of them, but it should be done where other children in the family have been shown to be affected. It is however Government policy to screen for phenylketonuria and this is done shortly after birth using the Guthrie Test (Yu, 1972). A filter paper is impregnated with a drop of the infant's blood collected from a heel prick and is sent dry to the laboratory where the level of phenylalanine is estimated by a bacterial inhibition assay method. A level above 4·0 mg per 100 ml indicates phenylketonuria.

The future

Intrauterine interference with the foetus is already practised in some cases of rhesus immunisation disease. Amniocentesis at 14 to 16 weeks gestation is now fairly easy (Rhodes, 1973) and the resulting chromosome and enzyme studies may detect genetic anomalies such as ovarian agenesis, Down's Syndrome (Stein *et al.*, 1973), Huntingdon's Chorea and some muscular dystrophies. Where a foetus is 'at risk' such a screening procedure will surely find a place in the future; though whether termination of the pregnancy would then necessarily follow is a question which will have to be discussed by those concerned with the ethics of modern medicine.

ACKNOWLEDGEMENT

I would like to thank Dr R.C. MacKeith for kindly reading through this chapter, and making several valuable suggestions.

REFERENCES

Council of Europe Report (1973). Collective results of mass screening for inborn metabolic errors in eight European Countries. Report of a working party set up by the Council of Europe to study hereditary metabolic diseases. *Acta Paediatrica Scandinavica,* **62,** 413–416.

DHSS (1969). *Screening for the Detection of Congenital Dislocation of the Hip.* Monograph prepared for the DHSS by the Standing Medical Advisory Committee of the Central Health Services Council, circulated to NHS general practitioners by the Executive Councils.

Hooper, P. D. & Alexander, E. L. (1971). Developmental assessment in general practice. *Practitioner,* **207,** 371.

Illingworth, R. S. (1971). *Development of the Infant and Young Child, Normal and Abnormal.* Edinburgh and London: E. & S. Livingstone.

Joseph, M. C. & MacKeith, R. C. (1966). *A New Look at Child Care.* London: Pitman Medical.

MacKeith, R. C., Egan, D. & Illingworth, R. S. (1969). *Developmental Screening 0–5 years.* London: Heinemann.

Mitchell, R. G. (1960). The Moro Reflex. *Cerebral Palsy Bulletin,* **2,** 135.

Prechtl, H. & Beintema, D. (1964). *Neurological Examination of the Newborn Full-term Infant.* London: William Heinemann.

Prechtl, H. (1965). *Proceedings of Royal Society of Medicine,* **58,** 3.

Rhodes, P. (1973). Obstetric prevention of mental retardation. *British Medical Journal,* **1,** 399.

Rogers, M. G. H. (1968). Risk registers and early detection of handicaps. *Developmental Medicine and Child Neurology,* **10,** 651.

Sheridan, M. (1960). *The Developmental Progress of Infants and Young Children,* London: HMSO.

Stein, Z., Susser, M. & Guterman A. V. (1973). A screening programme for the prevention of Down's Syndrome. *Lancet,* **1,** 305.

Yu, J. S. (1972). Screening tests for inborn errors of metabolism. *Modern Medicine* December, 753.

9 The Pre-School Child   *G.H. Curtis Jenkins*

'Any country that wishes to raise the quality of child care will do well to ensure competent periodic developmental paediatric screening examinations of all infants and young children.'

Egan, Illingworth and MacKeith, 1969.

It was 27 years ago that Gesell and Amatruda (1947) described for the first time a system they called developmental diagnosis. Their research programme involved first the construction of test procedures and then their painstaking application to the examination of great numbers of children. As the result of this work they claimed it was possible, using their system, to diagnose by the end of the first year of life nearly all cases of amentia, sensory and motor defects as well as most severe personality defects. No claims were made as to the prediction of intelligence. The diagnostic process was possible only after a large number of painstaking and unfailingly accurate examinations had been carried out under carefully controlled conditions, which enabled accurate norms or means of behaviour to be ascertained. Once the norms were established, it was possible to assess an individual child's development by showing if the child's performance in the tests for the particular age group of that child fell within the norms expected. If the child's performance showed deviations from the norm, it was then possible to predict if the deviations were significant in the overall picture of the individual child.

In principle the idea was simple, but subsequently many problems arose out of the application of the process. Correlation, for instance, proved very difficult to achieve. Workers attempting to reproduce the original work, found that if a child was seen in different environments, there was considerable variation in the child's performance of the tests. It was also found that sometimes there was

91

little correlation between tests carried out at different ages on the same child, because of natural variation in the rates of growth that can occur. Even the actual assessment process has been found difficult to structure and record. Problems have arisen in allowing for such extraneous factors such as deprivation and hunger, which are obviously very difficult to judge objectively.

In the search for further suitable criteria, research workers have often concentrated their attention on sensory and motor tests (which are easy to do) to the exclusion of equally important aspects of behaviour such as concentration and responsiveness, which are much more difficult to investigate and record. Illingworth (1972) reviews more fully the difficulties encountered, and short-comings of the various test systems. In spite of these drawbacks, justification for instituting such a screening programme arises out of the many studies that have been made of the health of children in the United Kingdom. Rutter, Tizard and Whitmore (1970) in a study of 3,200 children in the Isle of Wight, revealed something of the unsuspected handicap that exists in children in spite of local authority clinics, general practitioners and other services responsible for the care of the infant and young child. Only one in seven of the children discovered to have a handicap had previously been identified by parent, teacher or doctor. One in 10 of all the children had a learning handicap, which given an efficient screening programme could have been detected prior to school entry. Further studies of specific disorders have produced similar findings. In a review of the ophthalmological services in the Northampton area, Ingram (1973) has shown that only half the children with squint had reached an ophthalmologist by the age of seven years. The serious aspects of this are firstly that by this time all the children with amblyopia had lost sight in the lazy eye and therefore binocular vision was lost for ever, and secondly as many as 60 per cent of all children with squints have an associated loss of acuity in the remaining good eye that would probably have prevented them from seeing the blackboard clearly in school, and it is almost inevitable that this remained undiagnosed and untreated as well (Davie, Butler and Goldstein, 1972).

Studies such as these have shown the need for the institution of efficient screening. If it existed, all such children would have been detected, and the handicap produced by such disorders diagnosed and treated appropriately. In nearly every case early diagnosis can alter ultimate prognosis and management of the child.

Other reasons for offering an efficient screening programme are less dramatic in their effect. However it is as well to realise what can be achieved once a child has been identified as deviating from the accepted norms of growth and development. Disorder, especially when caused by brain damage, often presents as delay occurring in the normal development of the child. If the delay is recognised by a screening examination, the handicap so caused can be assessed comprehensively by the specialist to whom the child is referred. Usually the specialist works at an assessment centre as set up by many local authorities, although the hospital sector offers, in many parts of the country, similar service. On assessment, further handicaps are often found; for handicap, when it occurs, is often multiple. That maternal rubella induces a particular form of deafness in the child is well known. The associated visual disorder was detected only when an overall assessment began to be made of these children (Gregg, 1941).

A disorder can occur at any time and in any system of the rapidly growing infant and young child. Catarrhal deafness occurring at a critical time, unsuspected by parent or doctor not trained to look for it, can cause considerable problems in the acquisition of speech. So can the high tone deafness caused by haemolytic disease of the new born. Both are treatable, but only when first detected by an efficient screening system and then assessed by the appropriate specialist, so that an accurate diagnosis can be made and treatment instituted.

As has already been mentioned, major handicap in one system is often accompanied by handicaps occurring in other systems. The resulting disablement of the child can cause enormous problems. For the parents responsible for the child's care, the burden can be so heavy that siblings are deprived of love and affection because of the sheer impossibility of spreading out time and effort to beyond that of satisfying the needs of the handicapped child. Often, too, the marriage itself can become permanently affected. Initial detection of the damaged child and continuing multidisciplinary assessment and the provision for instance of nursery and day centre care can often prevent such disasters occurring, and can greatly help the families with handicapped children as well as the child affected.

Finally, efficient screening could detect those severe disturbances of behaviour that occur at any time in the first few years of a child's life. A hyperkinetic, non-sleeping destructive child can disrupt an already strained marital relationship, and even bring down on his or her head actual physical retaliation from parents at the end of their tether. Early recognition can often alleviate such problems with effective treatment of parent and child. Handled incorrectly by parent or doctor, more severe disability such as neurotic obessional rituals sometimes contribute to the establishment of a lifetime pattern of neurotic behaviour. Early detection and treatment has a much greater chance of success (Eisenberg, 1966).

With the need for screening established, problems now arise of organisation at a national level, and of allocation of scarce resources. To alleviate the latter Lindon (1961) and Sheridan (1962) introduced the concept of the 'at risk' register. Children with 'at risk' factors, preeclamptic toxaemia in the mother, foetal asphyxia, haemolytic disease of the new born with a serum bilirubin level rising above 15 mg/100 ml and a family history of deafness, and many other factors identified as possible causes of handicap, should be placed on the register and screened as a priority group; it was felt that children with no such 'at risk' factors could be safely left unscreened.

Problems of great complexity have arisen consequent to the introduction of this selective screening (Alberman and Goldstein, 1970). Over-enthusiastic application of the rules have placed more than half the new born children in some areas on 'at risk' registers. Davie et al. (1972) have shown too that only at very low resource levels was the optimal procedure that which allocated all to the high risk groups. At higher levels this became progressively more inefficient. In spite of the absence of reliable screening tests, many local authorities have installed elaborate computer controlled screening programmes. Because of the inherent unreliability of the screening tests, it is possible that many children without handicap are needlessly being followed up and many children with handicap are actually missed.

The unreliable nature of the screening tests has been highlighted by Richards and Roberts (1967), and again by Roberts and Khosla in 1972. Even the well established vision and hearing tests pioneered by Sheridan (1958, 1960) have never been statistically validated, nor have properly controlled trials of observer variability been carried out. That screening clinics were of doubtful benefit when the actual tests had not even been statistically validated is therefore not difficult to understand. Together with the problem of the self-selected nature of the group that attends local authority infant welfare clinics, and such factors as the fall in attendance after the child's second birthday, inadequate staff, inefficient deployment of resources, and both the uneven nature of the application of actual screening tests and the geographically uneven provision of the back-up specialist assessment centres, it becomes a matter of some surprise that the present system works as well as it does.

Having established that developmental diagnosis is possible, and that efficient screening would detect, if carefully instituted, a great deal of the presently undetected disorder, it is now worth considering the criteria that a screening programme would have to fulfil before its introduction at a national level, and into general practice in particular.

(i) Effective use of available time is of paramount importance. If an effective 15 minute screening examination, statistically validated, existed which could detect at the earliest possible moment most if not all disorders that cause handicap, then one doctor working 2 two-and-a-half hour sessions weekly could satisfy the screening needs of a practice population of 10,000 with a birth rate of 120 yearly. Each child could be screened six times in the first five years of life. That this is possible in present-day general practice has already been confirmed (Curtis Jenkins, 1973).

(ii) Any examination carried out should be painless in every sense to doctor, parent and child. Only with the complete trust and co-operation of parent and child can an adequate examination of all aspects of the child's behaviour be made, so as to make an assessment of the child's progress possible.

(iii) The disorders detected should be capable of amelioration, and the prognosis for the most part be improved by any treatment offered. Adequate provision of specialist assessment centres is therefore essential.

(iv) If the condition discovered cannot be significantly altered by treatment, then someone must be responsible for the co-ordination of services designed to lift some of the burden of care placed by society on the parents of children with handicap. Community care still all too often means just care by the parents in the home, with inadequate help. Intelligent co-ordination of the help that can be obtained from pressure group organisations, like the Spina Bifida Association, the Coeliac Society or the Spastic Society will often change an impossible situation to a bearable one. The informed well-motivated general practitioner with his knowledge of the family is ideally placed for such a role. Even intelligent interest and understanding can be of great psychological help.

Having established the criteria, how can the general practitioner screen his practice population of under-five-year-olds effectively? If a practice could state that every child in its care under five years old was efficiently screened at regular intervals, then on the basis of the improved detection rate of vision and hearing disorder, developmental delay of all kinds and even learning handicap, it could be reasonably assumed that the quality of care in that practice was better than in a practice offering no such screening. Once one doctor in a partnership started to gain experience of the screening tests now used, inefficient though they may be, then he would start to gain knowledge and insight into the development and variety of growth pattern that occurs in the normal child.

It is essential in my opinion that the doctor should carry out the entire examination, and delegate none of it to other workers. Successfully carried out, tests of vision and hearing are not just tests of vision and hearing; they also afford the doctor considerable insight into the whole picture of a child's development. To deprive himself of this is to diminish greatly his effectiveness. Nor is it fair to expect health visitors to be specialists in developmental paediatric medicine. They are not trained with this in mind. Their skills are of a totally different order, and their time far too valuable to be used in the wasteful testing of vision and hearing. The doctor with his skills is far more efficient in performing these tests when they are carried out as part of an overall screening examination. Studies made by Roberts and Khosla (1972) on the effectiveness of screening tests performed by the health visitor cast considerable doubt (not surprisingly) on their ability to pick up neurological visual and auditory handicaps anyway.

Continuing postgraduate education is very important. However, the hospital base of the technology taught is sometimes of doubtful benefit. Books, such as *Developmental Screening 0–5 years* (Egan, Illingworth and MacKeith, 1969) which offers a basis for a developmental screening system, are also extremely useful in the learning process. However, unallied as the suggested system is to any recording device, and lacking as it does a carefully constructed protocol, it remains a primitive tool, and partly because of the time factor not wholly suitable in a general practice screening situation. Nevertheless it offers an excellent framework on which to build skills of detection.

In the absence of any statistically validated screening system coupled to a standard record, a developmental paediatric research subcommittee of the practice organisation committee of the Royal College of General Practitioners has developed and is testing at this moment just such a screening tool. Prefeasibility studies already carried out have been encouraging enough for a 5,000 child survey to be actively planned. Observer variability, statistical validation, incidence of disorder, as well as the effectiveness of the actual screening tests used in detecting disorder, are all under scrutiny.

In the practice in which I work this system has been used for three years, after six years of unsystematic and, for at least some of the time, poor quality screening. I am personally responsible for the developmental paediatric care of approximately 1,300 children under five years old. With the help of a doctor from outside the practice who has received training in developmental paediatrics, and the invaluable assistance of three health visitors and a part-time programme secretary who organises the running of clinics, the maintenance of the birth book (an accurate register in birth order of all children in the 0–5 years age group) and the running of the appointment system, we have screened nearly all children at least five times in the first five years of life, using a standard examination and recording system. The children are examined routinely within three weeks of birth usually by me on a visit to the home (increasing my total visits by only 15 per cent a year), at seven months (when the responses to the Stycar hearing and vision tests have become much more reliable than at six months), one year, two years, three years (if indicated as necessary by parent, health visitor or doctor), and four and a half years. The 15 minute examination covers all aspects of a child's growth and development, and a full psychosocial history is obtained by the health visitor immediately before the examination.

The system gives early warning of any disorder that could lead to handicap, adequate surveillance of existing disorders and a tentative prediction of learning handicap. Children, who for any reason need to be followed up more frequently, are fitted in with no difficulty. Special care is taken to identify those children likely to be socially deprived for any reason. The health visitors are largely responsible for the surveillance, and for bringing any change in situation to the notice of the doctor in the partnership with whom the child is registered, so that he can become aware of the situation as well as the doctors responsible for the paediatric care programme. The separation between illness care and well care is easily understood by the parents, who ask automatically to see their own personal doctor in the partnership for any acute illness in their child. No pooling of patients occurs, and the other doctors in the practice do not feel that the running of the screening programme intrudes on their relationship with their patients.

As well as the increased detection rate of disorder, many influences are at work in promoting the positive health of the child in our care. The reasons are many. For instance, similar advice given to parents for the same disorder at infant welfare clinics, by health visitors and by general practitioners is unusual when parents and their children alternate between infant welfare clinic and general practitioner; it is not surprising that both lose credibility in a situation that allows this to happen. In a practice running a dynamic programme with the closest co-operation between attached health visitors and general practitioner, it is easy to prevent this situation occurring. Patient acceptance of advice is greatly enhanced, and obesity and dental caries both respond gratifyingly to such an approach. Hooper (1973) has shown that obesity can be virtually eradicated by such a programme. A near 100 per cent immunisation rate is easy to achieve. Natural fluctuations that occur in growth and development of children, which can cause so much heartache to parents, can be identified first of all, then honestly and authoritatively discussed with them. It is always worth remembering that a mother is nearly always right if she is worried about her child's growth and development, as she has ample time to compare her child with others of the same age group. Even though she ascribes the delay to 'laziness', she has often identified its presence long before the doctor or health visitor.

Finally, the impact on practice management and organisation is considerable, and dynamic shifts occur in patient usage as well as in the doctors' patterns of working in the practice. From provisional data obtained from the National Morbidity Survey 1970—71, shortly to be published, comparisons between the author's group practice and the other 50 practices taking part in the Survey show for our practice a consultation rate at least 25 per cent *lower* than the average for the 0—4 year age group, in spite of the inclusion of developmental screening examinations in the calculated figures. Yet our consultation rates for all other age groups are over 20 per cent *above* the norm. This indicates, I feel, a highly significant reduction of workload arising from our paediatric screening programme, as does the paediatric out-patient referral rate of the 0—4 year age group in our practice, which is 35 per cent lower than the average rate of other practices in the Survey. Moreover, increased detection rates of, for instance, eneuresis and all forms of behaviour disturbance point to the much closer involvement of the group practice in the preventitive aspects of paediatric care just as obviously as does the increased detection rate of such disorders as reduced visual acuity and hearing handicap.

In spite of the increased detection rates in all these disorders, the overall work load as measured by consultation rates for the 0—4 year olds is reduced substantially, and this enables the partners to spread the medical resources of the practice over other age groups, with consequent improvement in care quality. Last and by no means least, registration of new born babies with individual doctors occurs within days of birth, not weeks, months or even years, which was the disordered pattern before the introduction of the child care programme.

Nationally, such a programme as I have described is feasible; 4,000 doctors, suitably trained, could screen the under-five year old population of the United Kingdom six times in the first five years of life working only two sessions weekly, seeing nine or ten patients each session, as well as fitting in those children who need increased frequency of surveillance. The reservoir of skill is already present in part in the local authority sector and, with the addition of general practitioners already holding the DCH (some 5 per cent), more than enough doctors are available. Adequate realistic training is required, without its present hospital bias, and remuneration matching the responsibility and extra work entailed for the individual doctor.

In 1971 £13,000,000 was spent by local authorities running clinics and centres under sector 22 of the National Health Service Act 1946 in England and Wales. 246,000 sessions were worked in all, 171,740 by medical officers employed by the local authorities concerned, 73,569 by general practitioners, and 1,337 by hospital medical staff. With a new direction, adequate tools, and increased job satisfaction that a good working environment brings, a far greater cost effectiveness will be gained from the exercise by the introduction of an efficient screening system. General practitioners could contribute greatly to the existing manpower situation. 1,000 practitioners working two sessions a week could carry out nearly a million screening examinations in 96,000 sessions yearly. The consequent reduction in consultation rates and subsequent savings in money and time would contribute greatly to a slowing down in the continuing increase in the cost of the National Health Service, while actually increasing its effectiveness in preventive medicine. The participating general practitioners gain a whole new dimension in their skills and awareness by making themselves responsible for the wellcare of the children in their practice.

However, until efficient screening tests exist, and until a system is built up to ensure that every child is seen (our experience shows that non-attendance at first appointment running at 10 per cent is probably the best 'at risk' indicator of disorder existing in the child), and until there is a nation-wide implementation of the national policy to create specialist assessment centres fully staffed to provide the essential back up services to any such national screening programme, it is likely that money now spent on all such services is producing a poor return in proportion to the effort and time expended. Whether the reorganised National Health Service will allow central government to grasp this nettle remains to be seen.

REFERENCES

Alberman E. D. & Goldstein, H. (1970). The 'at risk' register. A statistical evaluation. *British Journal of Preventative and Social Medicine*, 24, 129–135.

Curtis Jenkins, G. H. (1973). Developmental paediatrics in general practice? *Medical Digest*, 6, 18.

Davie, R., Butler, N., & Goldstein, H. (1972). *From Birth to Seven* pp. 90–92, 186. London: Longman.

Egan, D. F., Illingworth, R. S., & MacKeith, R. C. (1969). *Developmental Screening 0–5 yrs. Clinics in Developmental Medicine.* London: Spastics International Medical Publications, in assoc. with William Heinemann Medical Books Limited.

Eisenberg, L. (1966). *Developmental Medicine and Child Neurology*, 8, 593.

Gesell, A., & Amatruda, C. S. (1947). *Developmental Diagnosis.* London: Hoeber.

Gregg, N. McA. (1941). Congenetial cataract following german measles in mother. *Transactions of Ophthalmological Society of Australia*, 3, 35.

Hooper, P. D. (1973). Personal communication.

Illingworth, R. S. (1972). *Development of the Infant and Young Child.* 4th Edition. London and Edinburgh: Churchill Livingstone.

Ingram, R. M. (1973). Role of school eye clinics in modern ophthalmology. *British Medical Journal*, 1, 278.

Lindon, R. L. (1961). The risk register. *Bulletin of Cerebral Palsy*, 3, 481–487.

Richards, I. D. G. & Roberts, C. J. (1967). The 'at risk' infant. *The Lancet*, 2, 711–713.

Roberts, C. J., & Khosla, T. (1972). An evaluation of developmental examination as a method of detecting neurological, visual and auditory handicaps in infancy. *British Journal of Preventative and Social Medicine*, 26, 94–100.

Rutter, M., Tizard, J., & Whitmore, K. (1970). *Education, Health and Behaviour*. London: Longman.

Sheridan, M. D. (1958). Simple clinical hearing tests for very young or mentally retarded children. *British Medical Journal*, 2, 999.

Sheridan, M. D. (1960). Vision screening of very young and handicapped children. *British Medical Journal*, 2, 453.

Sheridan, M. D. (1962). Infants at risk of handicapping conditions. *Monthly Bulletin of Ministry of Health and Public Health Laboratory Service*, 21, 238–245.

10 The School Child
R. Harvard Davis

'If prescriptive screening were developed logically the problem of assembling a balance sheet of benefits and costs would hardly arise until certain basic criteria be met.'

T. McKeown and E.G. Knox

There is a general obligation in screening groups of persons for disease to ensure:-

1 That a screening procedure is effective.
2 That it makes better use of limited resources than the available alternatives.

It is necessary to do this because in screening for disease, the doctor is placing himself in a different position from that which he usually holds. On the one hand, when a patient consults a doctor, the latter undertakes to do the best that he can within the limits of the knowledge and resources available to him. He does not and cannot be condemned if the state of medical knowledge or the limitations of his resources do not allow him to make an accurate diagnosis or to prescribe the necessary treatment. On the other hand, when a doctor or an authority goes to people and says 'we think that it is in your best interest to be investigated for a certain disease' then the person can reasonably demand that the doctor will not only be able to identify the abnormality accurately but will also be able to do something effective about it if this is found to be necessary.

From these obligations, certain criteria can be established by which all screening procedures can be measured. These are:-

1 The condition should be an important problem. The natural history of the condition must be established and there should be a recognisable latent period before symptoms appear.

101

2 It must be possible to identify the condition accurately at an early stage by an acceptable technique.

3 Methods of effective treatment of management must be available.

4 Screening must be economic in relation to other medical expenditure.

Before applying these criteria to the problems of school-children, it is worthwhile first to review briefly the way in which the school health services have evolved, and then to consider what should be the objectives of screening for school-children in the light of the criteria which have been outlined above. It is worth noting that the service is called the 'School Medical Service' rather than Health Service, implying thus a significant concern in the management of symptomatic disease rather than with pre-symptomatic conditions. Regular examination of children during their school years has been a prominent feature of child health care and the local health authority services for many years. The origin of this type of screening goes back to the era when medical care was not freely available for the majority of this section of the population. The practice served in its early years to uncover a great deal of ill-health which required treatment and which would undoubtedly have significantly affected the prospects of children by interfering with their education and employment capabilities. As a result of this experience, it became a statutory part of the school medical service that each child should be examined at certain times. These were at school entry, which is at the age of five years, and at school leaving, which was, until recently, between fifteen and sixteen years of age. Further examinations were undertaken at more frequent intervals, of those children who were found to have conditions which warranted this.

More recently, the school medical examination has come to be regarded as a method of multi-phasic screening of children of school age. But because of its origins, the process still retains a large element of the routine medical examination about it. For example, the statutory form which has to be completed for each child (Form 10M), lists not only hearing and vision, but also all the major systems of the body. The examining medical officer is expected to place a tick against those in which there is no abnormality and another symbol in those in which there is some abnormality.

Thus, for historical reasons, the school medical examination clearly does not fulfil the criteria generally regarded as applicable to methods of screening for pre-symptomatic disease. It is a mixture of screening and of the detection of established disease, the common objective being to ensure that neither shall impair the educational opportunities of the child.

Since the inception of the National Health Service medical advice, free at the point of delivery has become available to all, including school children through the medium of the general medical services. In practice, however, there still appear to be gaps in the clinical service. For example as late as 1967, Horner when comparing the results of school medical examinations with data obtained from a questionnaire circulated to general practitioners in Croydon, found that only 67 per cent of the defects that had been discovered at the school medical examination were apparently known to the general practitioner. These figures must be accepted with caution however, because only 63 per cent of the doctors replied to the questionnaire.

More recently, Wintle, Clay and Davis (1972) studied the position in a group practice which served a defined population, most of whom were registered with the practice, and in which the staff also undertook the school medical examinations. This group practice were also using a system of records designed to integrate the data of the doctor, the health visitor and the district nursing sister within the same record (Wallace and Davis, 1970). In these circumstances, which it is to be hoped will be those pertaining throughout the United Kingdom in the future, Wintle and his colleagues noted the abnormalities found at the school medical examination and then looked at the medical practice record to see whether the defect had been already defined. Eighty-seven per cent of all the defects which were found at the school medical examinations were not apparently known to the general practitioner, health visitor or district nurse, or at least had not been recorded. But on a more detailed analysis it was clear that the vast majority (81 per cent) of the defects that had been noted at school medical examinations could have been detected by suitably trained nurses, and that all except one of the defects were acute conditions which would almost certainly have been brought to a doctor in the course of a few days (Table 6).

It is only recently however, that the local health authority services and the general medical services have begun to be effectively integrated by the attachment of district nursing sisters and health visitors to group practices and the development of the concept of the primary health care team. Theoretically, with such a team it should not in the future be necessary to organise a service to deal with the unmet needs arising from acute illness and it should be possible to concentrate upon the chronic problems and thus to make the school health service a screening mechanism for those abnormalities which are likely to affect a child's education or occupational future. In any case, it would seem to be inappropriate to set up a screening programme to detect the inefficiency and ineffectiveness of a clinical service except as a research procedure.

Table 6. Findings at school medical examination of 90 children (Average age five years).

System	Defect	Total	Known to general practitioner	Not known to general practitioner	Could be detected by nurse	What nurse would have missed
Ears	Acute otitis media with hearing loss	4	1	3	0	4
	without hearing loss	4	0	4	4	0
Eyes	Poor visual acuity	2	0	2	0	0
	Strabismus	1	1	0	4	0
	Colour blindness	1	0	1	0	0
Skin	Warts	0	0	0	0	0
	Scabies	8	1	7	8	0
	Head lice	0	0	0	0	0
	Dry skin	0	0	0	0	0
Chest	Bronchitis	1	0	1	0	1
Heart	Systolic murmurs	3	0	3	0	3
Enuresis		15	1	14	15	0
Speech		3	1	2	3	0
Psychological	Head banging	1	0	1	1	0
	Schooltime urinary incontinence	1	0	1	1	0
Other	Maldescended testes Faecal incontinence	3	1	2	2	1
	Pectus excavatum	1	0	0	0	0
Total		48	6	41	38	9
		100 per cent	12·8 per cent	87·2 per cent	80·9 per cent	19·1 per cent

If we make the assumption that the school medical service will not continue as it is presently organised, but will be a service which is designed to screen school children with regard to their health then it is possible to consider what is needed, taking into account the criteria that have already been outlined.

The objective of screening school children is clearly to detect those conditions which will impair a child's educational ability or which will affect the nature of their future occupation. Some of the conditions will be congenital defects whilst others will be acquired defects.

The detection of congenital abnormalities is a major argument in favour of the establishment of developmental assessment of children from birth. Theoretically, therefore, all congenital abnormalities should be detected before school age, that is before the disability has resulted in any substantial hindrance to development, provided that the means of such detection exists. The only possible exception is maldescent of the testes in boys. If this state of affairs were to be achieved, then screening for congenital abnormalities would not be a problem in children of school age. That is, the frequency with which these conditions would occur undetected in the population would not be worth the expenditure of the resources necessary to detect them. In other words, screening for congenital conditions in school children is merely highlighting the deficiencies of the pre-school screening programme.

Some acquired conditions are important because they pose a substantial threat to development, education and future occupation and because they occur sufficiently frequently or may go undiagnosed for an appreciable length of time. Amongst these, the most important are deafness resulting from acquired disease. Fraser's studies (Fraser, Morgan and Trotter, 1960; Fraser, Froggart and James, 1964; Fraser, 1964), have shown that the great majority of cases of severe deafness arising from post-natal causes can be predicted upon the basis of a few readily recognised conditions, notably meningitis and otitis media. Deafness resulting from serous otitis media is however, less likely to be immediately recognised because pain is not a feature of this condition. Impacted wax is another condition that may give rise to unsuspected deafness.

Pure tone audiometry is probably the best method of detecting loss of hearing but it will be clear that auroscopic examination will be more effective in determining the cause of deafness. Further research is needed to determine the precise extent of the frequency of significant deafness in school children. Ideally, all children should be examined, and the examination needs to be repeated. There is, however, no evidence with regard to the frequency with which the examination should be repeated, but since upper respiratory tract infections are most common in the early school years, this would probably be the most profitable time.

As with deafness, defects of visual acuity and colour-blindness can be reliably and readily tested for. The examination, likewise, needs to be repeated at intervals.

Both deafness and visual defects can be tested for by suitably trained nurses in children of school age. There is an effective treatment which can be given in the majority of cases and certainly the educational process can be modified to give the child the best chance.

Further work needs to be undertaken in order to estimate the size of the problem, and until this is done, it is not possible to make a realistic assessment of the economic viability of screening for these defects.

There is no good evidence that any other condition justifies screening in children of school age. For example, the evidence that treating asymptomatic bacteriuria in young girls will prevent pyelonephritis is not conclusive, and although obesity which is probably determined at an early age could be detected by a nurse, the treatment involves such a major programme of health education that it would be almost certainly uneconomic even if it was effective.

The screening of school children represents an instance where screening, prevention and routine clinical work have in the past become confused. It is however, an area which is liable to raise emotive feelings and to be the subject of much influential lobbying to provide screening services upon a national basis. It is essential that a proper analysis of each problem in terms of effectiveness and efficiency be made before these pressures are acceded to. The screening of school children also provides an example of the importance of making sure that the data which is collected by screening is not being collected elsewhere. The organisation of multi-phasic screening even for a population such as children is expensive both in terms of the equipment that is needed and of the manpower that is required. It is therefore important to be certain that the same result cannot be achieved by grafting it on to routine clinical work. School children experience a high morbidity rate and are therefore taken to a doctor more frequently than the general population. This is particularly so in their early years at school. It is thus possible to screen such children on these occasions. This is what has been termed tactical screening as opposed to whole population strategic screening. This method of screening has been particularly effective in other fields such as cervical cytology, and has been advocated, for example, in screening for cancer of the breast.

The screening of school children presents a very good example of the confusion that can arise when pre-symptomatic screening is mixed up with clinical work. This is not to imply, however, that the two cannot go hand in hand. Indeed, to separate preventive medical care from curative care is illogical by any standards. It is important to ensure that screening for pre-symptomatic disease is incorporated into the existing clinical services in the most appropriate way. In the United Kingdom the general practitioner is peculiarly well placed to undertake a considerable amount of this work by virtue of his relationship with his patient and because he has a definable population of patients at any one point in time. These factors can have a significant effect both on the acceptance rate and upon the cost of providing the service. If however, these objectives are to be achieved, then general practitioners need to review and in some cases change their organisation and in some cases to be re-trained. This process is going to take time, but will be facilitated by the changes in the organisation of general practice, which are going on at a remarkable pace. We should therefore plan our future services upon the assumption that such changes will take place rather than attempting to provide a temporary expedience.

REFERENCES

Fraser, G. R. (1964). In *Research in Deafness in Children*, edited by L. Fisch. Oxford University Press.

Fraser, G. R., Froggatt, P. & James, P. N. (1964). Congenital deafness associated with electrocardiographic abnormalities, *Quarterly Journal of Medicine*, 33, 361.

Fraser, G. R., Morgan, M. E. & Trotter, W. R. (1960). The syndrome of sporadic goitre and congenital deafness, *Quarterly Journal of Medicine*, 29, 279.

Horner, J. S. (1967). The school medical service. *Lancet*, 2, 822.

Wallace, B. B. & Davis, R. H. (1970). A record system for general practice. *Journal of the Royal College of General Practitioners*, 20, 163.

Wintle, C. J., Clay, S. & Davis, R. H. (1972). The school medical examination in an integrated group practice. *Journal of the Royal College of General Practitioners*, 22, 327.

11 The Ante-Natal Clinic *Gareth Lloyd*

'If there be doubt about the effectiveness of mass screening of the general population in preventing disease or limiting disability, there can be none about the possibilities of careful scanning and care of the parents, the foetus, and the newborn.'

H. Rocke Robertson, 1973.

Optimal ante-natal care may be defined as the accomplishment of those measures which are necessary to achieve a state of physical, mental and social well-being and the maintenance of this state prior to planned confinement.

Such optimal care will include the following:

1 Early diagnosis of pregnancy.
2 Evaluation of the physical and mental health of the mother with application of preventive and corrective measures, including selection of the correct place for delivery.
3 Evaluation of the social circumstances of the family and the provision of adequate support.
4 Control of hazards to the foetus.
5 Avoidance of teratogenic influences.
6 Monitoring of maternal health and foetal development and the selection of the optimum time for delivery.
7 Nutritional supplementation and instruction.
8 Consultation with all necessary specialist services.
9 Provision of appropriate emotional support and childbirth education with opportunity for sympathetic and intelligent counselling on matters of parental concern.
10 An active programme of preparation for labour.

Such ante-natal care is achieved by means of organised ante-natal clinics either in hospital or in the community. It is customary for patients to attend ante-natal clinics each month up to the 28th week of pregnancy, each fortnight from the 28th to the 36th week and each week thereafter until confinement. In certain circumstances the frequency of attendance may be increased.

The general practitioner who has special training and maintains a special interest is well able to undertake optimal ante-natal care and should seek to do so in association with a registered midwife.

One of the main objectives of regular attendance at ante-natal clinics is the provision of screening procedures which permit the determination of the management of the pregnant woman and allow for the detection of pre-symptomatic abnormalities of pregnancy.

Three groups of screening procedures can be perceived in ante-natal care:

Group 1
Enquiries and tests which are normally undertaken only once in early pregnancy. Procedures of this kind are mainly concerned with establishing the state of the woman's health and determining the correct place for confinement. All pregnant women are included in these procedures.

Group 2
Enquiries and tests which are undertaken at each attendance at the ante-natal clinic. Such procedures are mainly concerned with the pre-symptomatic detection of abnormality, e.g. toxaemia of pregnancy. All pregnant women are included in these procedures.

Group 3
Enquiries or tests which are undertaken more than once but not at each clinic attendance. Procedures of this kind are associated with the evaluation of specific abnormalities, e.g. Rh incompatibility, or estimation of foetal maturity. All pregnant women are included in only some of these procedures.

Screening procedures undertaken during pregnancy are contained in three parts:

A The patient's health history.
B The clinical examination.
C Investigative procedures.

By combining the three kinds of procedures with the three containment parts, a descriptive analysis of screening during the ante-natal period is possible.

Selection of place for confinement

An important objective of screening during the ante-natal period is the determination of the most suitable place for confinement.

A choice of four possible places for confinement exists in the United Kingdom, and these require to be defined:

1 **The patient's own home.** There is considerable variation in the quality of homes in the United Kingdom. Many are so lacking in facility as to be considered wholly unsuitable for confinement. When the conditions are regarded as 'suitable' all additional facilities required at the time of confinement are provided by the midwife. The unpredictability of post-partum haemorrhage and neonatal asphyxia raises the question whether the home of any patient is suitable. In case of emergency, an obstetric 'Flying Squad' service is usually provided by a hospital obstetric unit.

2 **General Practitioner Maternity Home.** This is a place for confinement which is detached from the hospital obstetric unit, where the general practitioner has unsupervised responsibility for care during delivery; it may not be equipped with anaesthetic services and all the means for coping with complications, including blood transfusions and operative procedures. The findings of Hobbs and Acheson (1966), the reports of confidential enquiries into maternal deaths (Ministry of Health, 1957, 1960, 1963, 1966, 1969) and the perinatal mortality survey (Butler and Donham, 1963), all indicate that mothers who are transferred in labour from General Practitioner Maternity Homes constitute a high risk group, with a raised mortality for both mother and infant.

3 **General Practitioner Obstetric Unit.** Such a unit is in close association with a hospital obstetric unit (RCOG Report, 1968; Oldershaw and Brudenell, 1968; Rhodes, 1968). The consultant obstetrician has over-riding responsibility (RCOG Report, 1968; Barnard, Hall, Woodward and Quickenden, 1970). The general practitioner unit should share the same equipment as the hospital unit (Brudenell, 1968) and have equal facility for expert help.

It is expected that the integration of the general practitioner into the hospital obstetric team will effectively reduce the mortality associated with the General Practitioner Maternity Home (Report of Maternity Services Committee, 1969). There is also evidence that certain 'at risk' patients such as the grand multipara and the older patient, may be suitably confined in the General Practitioner obstetric unit (Law, 1968).

4 **Hospital Obstetric Unit.** Most hospitals which meet the criteria of a District General Hospital (DHSS, 1969) contain a specialist obstetric unit. The unit has adequate facility to deal with all manner of normal and emergency obstetrics. The hospital medical team

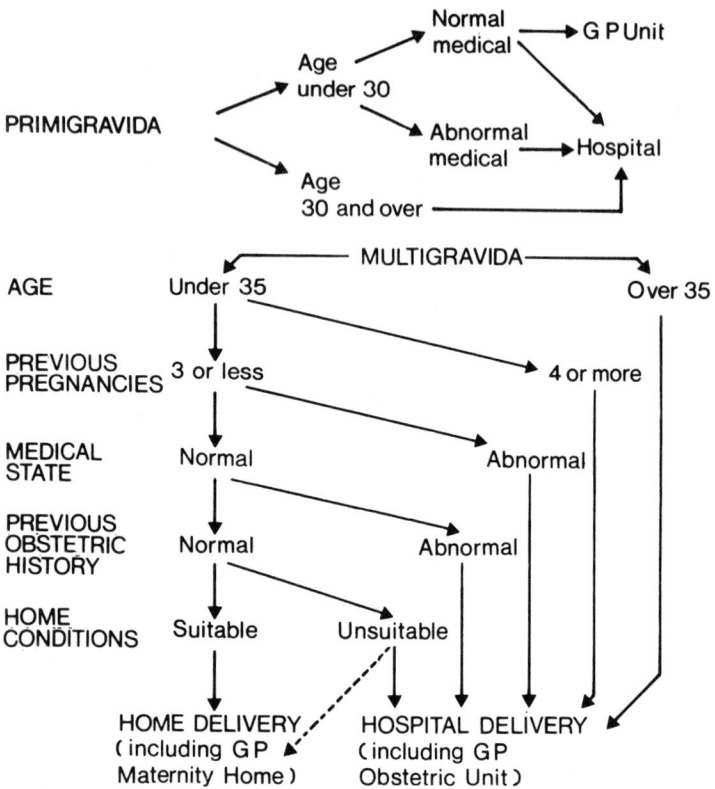

Figure 5. The extent to which abnormal conditions permit booking for the General Practitioner Obstetric Unit will vary according to agreed procedure between local consultants and general practitioners.

consists of a consultant, medical staff in training, together with midwives, usually a social worker, and sometime a dietician.

Screening procedure (Group 1)

In broad terms, the screening process relating to determining the choice of the place of confinement is shown in Figure 5.

The broad programme of screening shown in Figure 5 contains a very large number of items of enquiry or test. The commonly agreed items are shown in Appendix A (p. 118), together with an indication of the reason for each individual enquiry or test.

All the information contained in Appendix A should be secured, as far as is practicable, at the first ante-natal attendance. The general practitioner may already be aware of the greater part of the history.

All the factors described are of sufficient significance as to make special enquiry necessary when information is lacking.

The practitioner who lacks the confidence or experience necessary to determine all the factors indicated in the clinical examination should ensure that someone else has the opportunity to do so. Similarly, the patient should be offered access to resources for obtaining the investigative procedures.

Screening during continuing ante-natal care

The usual frequency of attendance by the patient for continuing ante-natal care has already been described. Screening procedures at these attendances have two objectives. The first, directed to all pregnant women, is the presymptomatic detection of abnormality and the recognition of symptomatic changes in physical, mental or social wellbeing (Group 2 procedures). The second objective is directed at selected groups of women and the purpose of screening is the evaluation of the progress of special 'at risk' characteristics such as rhesus incompatibility, dysmaturity or heart disease (Group 3 procedures).

At each ante-natal attendance the following information should be obtained for all women and the results recorded:

1 The general well-being of the mother.
2 Any amount of vaginal bleeding or discharge.
3 Emotional and social difficulties.
4 The weight of the mother.
5 The blood pressure.
6 The urine for sugar and protein.
7 The ankles for oedema.
8 The legs for varicose veins.
9 The abdomen for the height of the fundus of the uterus.

From the 15th week, foetal parts may be ballotted. From the 26th week, the foetal heart may be heard. From the 28th week, the presenting part should be discernible and from the 32nd week, the presenting part should be stable.

The screening procedure at the ante-natal clinic should include these clinical evaluations for the respective duration of pregnancy indicated. The results should be recorded in each instance. An awareness of common abnormalities helps to make their early and more frequent detection possible, and emphasises the logic of screening procedures. A list of common ante-natal abnormalities is shown in Appendix B (p. 121).

A number of special circumstances encountered during pregnancy attract special screening needs. Three examples are offered for consideration.

1 **Anaemia in pregnancy.** A good review of anaemia in pregnancy is given by Steingold (1966). It is generally agreed that a haemoglobin value of less than 10·2 g/100 ml is unacceptable, even allowing for possible physiological phenomena.

It should be the aim during the ante-natal period, to ensure that anaemia is detected and adequately treated, so that at the time of delivery, the highest possible haemoglobin level is attained. Jacobs and Greenman (1969) have shown that only half the iron available in 25 common foods is released into solution under conditions similar to those prevailing in the stomach. The maximum quantity of iron normally available from food is 2·4 mg per day (Finch, Haskins and Finch, 1950). Iron deficiency anaemia is not an uncommon event in pregnancy and the risk is increased by inadequate diet or failure to take prophylactic medicinal iron.

Megaloblastic anaemia in pregnancy, due to a deficiency of folic acid, is reported to have an incidence of about four per cent in the United Kingdom (Giles and Shuttleworth, 1958; MacKenzie and Abbott, 1960). Addisonian pernicious anaemia is extremely rare in pregnancy. An instance was recently reported by Armstrong, Davis, Martin and Woodliff (1968). In Liverpool, Hibbard failed to find an instance among 30,000 pregnancies (Hibbard and Hibbard, 1968). A daily oral intake of medicinal iron of the order of 100 mg per day and of folic acid of the order of 300 mg per day provides good prophylaxis. The significant role of ascorbic acid in the metabolism of folic acid is emphasised by Steingold (1966).

Ratten and Beischer (1972) have drawn attention to the increased significance of anaemia in association with chronic renal disease in pregnancy.

Possession of the sickle-cell tract Hb AS by the African mother has been shown to be associated with a significant increase in perinatal mortality when there is anoxic stress (Platt, 1971). An increase in the African immigrant population of the United Kingdom creates a need for special screening.

Screening procedure (mainly Group 1 and Group 3)

1 Determine as closely as possible, the dietary habits of all pregnant women.
2 Estimate the haemoglobin value of all pregnant women at the first attendance, and at least twice again between the 28th week of pregnancy and confinement.

3 Estimate the sickle-cell trait of all African women at the first ante-natal attendance.

4 Investigate more fully all women who have a haemoglobin value of 10·2 g/100 ml or less.

5 Ensure increased frequency of haemoglobin estimations of all women with anaemia in pregnancy, particularly following treatment. Additional screening should continue until an acceptable level of haemoglobin is achieved.

2 **Rhesus incompatibility.** 'It is a rarity in clinical medicine that in a single generation, a disease process is discovered, successfully treated, and finally prevented' (Commentary, Clinical Paediatrics, 1968).

Erythroblastosis foetalis was first related to isoimmunisation to the Rh antigen in 1941 (Levine, Burnham, Katzin & Vogel, 1941). This illness of the new-born can be anticipated by screening all pregnant women for the Rh factor. 15 per cent of women are Rh negative and are at risk of reacting with an Rh positive foetus to the point of producing an adverse iso-immunisation of the foetus.

The mother is rarely sensitised to the Rh antigen in her first pregnancy. Woodrow *et al.* (1965), using the Kleihauer Braun and Betke (1957) acid-elution technique for demonstrating foetal red blood cells in the maternal circulation, showed that in most instances the sensitising transplacental haemorrhages occurred during, or shortly after, labour.

An Rh incompatible blood transfusion of a woman produces a severe sensitisation and is much more likely to be associated with erythroblastosis foetalis than sensitisation by an Rh positive foetus. Sensitisation can also occur as a result of abortion (Murray and Barron, 1971).

Screening procedure (mainly Group 1)

1 Enquire of all pregnant women about blood transfusions prior to pregnancy.

2 Obtain relevant previous obstetric history.

3 Test the blood of all pregnant women for Rh grouping at the first ante-natal attendance. Previous Rh tests should not be accepted as absolute evidence.

4 Test the blood of all pregnant women for Rh antibodies at the first ante-natal attendance. This permits the early anticipation of iso-immunisation in Rh negative women who may have had a previous incompatible blood transfusion or who may be concealing information about a previous pregnancy.

E

5 Test the blood of all Rh negative women for Rh antibodies at the 30th week.

Special attention will need to be given to women who have a history of previous rhesus iso-immunisation and the frequency of tests for antibodies will depend on individual circumstances. Whilst erythroblastosis foetalis is now largely preventable, the screening procedure needs to be carefully observed if the occasional stillbirth or neonatal tragedy is to be avoided (A Combined Study from Centres in England and Baltimore, 1971).

3 **Foetal maturity**. Foetal maturity is traditionally predicted by calculation of the expected date of confinement (EDC), using Naegele's rule, from the date of the last menstrual period (LMP). Beazley and Underhill (1970) have shown that in about 22 per cent of pregnant women, calculation of the EDC by this method is unreliable and that for the infants of these women the perinatal mortality is higher.

Measurement of the fundal height has been shown by the same authors (Beazley et al., 1970) to be an unreliable measure of maturity. Though this measurement continues to be a part of the screening procedure at each ante-natal attendance, it provides only a crude estimate, and at best, can be justified as an indicator for further investigation.

More accurate estimation of maturity can be made by means of ultrasound cephalometry (Underhill, Beazley and Campbell, 1971). Ian Donald (1963) first showed interest in determining uterine content by means of 'sonar'. His work has been developed to a stage where sophisitcated ultrasound equipment is available for the measurement of the biparietal diameter of the foetal skull in utero.

The measurement is accurate between the 20th and 30th week of pregnancy (Campbell and Newman, 1971: Lee, Major and Weingold, 1971). This facility is not yet universally available. The method is considered to be safe and does not have the genetic hazard of radiography (Watts and Stewart, 1972). Serial ultrasound cephalometry allows the separation of those patients 'at risk' with a small-for-dates foetus from those with uncertain maturity (Varma, 1973).

Screening procedure—ultrasound cephalometry (Group 3)

1 Screen all women between the 20th and 30th week of pregnancy, who have an unpredictable EDC as calculated by Naegele's formula.
2 Screen all women between the 20th and 30th week if the

EDC is predictable by Naegele's formula and if they appear clinically to have a smaller-for-dates pregnancy.

3 Screen all women at intervals of one or two weeks, after the 20th week, if there is suspicion that the foetal growth is retarded, or if the mother fails to gain weight, or loses weight.

Examples have been offered in this chapter of screening procedures at the ante-natal clinic and the reasons for them. Other procedures relating to urinary infection, emotional behaviour, placental location, maternal cigarette smoking, or other specific aspects of ante-natal care, can be determined along similar lines.

Urinary infection and asymptomatic bacteriuria in pregnancy create a need for the routine screening of urine beyond the mere estimation of proteinuria. There is not yet an agreement on the most suitable screening procedure and the existing situation is well summarised by I.R. McFadyen and his associates at St Thomas's Hospital, London (McFadyen *et al.*, 1973).

A clean specimen of urine is however required and such a specimen may be submitted to bacterial count, leucocyte count and/or culture. There is not yet general agreement on the criteria of abnormality for these tests.

B.G. Wren (1971) has shown that when the leucocyte excretion rate is elevated above 8×10^5 per hour during the last four weeks of pregnancy, the incidence of prematurity rises by 21 per cent and perinatal mortality by eight per cent. The observations of Ratten and Beischer (1972) suggest that pregnant women who have both anaemia and chronic renal disease are at particular risk of increased perinatal deaths.

Heavy smoking by pregnant women has been repeatedly reported to be associated with a decrease in the average birth weight of infants (Simpson, 1957; Butler, Goldstein and Ross, 1972; Andrews and McGarry, 1972). It is suggested by Cole, Hawkins and Roberts (1972) that the effect on the foetus is the result of diminished oxygen availability at tissue level.

Summary

The ante-natal clinic is an example of a clinical environment which contains a very large screening element. The population at risk is defined, a very high proportion attend an ante-natal clinic and the necessary procedures can be identified and largely applied fairly easily.

Variations in screening procedures can be expected between

different hospitals, health centres and individual doctors. The development of new understanding about pregnancy modifies the needs for screening and the nature of the screening programmes.

The precise nature of the overall screening programme of the ante-natal clinic has to be determined by individuals or groups of practitioners, bearing in mind the facilities available.

Appendix A. Information to be sought at first ante-natal attendance, and its significance in management of pregnancy and confinement.

FACTOR	POSSIBLE SIGNIFICANCE
HISTORY	
Personal History	
Rheumatic fever	Possible cardiac lesion.
Chorea	Worse during pregnancy.
Fits	Confusion with eclampsia.
Mental Illness	Complicates puerperium.
Urinary infection	Recurs during pregnancy.
Thyrotoxicosis	Worse during pregnancy.
Asthma	Complicates labour.
Chronic chest disease, pulmonary surgery	Risk of acute respiratory failure in labour. Anaesthetic risk.
Tuberculosis	Consideration of BCG and breast feeding.
Heart disease	Worse during pregnancy.
Orthopaedic conditions of spine and pelvis	Abnormal pelvic shape.
Diabetes	Serious foetal risk.
Neurological conditions	Multiple sclerosis and myasthenia may be worse during pregnancy.
Psoriasis	Better during pregnancy.
Depression or other psychiatric illness	Recurrence during pregnancy.
Family History	
Diabetes, maturity onset type in pregnant woman's parents	Associated with pre-diabetic state in pregnancy.
Hypertension	Possible inheritance.
Pulmonary tuberculosis	Need for BCG.

Gynaecological History

Irregular menstrual rhythm	Confusion concerning duration of pregnancy.
Infertility	Increases 'value' of infant.
Cervical operations	Incompetent cervix.
Pelvic floor repair	Avoidance of vaginal delivery.
Vaginal discharge	Recurrence in pregnancy.
Myomectomy, hysterotomy	Weakened uterus.
Fibroids	Degeneration.
Curettage of the uterus	Possible perforation.

Previous Obstetric History

Habitual abortion (3 or more), no living issue	Increased 'value' of infant.
Toxaemia	All these factors are associated with a tendency to recurrence and are indications for confinement in a hospital maternity unit.
Hydramnios	
Ante-partum haemorrhage	
Premature labour	
Prolonged or precipitate labour	
Rhesus negative with antibodies	
Forceps delivery	
Breech	
Twins	
Caesarian section	
PPH or retained placenta	
Stillbirth	
Neonatal death	
Congenital abnormality	
Inherited metabolic disorder	
Premature infant	
Immature infant	
Unstable lie	

Present History

Age, primigravida over 30	Increased foetal risk.
Age, primigravida over 35	Increased risk of PPH and foetal abnormality.
Over 5 years since last confinement	Increased 'value' of infant.
Attitude towards pregnancy	Need for counselling. Possible immature baby.
Smoking habits	Possible obesity and anaemia.
Diet	

CLINICAL EXAMINATION
General Examination

Height	Less than 5 ft associated with small pelvis.
Weight	Overweight tend to develop hypertension.
Teeth and gums	Oral sepsis-puerperal sepsis.
Thyroid gland	Thyrotoxicosis.
Other glands of neck	Rubella, foetal abnormality.
Vertebral column	Pelvic size and shape.
Breasts	Infant feeding.
Chest	Chronic disease—need for X-ray.
Heart	Significant murmurs. Need for specialist opinion.
Blood pressure	Essential hypertension.
Legs	Varicose veins.
Abdomen	Size of uterus and renal angle abnormalities.

Pelvic Examination

Vaginal discharge	Treatment.
Size of uterus	Assessment of duration of early pregnancy.
Position of uterus	Correction of retroversion.
Pelvic tumours	Surgical treatment.

INVESTIGATIONS
Blood

Haemoglobin or full blood count	Anaemia.
Blood group	ABO incompatibility.
Rh factor	Rh incompatibility.
Rh antibodies	Rh Iso-immunisation.
Specific tests for syphilis	Previous infection, risk to infant.

Urine

Sugar	Diabetes.
Protein	Pyelonephritis or renal hypertension.
Ketones	Hyperemesis, diabetes
Organisms	Urinary infection.
WCC excretion	Kidney infection.

Other

Vaginal swab and/or cervical smear	Infection, trichomonal or monilial.
	Cancer of cervix.

Appendix B. Common ante-natal abnormalities

9th to 11th weeks	Threatened abortion.
9th to 14th weeks	Hyperemesis. Disparity between dates and size of uterus.
14th to 24th weeks	Hydatidiform mole—toxaemia. Abortion due to incompetent cervical os. Torsion of ovarian tumours. Hydramnios—multiple pregnancy.
24th to 32nd weeks	Anaemia. Pyelitis. Hydramnios—multiple pregnancy or foetal abnormality. Rhesus antibodies appear. Excessive weight gain Oedema of ankles First 'bleed' of placenta praevia.
From 32nd week	Anaemia. Pyelitis Toxaemia. Pre-diabetes. Ante-partum haemorrhage. Breech pesentation. Unstable lie of foetus. Multiple pregnancy. Hydramnios—foetal abnormality. Premature labour. Failure of descent of presenting part.

REFERENCES

Andrews, Joan & McGarry, J. M. (1972). A community study of smoking in pregnancy. *Journal of Obstetrics and Gynaecology of the British Commonwealth,* 79, 1057.

Armstrong, B. K., Davis, R. E., Martin, J. D. & Woodliff, H. J. (1968). Pregnancy and untreated Addisonian pernicious anaemia. *British Medical Journal,* 4, 158–159.

Beazley, J. M. & Underhill, Rosemary, A. (1970). Fallacy of the fundal height. *British Medical Journal,* 4, 404.

Barnard, M. J., Hall, D. S., Woodward, J. W. & Quickenden, D. R. J. (1970). A combined maternity unit. *Journal of the Royal College of General Practitioners,* 19, 211.

Brudenell, M. (1968). Opening the hospital door. *Proceedings of the Royal Society of Medicine,* 61, 1034.

Butler, N. R. & Donham, D. G. (1963). *First report of 1958 British perinatal mortality survey under the auspicies of the National Birthday Trust Fund.* Edinburgh: Livingstone.

Butler, N. R., Goldstein, H. & Ross, E. M. (1972). Cigarette smoking in pregnancy: its influence on birth weight and perinatal mortality. *British Medical Journal,* 2, 127.

Campbell, S. & Newman, G. B. (1971). Growth of the foetal biparietal diameter during normal pregnancy. *Journal of Obstetrics and Gynaecology of the British Commonwealth,* 78, 513.

Combined Study from centres in England and Baltimore (1971). Prevention of Rh haemolytic disease: final results of the 'high risk' clinical trial. *British Medical Journal,* 2, 607.

Cole, P. V., Hawkins, L. H. & Roberts, D. (1972). Smoking during pregnancy and its effects on the foetus. *Journal of Obstetrics and Gynaecology of the British Commonwealth,* 79, 782.

Commentary. Clinical Paediatrics (1968). Prevention of Rh isoimmunisation. November. 643.

Donald, I. (1963). Ultrasonics in the diagnosis of abdominal swellings. *British Medical Journal,* 2, 1154.

Department of Health and Social Security (1969). *The functions of the District General Hospital: report of the Committee.* London: H.M.S.O.

Finch, S., Haskins D. M. & Finch, C. A. (1950). Iron metabolism. Hematopoiesis following phebotomy. Iron as limiting factor. *Journal of Clinical Investigation,* 29, 1078–1086.

Giles, C. & Shuttleworth, E. M. (1958). Megaloblastic anaemia of pregnancy and the puerperium. *Lancet,* 2, 1341.

Hibbard, B. M. & Hibbard, E. D. (1968). Folate metabolism and reproduction. *British Medical Bulletin,* 24, 10.

Hobbs, M. S. T. & Acheson, E. D. (1966). Perinatal mortality and organisation of obstetric services in Oxford area in 1962. *British Medical Journal,* 1, 499–505.

Jacobs, A. & Greenman, D. A. (1969). Availability of food iron. *British Medical Journal,* 1, 673.

Kleihauer, E., Braun, H. & Betke, K. (1957). Demonstration von fetalem haemoglobin in den erytrochyten eines blutausstrichs. *Klinische Wochenschrift,* 35, 637.

Law, R. G. (1968). Domiciliary confinement in three high risk obstetric groups. *Proceedings of the Royal Society of Medicine,* 61, 1029–1032.

Lee, B. O., Major, F. J. & Weingold, A. B. (1971). Ultrasonic determination of fetal maturity at repeat cesarean section. *Journal of Obstetrics and Gynaecology,* 38, 294–297.

Levine, P., Burnham, L., Katzin, E. M. & Vogen, P. (1941). Role of isoimmunisation in pathogenesis of erythroblastosis fetalis. *American Journal of Obstetrics and Gynaecology,* 42, 925.

MacKenzie, A. & Abbott, J. (1960). Megaloblastic erythropoiesis in pregnancy. *British Medical Journal,* 2, 1114.

McFadyen, I. R., Eykyn, S. J., Gardner, N. H. N., Vanier, T. M., Bennett, A. E., Mayo, M. E. & Lloyd-Davies, R. W. (1973). Bacteriuria in pregnancy. *Journal of Obstetrics and Gynaecology of the British Commonwealth,* 80, 385.

Ministry of Health (1957; 1960; 1963; 1966; 1969). *Reports on confidential enquiries into maternal deaths in England and Wales.* London: H.M.S.O.

Ministry of Health (1959). *Cranbrook. Maternity Services Committee report.* London: H.M.S.O.

Murray, Sheilagh & Barron, S. L. (1971). Rhesus isoimmunisation after abortion. *British Medical Journal,* 3, 90.

Oldershaw, K. L. & Brunedell, J. M. (1968). Use by general practitioners of obstetric beds in a consultant unit: report of first 500 cases. *British Medical Journal,* 3, 112–116.

Platt, H. S. (1971). Effect of maternal sickle-cell trait on perinatal mortality. *British Medical Journal,* 3, 334.

Ratten, G. J. & Beischer, N. A. (1972). The significance of anaemia in an obstetric population in Australia. *Journal of Obstetrics and Gynaecology of the British Commonwealth,* 79, 228.

Rhodes, P. (1968). General practitioner obstetric beds in a consultant unit. *British Medical Journal,* 4, 509.

Robertson, H. Rocke (1973). *Health Care in Canada—A Commentary.* Background Study for the Science Council of Canada. Special Study No. 29, p. 138.

Royal College of General Practitioners Report (1968). *Report of Council on hospital obstetrics for the general practitioner.* July 1968.

Simpson, W. J. & Calif, L. L. (1957). A preliminary report on cigarette smoking and the incidence of prematurity. *American Journal of Obstetrics and Gynaecology,* 73, 808.

Steingold, L. (1966). *Recent Advances in Obstetrics and Gynaecology.* p. 96. 11th edition J. A. Churchill Ltd. London.

Underhill, Rosemary A., Beazley, J. M. & Campbell, Stuart (1971). Comparison of ultrasound cephalometry, radiology and liquor studies in patients with unknown confinement dates. *British Medical Journal,* 3, 736.

Varma, T. R. (1973). Prediction of delivery date by ultrasound cephalometry. *Journal of Obstetrics and Gynaecology of the British Empire,* 80, 316.

Watts, P. L. & Stewart, C. R. (1972). The effect of foetal heart monitoring by ultrasound on maternal and foetal chromosomes. *Journal of Obstetrics and Gynaecology of the British Commonwealth,* 79, 715.

Woodrow, J. C., Clarke, C. A., Donohoe, W. T. A., Finn, R., McConnell, R. B., Sheppard, P. M., Lehane, D., Russell, S. H., Kulke, W. & Durkin, C. M. (1965). Prevention of Rh haemolytic disease: a third report. *British Medical Journal,* 1, 279.

Wren, B. G. (1971). The value of leucocyte excretion rates in determining 'at risk' patients with asymptomatic bacilluria *Journal of Obstetrics and Gynaecology of the British Commonwealth,* 78, 130.

12 Women in the Middle Years I.F.W. Kerr

Women in their middle years provide the doctor interested in screening with a considerable problem. The younger woman, primarily from contraceptive and post-natal care, and later through the continuing care of her children with their infant ailments, is often rendered amenable to a screening programme by the enthusiastic doctor's progressive indoctrination. The middle-aged woman, however, often with a grown up family, no longer finds any regular medical liason necessary, and may lament the passing of the old standard of medicine without accepting the benefits of its successor.

No longer tied to the responsibility of young children, the middle-aged woman may pursue her intended career, which may widen the generation gap. Her duty as an employee may be in conflict with the time schedule of the screening clinic. This and the approaching menopause with its multiple symptomatology may induce in the unfortunate woman an overwhelming barrier against interventionist medicine.

For the patient prepared to accept a screening programme it is essential that it be of maximum benefit to that patient, while preserving a financial and temporal economy. Each section of a comprehensive programme should make possible the detection of an important but treatable disease in an early or latent state (Wilson, 1966). Any programme requires administration and adequate ancillary help and might include urinalysis, measurement of weight, detection of possible anaemia or raised blood pressure, breast examination, pelvic and cytology study. Positive or equivocal findings frequently involve the patient in further screening tests.

Urinalysis offers simple tests for the detection of albumen and sugar. The presence of albumen justifies microscopy and bacteriological culture of the urine, thus making possible the treatment of

123

asymptomatic urinary infection. Sensitivity tests to various anti-bacterial agents ensure thorough treatment and failure to eradicate infection under these conditions justifies a full renal survey.

The detection of glycosuria would call for further biochemical tests, and ketosis should especially be excluded in the patient with glycosuria. The weight of the patient should be estimated and the relationship between obesity, pruritis, diabetes and hypertension should always be borne in mind. The integration of a dietician into the clinic is of obvious value.

The detection of anaemia involves organisational problems concerning the bleeding of patients and transporting samples. However, as observation is notoriously unreliable, blood testing may be feasible if adequate ancillary help is available. A possible screening test was the Ferrotest 80 where haemoglobins below 80 were detected from a sample obtained from the thumb. Unfortunately this appears not to have been marketed by the manufacturers. In the event of detecting anaemia, further screening tests will be required to elucidate the cause of the anaemia.

The unrecognised hypertensive is at risk from various crises and the measurement of blood pressure can identify a disease which, unrecognised, carries both a high mortality and morbidity.

Shown in Table 7 is a random study of raised diastolic pressures in 1,000 women attending a screening clinic, none of whom were previously recognised hypertensives.

Table 7. The incidence of occult hypertension in women attending a screening clinic (Kerr, 1972).

| | | Diastolic BP | |
Age of Women	Total	>95 mm Hg	>110 mm Hg
Under 26	206	2	1
26 – 35	344	16	1
36 – 45	210	22	11
46 – 55	156	23	7
56 – 65	59	19	5
Over 65	25	5	6

While it is accepted that there is a physiological elevation in blood pressure with age, it can be observed that there is an increased risk dependent on age. Whilst steps should be taken to exclude a renal or supra-renal cause by pyelography and serum potassium estimation, most cases identified will finally be classified as essential hypertension.

The potential of thermography and mammography as diagnostic tools is recognised (Gershon Cohen, 1963), but both precedures are time consuming and financially not feasible for random screening, although cancer of the female breast is four times more common than either lower colonic or cervical lesions. In contrast to these latter conditions, the radiological methods used for investigating the female breast are still able to identify only frank carcinomas; however it might be justifiable to utilise such facilities for high risk groups, though the groups themselves are poorly defined. Such women might include those with a previous history of breast disease or a family history. In addition it seems that there is a relationship between low androgen levels in multipara or those who conceive later in life, and cancer of the breast (Ghosh et al., 1973; Bulbrook et al., 1960). Palpation and teaching the patient self examination still plays an important role as early lesions, detected while still asymptomatic, carry a better prognosis following treatment.

Cervical cytology is the nucleus of most female screening programmes, and while it is not certain that all carcinomas of the cervix pass through a latent pre-invasive stage it is certainly true that frequent screening will enable diagnosis to be made in its infancy or in situ stage, thereby improving prognosis (Fidler et al., 1962, 1968). At present the middle-aged woman is most at risk, but it will be interesting to observe the effects of altered moral standards in the future.

Cytology necessitates the performance of a full pelvic examination, and it is possible to identify several abnormal clinical situations, often asymptomatic, by this combined procedure, as shown in Table 8.

Table 8. The range of gynaecological disorders detected at a screening clinic (Kerr, 1972).

Diagnoses	Age of the women						Total
	Under 26	26—35	36—45	46—55	56—65	Over 65	
Trichomonas vaginalis	10	16	4	5	—	1	36
Monilia	5	13	8	6	2	1	35
Erosion (treated)	—	16	12	—	—	—	28
Senile vaginitis	—	—	—	3	9	9	21
Cervical polyp	—	1	8	6	5	1	21
Prolapse (treated)	—	2	2	3	3	2	12
Fibroids (operation)	—	—	5	4	1	—	10
Fibroids (untreated)	1	1	1	4	—	—	7
Ovarian cyst	1	1	4	—	1	—	7
Leukoplakia/kraurosis	—	—	—	2	4	—	6
Positive smear	—	3	2	1	—	—	6
Carcinoma of body of uterus	—	—	—	—	3	1	4
Extravaginal infection	1	1	1	—	—	—	3
Carcinoma of cervix	—	—	2	—	—	—	2
Dysplasia	—	2	—	—	—	—	2
Suspicious smear (negative biopsy)	—	—	—	—	—	—	0
Total Patients Screened	206	344	210	156	59	25	1,000

Further correlation of these results is sometimes significant. Thus vulval abnormalities may be associated with iron deficiency anaemia, or alternatively fibroids may have induced an anaemia. The importance of asymptomatic presentation is shown further in Table 9.

Table 9. Asymptomatic presentation of major gynaecological disorders in 1,000 patients attending a screening clinic (Kerr, 1972).

	Total	Asymptomatic
Positive smears and carcinoma of cervix	8	6
Fibroids treated	10	3
Ovarian cysts	7	4
Carcinoma of body of uterus	4	1
Carcinoma of breast	2	2

Other screening procedures should also be considered. While rectal examination is mandatory in the presence of anaemia or rectal symptoms, there appears also to be a strong case for its inclusion in routine screening projects, as rectal examination makes possible identification of over 50 per cent of neoplasms in the rectum and recto-sigmoid region, which together account for more deaths in a year than carcinoma of the cervix. In addition rectal examination may reveal an occasional bladder or ovarian tumour. Sigmoidoscopy is best left in the hands of the expert.

Other screening procedures of debatable value include chest radiology, which depends on local hospital facilities. The benefits of this are arguable; for instance it appears that those neoplasms picked up routinely fare no better than those presenting with symptoms (Brett, 1968).

As we have the potential to offer the patient the advantages of early detection of disease and thereby prolonged life expectancy, it rests with us to persuade the middle-aged woman to accept our programme, occasionally no mean task. Often she is no longer in need of postnatal or contraceptive advice, and so a valuable means of communication is lost. Also, with her grown up family no longer dependant on her, frequently she pursues outside work where her hours of employment coincide with surgery hours, thus widening the generation gap even further.

Various advertising media appear to have little influence; even occasional television and radio coverage produce little response. (In a personal series only three per cent of those screened admitted being influenced primarily by such means.) What a boon it would be if Elsie Tanner in Coronation Street were involved in a few episodes concerning cytology!

Despite these pitfalls it is fortunate that many attend of their own volition, the patient often regarding screening as an insurance policy, covering herself as an essential part of the family unit.

There seems little doubt that the doctor himself has a major role to play in canvassing a screening programme, and the enthusiast will find the time taken persuading the patient of its benefits pays dividends. Some may be relieved of the fear and embarrassment sometimes associated with attendance at a clinic, especially in the menopausal patient, by the doctor's tactful approach, while others accept the authority of the doctor who makes an appointment for her, though such an autocratic attitude must be pursued with caution and judgement.

There remains a large number of patients who have not undergone screening, failing to find the time to get around to it. Usually working women, they find the clinics coincide with their hours of employment. However, with the increasing tendency for firms to make cytology available to their workforce at their place of employment, there appears every chance that this group will be able to benefit. An added advantage of the medical team moving into the industrial field is the possibility that some will undergo screening rather than differ from their working companions.

The recent use of a mobile caravan in Salford offering screening programmes to various areas has been more successful than could have been envisaged at its onset. Though the computer data is not yet available the scheme has been enthusiastically received by those most at risk, the lower social classes, possibly because it did not necessitate the use of appointments, and the available screening time did not coincide with normal working hours.

There are a few patients who admit ignorance of the existence of screening, but they are usually loath to undergo screening due to coincidental fear and embarrassment. Occasionally middle-aged women believe that screening projects are not for their benefit, considering either they are too old for such surveys, or that the lack of symptoms removes the need for their attendance. Sometimes there is a belief that only parous or married women are at risk. Post-hysterectomy patients, as well as doctors, rarely consider the possibility of carcinoma *in situ* recurring within the vaginal vault.

In conclusion, the need for the family doctor to play an active role in screening is plainly essential. Lest we become complacent we should remember that for every 1,000 failing to be ensnared in our screening net, eight of these statistically will develop carcinoma of the cervix with its associated morbidity and final mortality, invariably leaving the bereaved family in total disruption (Wookey, 1971).

REFERENCES

Brett, G. Z. (1968). The value of lung cancer detection by six monthly chest radiographs. *Thorax*, 23, 414.

Bulbrook, R. D. et al. (1960, 1962). Relationship between urinary androgen excretion and subsequent breast cancer. *Lancet* 1960, 1, 1154; 1962, 2, 1235 and 1238.

Fidler, H. K., Boyes, D. A. & Lock, D. R. (1962). Significance of *in situ* carcinoma of uterine cervix. *British Medical Journal*, 1, 203.

Fidler, H. K., Boyes, D. A. & Worth, A. J. (1968). Cervical cancer detection in British Columbia. *Journal of Obstetrics and Gynaecology of the British Commonwealth*, 75, 392.

Gershon-Cohen J. (1963). Breast Roentgenology; a historic review. *American Journal of Roentgenology*, 86, 874.

Ghosh, P. C., Lockwood, E. & Pennington, G. W. (1973). Abnormal excretion of corticosteroid sulphates in patients with breast cancer. *British Medical Journal*, 1, 328–330.

Kerr, I. F. W. (1972). A well women clinic in Ashton under Lyne. *Journal of the Royal College of General Practitioners*. 22, 108.

Wilson, J. M. G. (1966). Some principles of early diagnosis and detection. *In Surveillance and Early Diagnosis in General Practice*. Edited by G. Teeling-Smith. London: Office of Health Economics.

Wookey, B. E. P. (1971). A well-woman clinic in general practice. *British Medical Journal*, 1, 396.

13 Men in the Middle Years *L.A. Pike*

'The man in middle life is not isolated but is affected by what went on before and what is coming to him later'.

Prof. Otto Klineberg, 1970.

Definition of the problem

Young people look forward to a future, old people look behind them at the past, whilst the middle-aged are concerned with the here and now. A suggested definition of middle-age is the years 45—55 inclusive. The middle-aged man is a most important member of our society. Much of the expertise and drive, dependability and responsibility come from this age group.

Some schemes for screening this age-group have been described: business executives (Beric Wright and Bailey, 1973); middle-aged men in a general practice (Pike, 1972; Coope, 1974); a population of men and women between 45 and 65 years in Eskilstuna, a Swedish town (Rigner *et al.*, 1969), and a middle-aged population in South East London (Trevelyan, 1972). During these programmes middle-aged populations have been subjected, when apparently well, to questionnaires, interviews, physical examinations, clinical, biochemical and haematological tests in an endeavour to keep them healthy and prevent disease.

In middle-aged men, the main causes of death and morbidity are ischaemic heart disease and cerebrovascular disease, these accounting for a little over half the male deaths, followed by cancer, particularly lung cancer. Coronary artery disease has reached epidemic proportions in the middle-aged men of our society, particularly in the higher classes of the Registrar General's classification. In the lower categories of this classification chronic bronchitis is a major cause of morbidity and mortality.

Is it possible that the course of these diseases can be modified if they are detected early by the medical worker, and if advice and treatment is accepted by the patient? We know that health education to effect a reduction or cessation of smoking cigarettes, for example, may prevent the onset of disease.

Certainly some change of attitude and method by medical workers in dealing with middle-aged men and their diseases is needed, for since the advent of the National Health Service in 1948 the number of doctors, nurses and other health workers has increased whilst the expectation of life at the age of 45—55 in the male has not improved, as is apparent from Table 10.

Table 10 Expectation of life in years for males aged 45 and 55, 1948—1967. (Digest of Health Statistics for England and Wales).

Age	1948—50	Year 1957—9	1965—7
45	27·0	27·0	27·2
55	18·8	18·6	18·8

Also the standardised morbidity ratios (base year 1968 = 100) for the years 1959 to 1969 have worsened for coronary artery disease and malignant neoplasms of the trachea, bronchus and lung, as can be seen from Table 11.

Table 11. Standardised morbidity ratios for coronary artery disease and malignant disease of trachea, bronchus and lung, 1959—1969 (1968 = 100). (Registrar General's Statistical Review of England and Wales 1969, Part 1).

	1959	1961	1963	1965	1967	1969
Coronary artery disease	83	89	98	98	95	100
Malignant disease of trachea, bronchus and lung	84	88	93	97	99	102

It is assumed that we wish to prolong the life expectancy and improve the health of this group, as well as other sections of our society. To make sense of this suggestion, as Cochrane has pointed out, such a policy must go hand in hand with an attempt at limitation of the size of family and the use of conception control methods, if necessary backed by financial encouragement from governments.

What has to be determined before the widespread application of screening techniques to the healthy population in this age group is whether such efforts would lead to a greater expectation of life, a reduction in mortality and morbidity. Present methods of management have failed, despite the great use of coronary care units and coronary care ambulances, and the availability of new drugs such as beta blockers; and there has been singular lack of success in persuading the population to stop or never start smoking.

One possible method of screening is from the basis of the general practice 'list', using the practice age-sex register. It is increasingly clear in any screening programme that the central figure must be the general practice team, with health workers in laboratories, hospitals and local authority departments in support. The reasons for this are:-

(1) There is no clear dividing line between health and disease, and those just above or below the borderline will need long-term surveillance by the general practitioner.
(2) The patient, after screening, will have to be contacted by his doctor to assess the results, and be given advice as to the significance of abnormal findings, and when appropriate their subsequent management.
(3) Evaluation of screening procedures should be done in normal populations who do not volunteer themselves for examination as during 'health weeks' or by attending hospital out-patients.

All the partners in the health care team such as health visitors, nurses and doctors can be involved in screening middle-aged men. There must be an attempt to balance the time available for the team to manage existing problems of diagnosis and therapy, against such time as can be spared to prevent and modify disease, and accurate recording and evaluation of the methods to be employed is necessary before over-enthusiastic attempts at nationwide application of screening.

Possible screening procedures in the middle-aged

Screening procedures in middle-aged men aim at detection at three levels:

1 **Preventive** Detecting and remedying some of the predisposing causes of:
(a) *Coronary artery disease;* i.e. smoking, obesity, lack of exercise, diabetes, hypercholesterolaemia, hypertension and possibly hyperlipidaemia.
(b) *Chronic bronchitis;* smoking, obesity, alcohol abuse, occupational hazards.

(c) *Carcinoma of bronchus;* smoking, occupational hazards.

(d) *Cerebral and renal vascular disease;* hypertension and diabetes.

2 **Presymptomatic** Detecting presymptomatic features of:

(a) *Coronary artery disease.* Oliver has categorised these into *clinical features*—tiredness, absent peripheral pulses, arcus senilis, xanthomata, systolic or diastolic hypertension; *social history*—history of ischaemic heart disease in siblings or parents, heavy cigarette smoking, rapid gains in weight; *the result of investigations*—positive changes in the electrocardiograph before or after exercise, abnormal glucose tolerance, hyperuricaemia, coronary calcification on X-ray, hypercholesterolaemia.

(b) *Chronic bronchitis.* A history of winter cough productive of mucopurulent or purulent sputum, with gradual loss of pulmonary reserve as detected by the Peak Flow Rate, FEV_1 and FVC, leads to the presymptomatic diagnosis of chronic bronchitis.

(c) *Lung cancer.* Presymptomatic diagnosis is unsatisfactory since early identification of the disease by mass radiography or sputum cytology is not likely to affect the prognosis. More of these patients are operable, however, than those in whom the disease presents with symptoms and signs (Brett, 1968).

(d) *Other cancers in this age group.* A questionnaire to be answered by the patient is likely to provide the earliest evidence of departure from normal function. Disturbances of bowel habit, blood in the stools or urine, and digestive symptoms occurring for the first time in middle-age all merit early attention. Abnormal blood reports such as unexplained anaemia or raised sedimentation rate may alert the doctor to perform further tests, though future developments in the biochemical diagnosis of early malignant disease may produce a diagnostic pattern from clusters of tests.

3 **Symptomatic**

It is unlikely that much more benefit will accrue from slightly earlier diagnosis than occurs already when the disease is presented to the doctor by the patient during normal consultation sessions, though possibly some men will attend by invitation to a special clinic earlier than otherwise.

It must not be forgotten that men in the middle years are affected by the take-over of companies, redundancies, and the introduction of new technologies such as computerisation into the most routine of jobs. Such situations should be sought for during screening, using a questionnaire incorporating such questions as 'Are you under stress at work?' and 'Is there any question you wish to discuss with the doctor during your visit to the clinic?' Pike (1972) reports that over half the men attending screening clinics had some question for discussion, though men in this age group are among the least frequent visitors for routine surgery consultation. This is part of prevention and will help to relieve worry, reactive depression and family tensions.

Present status of screening for disease in men of middle-age

There is controversy over the merits of screening individuals in a population with the aim of preventing individual diseases, and whether the early detection of disease is beneficial to the patient is still not established. Whether or not money and the time of skilled medical personnel should be spent on screening well populations when there is still the mass of established illness to deal with has yet to be decided.

Coronary artery disease. It would seem that preventive measures are more important than the early detection of cardiovascular abnormalities, because little can be done to alter the course of arteriosclerotic heart disease. On consideration of the predisposing causes, then, it would seem that treating hypertension, persuading middle-aged men to take more exercise and not to smoke, detecting high serum cholesterol, and keeping weight within 10 per cent of the average for body configuration may be preventive measures, though whilst these factors predict increased risk they are likely to produce false negatives in some patients, who will be wrongly reassured by the findings, and false positives in others, who may well be prescribed treatment to last the rest of their lives.

Hypertension. When to treat hypertension is still a problem. Grimley Evans and Rose (1971) suggest an operational definition of hypertension as 'a blood pressure level above which investigation and treatment do more good than harm'. Pickering (1970) has recommended treatment for males over the age of 40 where the diastolic pressure on at least three visits is 105 mm Hg, though he states that this is purely a guess. The Veterans' Administration Co-operative Study Group (1967) and Hamilton et al., (1964) confirm that for men between the ages of 45 and 70 admitted to hospital for treatment of hypertension, life expectancy can be increased by lowering the blood pressure, where the diastolic pressure is above 100 mm Hg.

The role of cigarette smoking. Pickering (1970) states that the greater the number of cigarettes smoked per day the greater the risk in developing a myocardial infarction. It would seem extremely important from the point of view of prevention of peripheral vascular and coronary artery disease, chronic bronchitis and carcinoma of the lung for the personal physician to do all that he can to deter his patients from smoking. The screening clinic, where health promotion is self-evident, provides the ideal opportunity for such advice, and this is reinforced if the doctor can state that he himself is a non-smoker.

The value of dieting. The Veterans Administration Study has demonstrated the greatly increased risk of developing myocardial infarction in patients over the age of 50 with serum cholesterol estimations above 260 mg/100 ml. There is a gradient of increasing risk of myocardial infarction parallel with increasing serum cholesterol. However, Slack (1972) states that for the majority of individuals in the population, the contribution of hyperlipidaemia to the risk of death from coronary heart disease is reassuringly small. One in 12 men in the population have cholesterol levels above 300 mg/100 ml, but only one in 25 of these men die of coronary heart disease between 45 and 54 years. Any diet which is subnormal in calorie content will lower serum lipid levels, so that by dieting those patients with a greatly raised serum cholesterol (i.e. in excess of 350 mg/100 ml), who may have in addition a raised triglyceride level (in excess of 150 mg/100 ml), a reduction should be anticipated. Adequate trial of diet should be made before resorting to drugs such as clofibrate or cholestyramine, since having accepted the need for the use of such drugs the patient and physician have to face the lifelong use of this therapy by the patient. There is some, but not yet conclusive, evidence that substituting polyunsaturated fats for saturated fats in the diet will reduce mortality and morbidity from coronary artery disease.

A low calorie diet will result in weight reduction, as well as lowering serum lipids. There is evidence that obesity has an effect on the blood pressure, and Hummerfelt and Wedervang (1957) found that there was a 3 mm systolic and 3 mm diastolic rise in pressure for every 10 kg increase in weight. It is common experience in practice, and in the screening clinic, that diet alone will be successful in reducing the blood pressure in a proportion of hypertensive middle-aged men, and it should be prescribed before the exhibition of hypotensive drugs.

The value of exercise. The harder the physical work, the lower the blood pressure in males (Miall and Oldham 1958). Conversely the lack of physical exercise in sedentary workers such as bus drivers and post office clerks is related to the fact that they have a greater incidence of myocardial infarction than is encountered in bus conductors and postmen who deliver the mail.

The role of electrocardiography. Preinfarction has been discussed by Hudson (1971) and various premonitory symptoms and electrocardiographic signs detailed. He states, however, that there are at the moment no effective measures to prevent infarction and that further research is urgently needed.

In addition to this, doctors will have encountered cases where coronary death has occurrred even when the electrocardiograph standard tracing was normal, and the predictive value is not always increased when exercise tests are added to the standard tracing.

Lung disease. To some extent screening for chronic bronchitis and carcinoma of the lung are similar, in that a questionnaire concerning smoking habit is the only effective measure, providing that health education is applied to correct the habit soon enough, and is successful. Screening for established chronic bronchitis and carcinoma of the lung, though leading to action such as influenza vaccination in the case of bronchitis or bronchoscopy for lung cancer, is of no use as a preventive method. An MRC trial (1966) demonstrated that treating early bronchitis with prophylactic antibiotics throughout the winter, or immediately an attack commenced, did not improve the underlying lung function tests. Pulmonary function tests will only reveal gradual worsening, and provide a baseline from which this worsening can be measured.

In a randomised controlled trial (Brett, 1968) no significant difference in mortality from lung cancer was found between subjects screened by mass radiography at six monthly intervals and a control group, though more of the screened cases were operable.

In the cases of other diseases discovered during the screening of men in the middle years such as diabetes and cancer of organs other than the bronchus, although the immediate comfort and well-being of the patient can sometimes be improved, there is little evidence that longevity will be increased.

There are situations which rarely threaten life such as chronic suppurative otitis media, hearing defects, eye disorders, alcoholism and mental health problems which are capable of detection at screening clinics and may be remedied, thus improving the well-being of the man and that of his family who are secondarily affected when the head of the household becomes ill.

In those clinics where screening of middle-aged men has been carried out, it has been difficult to quantify the benefit. Beric Wright and Bailey do not work with a random population and cannot provide a control group for their study, though they find unsuspected disease during screening at the BUPA medical centre. Pike (1972) found that his clinic was acceptable to the patients of his practice, that approximately half the age group attended, that the questionnaire was a valuable part of the session and that treatable conditions such as obesity, anaemia, diseases of the ear and hypertension were detected. In the male population of Eskilstuna, aged between 45 and 65, it was estimated that gains were attainable in 20 per cent of subjects as a result of the screening programme, these gains being along the lines of life improvement rather than life prolongation. In the South East London screening study there was a yield of 1·2 conditions per person screened; 56 per cent were minor and only 10 per cent were life threatening, the majority of the latter being known already to the medical service.

It would seem from these studies that critical evaluation of such clinics should be made before their wide adoption as general policy. The primary aims should be preventive, towards the prolongation of life by the avoidance, as far as this is possible, of ischaemic heart disease, chronic bronchitis and lung cancer. Secondary aims are to improve the quality of life by detecting physical and mental ill health at an early stage and remedying the situation. It is assumed that there are facilities for such treatment, otherwise screening itself is not appropriate. It cannot be assumed that there are sufficient medical workers available to carry out such screening at the present time, in the face of increasing demands for medical attention for established conditions of all sorts from trivia to serious illness.

The organisation of a screening clinic for middle-aged men in a general practice

The essential document is the age-sex register. Men between the ages of 45 and 55 if accepting an invitation to attend, are sent a health questionnaire (Appendix A), a form for mass radiography instructing the men to have the X-ray performed one week before attending the clinic, and an appointment. They are instructed to bring a urine sample when they attend. The following tests are carried out by the practice team.

1 Weight, Snellen test type—receptionist/secretary.
2 BP, examination of the eyes and ears, PFR, skinfold, review of the questionnaire, mental assessment and physical examination as indicated—doctor.
3 ECG and urinalysis—nurse.
4 Haematology and biochemistry—technician.

The results are entered on a recording sheet, reviewed by the doctor, and the results made known to the patient at a subsequent appointment, when further action, e.g. hospital referral, reappointment with doctor, health education regarding smoking, etc. is arranged. If no abnormality is detected the patient is told that he is to regard the results as normal as of this time, but that he is not to regard them as permanent reassurance. Any departure from what he regards as normality is to be reported to the doctor; he will be sent a further appointment to attend the clinic in 1—2 years time.

A control group should be established from the age-sex register of those who do not attend, so that subsequent mortality and morbidity can be compared.

APPENDIX A. Questionnaire in use at a pilot screening clinic for middle-aged men in a general practice

NAME   ADDRESS

DATE OF BIRTH   OCCUPATION

1 Have you any particular health problem you would like to discuss at your visit?

2 Have you a persistent cough?
  If so, do you cough up phlegm?
  Have you noticed any blood in the phlegm?
  Do you smoke, and if yes, how many per day?

3 Are you short of breath on climbing stairs?
  Have you swelling of the ankles?
  Have you shortness of breath during the night?

4 Is there any family history of heart disease or high blood pressure?
  Have you had any chest pain in the past year?
  Are you excessively tired in the evenings lately?
  Have you any pain which you cannot satisfactorily explain?

5 Are your bowels regular?
  Do you pass blood with the motions?

6 Have you any pain or difficulty when you pass urine?
  Is there any blood in the urine?

7 Do you have headaches? (Please tick)

> Regularly
> Occasionally
> Never

8 Do you take alcohol? (Please tick)

> Regularly
> Occasionally
> Never

9 Do you sleep well at night?

10 Have you any hearing difficulty?

11 Do you consider yourself fit?
What is your height?
What is your weight?

12 Are you under pressure at work?

Please complete the above questionnaire and bring it with you together with a urine sample.

I should be grateful if you would take the attached form to the Chest Radiology Centre, 161 Corporation Street, and have a Chest X-ray taken at least one week before your appointment for your examination here.

REFERENCES

Beric Wright, H. & Bailey, A. (1973). Business executives. *Medical News,* 5, No. 9.
Brett, G. Z. (1968). The value of lung cancer detection by six-monthly chest radiographs. *Thorax,* 23, 414.
Cochrane, A. L. (1972). *Effectiveness and Efficiency; Random Reflections on Health Services.* Oxford: The Nuffield Provincial Hospitals Trust.
Dawber *et al.* (1962). *Procedings of the Royal Society of Medicine,* 55, 265.
Evans, Grimley J. & Rose, G. A. (1971). Hypertension. *British Medical Bulletin,* 27, 1, 37.
Hamilton, M., Thompson, E. N. & Wisniewski, J. K. M. (1964). The role of blood pressure control in preventing complications of hypertension.
Hudson, W. A. (1971). Pre-infarction. *Update,* Sept., 1083.
Hummerfelt, . & Wedervang, . (1957). A study on the influence of blood pressure marital status, number of children and occupation. *Acta Medica Scandinavica,* 159, 489.
Klinberg, O. (1970). The middle-aged men in contemporary society. Report of Proceedings 'The Middle-Aged Man'. Health Education Council Seminar.
Medical Research Council (1966). The value of chemoprophylaxis and chemotherapy in early chronic broncitis. *British Medical Journal,* 1, 1317.
Miall, W. E. & Oldham, P. D. (1958). Factors influencing arterial blood pressure in the general population. *Clinical Science,* 17, 409.

Pickering, G. (1970). *Hypertension.* 3rd Edition. Edinburgh and London: Churchill Livingstone.
Pike, L. A. (1972). Screening middle-aged men in a general practice. *The Practitioner,* 209, 690-695.
Rigner, K. G. *et al* (1969). A population study Eskiltuna (1964) with an attempt to evaluate the possible gains of health screening. *Acta Soc. Med. Scandinavica.* Supplement.
Slack, J. (1972).   Lipid abnormalities and coronary artery disease, detection and management. (Report on symposium held at the Royal Society of Medicine 21 March 1972).
Trevelyan, H. (1972). The yield of disease obtained at screening a middle-aged population. *British Journal of Preventive and Social Medicine,* 26, 54–55.
Veterans' Administration (1967). Co-operative study group on anti-hypertensive agents. *Journal of the American Medical Association,* 202, 1028.

14 Geriatric Screening   M. Keith Thompson

'La cigogne nourrit ses père et mère en leur vieillesse,
et les petits sachant voler aident aussi,
et supportent ceux d'entre eux
qui ne peuvent pas encore bien voler.
Par ainsi, ils ne sont pas seulement humains
envers leur père et mère,
mais aussi entre eux, comme frères et soeurs,
les uns envers les autres.'

Ambroise Paré (1510—1590)

The elderly population exists as the group *par excellence* in which disease, both latent and overt, in conjunction with varying degrees of social incapacity, can be revealed by screening programmes. It might be argued, however, that despite a rich harvest of morbidity, only marginal improvement in prognosis could be expected when people have reached late age, and that the economic importance to the community of the diseases found to be treatable would be small. Yet it is only relatively recently that medicine has had any real impact on the health of populations, and no change can be envisaged so long as family medicine remains essentially a treatment service depending on patient-motivated contact which, particularly in the elderly, results in diseases becoming known too late in their course for effective therapy. Nor can preventive geriatrics be envisaged in the type of *laissez faire* systems of health care in which family physicians develop as rugged competitive individualists. In the more structured National Health Service the evolution of health teams, working from purpose-built premises, responsible for a registered practice population of defined proportions, analysed to show its age-sex structure, with indices for various chronic disease entities, offers excellent conditions and opportunities for geriatric screening.

141

Although there is not as yet any hard evidence from comparative studies of screened and unscreened groups to indicate that the early detection and treatment of disabilities is effective in helping elderly people to continue living comfortably and independently in their own homes, there are impressive claims that the offer of a routine assessment to high risk groups is of benefit (Lowther, MacLeod and Williamson, 1970; How, 1973; Williams, 1974). It would seem from all points of view more desirable to control a patient's congestive cardiac failure, and so enable her to continue living at home, rather than to rehouse her at ground-floor level to avoid climbing the stairs up to her present dwelling.

Desiderata gerontologica

Geriatric medicine and the cases accorded to it are difficult and complex, not only because of the accumulation of pathologies with age, but also because the assessor of such patients needs to recognise the distinction between primary biological ageing and the effect of pathological processes imposed on the individual. If most chronic diseases are associated with changes, often demonstrable post mortem, not all are recognised during life largely because knowledge of their natural history is incomplete. Arteriosclerosis may be present in the absence of symptoms, but offers no recognisable latent stage; nor can one doubt, despite their being incapable of pre-symptomatic demonstration, that biological changes precede the clinical manifestations of a disease like rheumatoid arthritis. Furthermore, the studies of Bourlière et al. (1966) have shown that the rate of ageing of a well-to-do urban population differs in marked respects from a rural population sampled in the same country.

The physician's primary duty to avoid doing harm—the *primum non nocere* of Hippocrates—must be considered in any screening programme; but while this consideration is massively relevant to programmes of pre-symptomatic screening, it is lightweight in respect of case-finding in the older section of society which has not only reached unprecedented proportions, but consists of large numbers of *nouveaux pauvres* accustomed to low expectations and minimal requirements in health care.

Sound reasons exist why the general practitioner should be the central figure of any screening programme, with support from the hospital and local authority. He is the person best able to provide the long-term supervision required in a cohort of people who show no clear distinction at first sight between health and disease, and he is highly aware of the local and regional factors influencing a potential ability to progress to normality or regress into overt disease. He is in a favourable position to arrange for further investigations, or to provide the reassurance granted by normal screening findings. Again, the practice age-sex register forms a highly satisfactory basis on which systematic care of this kind can be organised, for non-participants in the programme can be noted for follow up when they attend for incidental reasons. The three phases of the programme will be:

1 Selection and identification.
2 Medico-social assessment.
3 Follow up and evaluation.

Selection and identification

The first question to be decided is who shall be included in a geriatric screening programme. Is universal screening to be offered to all who have reached a certain age? If so, at what age? Should screening be more selective and directed at arbitrarily defined 'at risk' groups within an age range? The answers will depend on many factors, such as the type of practice, the degree of co-operation of partners and staff, the accessibility of patients, and whether the findings are to be used for research. One thing is certain; geriatric screening is no light undertaking. The socio-medical survey of 297 patients, undertaken by Williams and his colleagues on all patients over the age of 75, proved to be a major administrative enterprise (Williams *et al.*, 1972). Allocating one hour for each patient, the survey took one year to complete, and involved four doctors, and a full range of ancillary and attached staff, with additional volunteers who helped with transport. This admirable study is open to the one criticism that it might have been carried out too late for the effective treatment of serious malignant diseases. Thomas (1968), on the other hand, has advocated universal screening at or before the age of 65, on the basis of assertion that the pattern of future disability is already determined by that age. Apart from the reason that it would not be possible in the average practice to screen such large numbers, it is difficult to accept his hypothesis, convenient as it would be to find all the disorders likely to give trouble in later life already present at retirement age, when major social readjustment is also called for. Andrews, Cowan and Anderson (1971) in the Kilsyth study, found that disease was much more common in people over 75 than in those aged 65—74. Thus, a selection based on the age attained would seem more realistic and practicable at 70.

The point is sometimes made, and with justification, that the doctor is frequently in contact with his older patients, and proper attention to their needs leaves nothing to be desired from a screening programme. In this instance, those patients who had not been seen within a period of one year might be considered to be at special risk, so that a programme to assess them selectively would be reasonable. The chief difficulty lies in the identification of this 'unknown' group.

Forbes (1969) has pointed out that identification and knowledge of patients' whereabouts must be 90 per cent complete for a successful programme because the unidentified will tend to be those most in need of help. A Geriatric Register compiled from the manual clerical systems of Area Health Authorities will be very inaccurate, containing about 10 per cent of names of people who have moved away, and 13 per cent who have died. Some improvement in accuracy so far as addresses are concerned can be achieved by checking against the Electoral Register. Forbes carried out weekly modifications of information relating to patients, but was fortunate in being able to avail himself of processing by business machines under the aegis of the Oxford Linkage Study. Furthermore, only 7·6 per cent of his patients were over 65, whereas the average for the country as a whole is 13·5 per cent, and in retirement areas considerably more. To compile a Geriatric Register, including identification data of name, NHS number, date of birth, and statistical data, including age, sex and geographical zone within the practice, and the full postal address, demands a considerable initial effort and continuous monitoring thereafter, best performed by computer storage, or an efficient punch-card system.

Organisation

A screening programme should not distort normal practice working, so that it would be advantageous to concentrate effort during a period when normal work load might be expected to be reduced. A study of the practice audit may show that, for most items to be covered, there is a sag in the level of demand in the early autumn. This is a good time in other respects: climatic extremes, which adversely affect the elderly, are avoided, and it is an opportune time to offer prophylaxis against winter hazards.

Various times may be selected for holding the clinic, but the time most convenient is usually the late morning, for this does not interfere with the afternoon sleep enjoyed by many elderly patients, and also specimens for pathological examination can be delivered to the laboratory in good time.

Once the preliminary briefing and measures of agreement have been worked out along the lines discussed in Chapter 4, patients may be invited into the programme. This is best done by a personal letter, rather than by a general notice. Each letter should be personally signed. Details should be given of the time and place at which the clinic is held; advice on the collection of a urine specimen, and the suggestion that clothing should be worn that is easy to remove and replace. Nothing is to be gained by the use of euphemistic appellations such as 'Senior Citizens'; being called 'old' or 'older' does not normally give offence. Delivery of letters by volunteers, or other patients living in the same area will reduce postage costs. A response within seven days should be requested, for if none is received within 14 days it may be assumed either that information about the patient is incorrect, or that the recipient is unable to reply because of depression, mental failure, poor vision or illiteracy. Acceptance rates vary quite considerably among different investigators.

The screening programme may be carried out by a specially interested practitioner, able and willing to devote all his time to it, or by a team with each member responsible for one part of the assessment. (Miller, 1963; Thompson, 1968; Elliott and Stevenson, 1973). It has been claimed that health visitors can elicit the more important signs and symptoms of disease with a degree of accuracy that correlates well with the findings of doctors so far as physical disorders are concerned, so that presumably they could carry out preliminary screening in the home, using a questionnaire (Williamson and Lowther, 1966). Chamberlain (1973) studied the use of a multiple screening questionnaire administered by geriatric visitors in Greater London. The false negative and false positive rates were such that the screening questions missed more than half of those with significant hearing loss, and was highly inaccurate in the classification of people with visual disability, locomotor disorders, and those in economic need eligible for supplementary pension.

At the centre

The requirements here are simple. Patients should progress through several stations where observations are made and recorded on a standardised case sheet. A basic model would consist of four stations, each manned by a member of the general practitioner team.

On arrival the patient is received by the medical secretary who enters identification data, and then records height and weight. She may also measure the Peak Expiratory Flow rate, and test the near and distant vision, using Snellen type. The patient then passes to the nurse, who tests the urine and takes the blood pressure, and a blood sample. Using the Spencer ABO or grey wedge photometer she may measure the haemoglobin, retaining samples for estimation of the MCHC, ESR and blood urea, where indicated. The patient may then move on to see the doctor in such a way that he can observe the patient's gait. In taking the history a prepared list of about fifteen standard questions is useful, including symptoms such as cough, chest pain, breathlessness, weight change, and control of micturition; but, first of all, the patient should be given the opportunity to give his own account of his health with an opening question such as 'Are you satisfied with the state of your health?' The examination should follow the routine outlined on the case sheet, and be directed to those areas where pathological change is most likely to be met in the elderly. The author has suggested elsewhere a method of geriatric examination, and some of the pitfalls that may deceive the unwary (Thompson, 1972). With practice, the full assessment can be done in 20 minutes. If the haemoglobin is below 85 per cent, a faecal smear taken at rectal examination can be tested for occult bleeding (Occultest). It is desirable to examine the eyes with the ophthalmo-scope and, if possible, the hearing by an audiometer measuring from 0 to 60 Db. Further tests, such as tonometry, dipslide, etc. may be added or deleted as experience of their value is gained. Further investigations, such as diagnostic radiography, are arranged where these are suggested by the clinical examination.

Certain patients will be earmarked for mental testing. It has been shown that the mental status questionnaire (MSQ), consisting of 10 questions, will disclose and roughly measure intellectual impairment at one point in time, powerfully and effectively, without provoking anxiety or embarrassment, since half of the questions relate to personal information that may not appear to constitute a formal test to the patient (Wilson and Brass, 1973). This important matter of mental screening in old age is discussed further by Dr Brian Harwin in Chapter 15.

The final, and in some ways the most important stage, is the social assessment to be carried out by the health visitor. If she has not already visited the patient's home, she may arrange for a home assessment visit for the purpose of discussing home safety and improvements, and the important matter of the patient's drugs. The unified control of the social services since the implementation of the Seebohm Report has made the detection of social problems more worthwhile.

The interpretation of results

It has to be understood that some screening tests may be poorly correlated with the presence or absence of the disease they purport to indicate. While the haemoglobin level is a direct indication of the presence or absence of anaemia, the blood sugar level in diabetes and the ocular tension in chronic glaucoma, are both indirect tests complexly related to the diseases of which they are indices. Care must therefore be exercised in distinguishing 'patients' from normals, and consultant advice obtained in doubtful cases. It is essential to acquire knowledge of the way in which biochemical and other values may be modified by age, and also how the natural history of certain conditions is similarly affected (Jeffereys, 1972). For instance, urinary tract infection in the elderly is often asymptomatic, and often runs a benign course; but attempts to eradicate infection are often subject to failure, and vigorous therapy may produce the hazards of drug toxicity, so that there is much wisdom in a conservative approach. This only underlines what was said earlier regarding the difficulties and complexities of geriatric medicine, and they should be much in the mind of anyone who sets up a geriatric screening programme.

Discussion and evaluation

The question of prevention can never arise, nor can any rational therapy be instituted, unless a diagnosis has been made at a prior stage. Incidental to any screening programme will be the discovery of a small number of severe conditions no longer amenable to treatment. The aim of geriatric screening is to provide the opportunity for disabilities to be reported to a skilled observer, who can decide what, if anything, needs to be done about them. Management is directed to four aims: to treat what is treatable, to restore function, to relieve symptoms, and to offer social support. Practitioner awareness is relatively high for sufferers with cardiac, respiratory and CNS symptoms, but less so for urinary, locomotor, foot problems, anaemia, and chronic cerebral failure. Table 12 (p. 148) indicates various conditions that can be expected to be found in a screening programme, listed in a descending order of incidence.

The main charges against the validity of a geriatric screening programme are:

1 A low response rate resulting from refusals, and inability to trace patients.
2 Recommendations for treatment as a result of screening are commonly not taken up.

These are administrative matters, and deficiencies that can be rectified. They do not invalidate the principle of preventive geriatrics—that early assessment of disability can prevent deterioration; nor reduce the hope that the general practice centre of the future will represent all the services which an old person might require.

Table 12. Incidence of disease expected in a screening programme.

Remediable conditions	Conditions which may be alleviated	Conditions requiring symptomatic relief and social support
Depression	Deafness	Carcinomatosis
Anaemia	Chronic respiratory	Dementia
Cardiac failure	impairment	Hemiplegia
Hernia	Foot defects	Vertebro/basilar ischaemia
Uterine prolapse	Arthritis	Gangrene
Urinary infection	Anxiety	
Prostatic hypertrophy	Visual defects	
Diabetes	Dyspepsia	
Faecal impaction	Parkinson's disease	
Gout	Varicose veins	
Thyroid disorders	Prostatic carcinoma	
Osteomalacia	Cervical spondylosis	
	Diverticulitis	
	Postural hypotension	
	Trigeminal neuralgia	
	Paget's disease	

REFERENCES

Andrews, G. R., Cowan, N. R. & Anderson, W. F. (1971). The practice of geriatric medicine in the community. In *Problems and Progress in Medical Care*, p. 58. Oxford University Press. Essays on Current Research, 5th Series, ed. G. McLachlan.

Bourlière, F. (1966). Le vieillissement individuel dans une population rurale française. Etude de la commune de Plozévet, Finistere. *Bulletins et Mémoires de la Société D'Anthropologie*. Paris: Masson et Cie. X1, 10, 41.

Chamberlain, J. (1973). Screening elderly people. *Proceedings of the Royal Society of Medicine*. In the press.

Elliott, A. E. & Stevenson, J. S. K. (1973). Geriatric care in general practice. *Journal of the Royal College of General Practitioners*, 23, 615.

Forbes, J. A. (1969). Locating the elderly in a general practice. *British Medical Journal*, 2, 42.

How, N. M. (1973). A team caring for the elderly at home. *Journal of the Royal College of General Practitioners*, 23, 627.

Jeffereys, P. M. (1972). The prevalence of thyroid disease in patients admitted to a geriatric department. *Age and Ageing*, 1, 33.

Lowther, C. P., MacLeod, R. D. & Williamson, J. (1970). Evaluation of early diagnostic services for the elderly. *British Medical Journal*, 3, 275.

Miller, R. C. (1963). *The Ageing Countryman*. London: National Corporation for the Care of the Old People.

Thomas, P. (1968). Experiences of two preventive clinics for the elderly. *British Medical Journal*, 2, 357.

Thompson, M. K. (1968). Care of the aged in general practice. *Transactions of the Hunterian Society*, XXVII, 115.

Thompson, M. K. (1968). Examination of the elderly patient. *Update*, 4, 8, 1,005.

Williams, E. I., Nicholson, M. R. & Gabert, J. (1972). Sociomedical study of patients over 75 in general practice. *British Medical Journal*, 2, 445.

Williams, E. I. (1974). A follow-up of geriatric patients after sociomedical assessment. *Journal of the Royal College of General Practitioners*, 24, 341-346.

Williamson, J. & Lowther, C. P. (1966). The use of health visitors in preventive geriatrics. *Gerontologia Clinica, Basel*, 8, 362.

Wilson, L. A. & Brass, W. (1973). Brief assessment of the mental state in geriatric domiciliary practice. The usefulness of the Mental Status Questionnaire. *Age and Ageing*, 2, 92.

15 Psychogeriatric Screening   *Brian Harwin*

'Let us hope that the heritage of old age is not despair'.

Disraeli.

Psychogeriatric morbidity

1 Extent of the problem

In Britain, as in many other countries, the prevalence of psychiatric disorder in the population reaches a maximum in old age. This is reflected in the increase with age of mental hospital admission rates (PEP, 1966), and in the evidence shown by large-scale surveys in general practice (Shepherd *et al.*, 1966; Watts *et al.*, 1964). The majority of the elderly mentally ill are not in hospital but at home, with their condition often unknown and untreated, although, in many instances, the clinical severity and social distress of their illness matches those cases being cared for in hospitals. The total amount of psychogeriatric morbidity is high and is likely to increase even further over the next decade as the numbers of elderly people in the population grow (Brooke, 1965). In the comprehensive psychogeriatric survey in Newcastle by Kay and his colleagues (1964), 30 per cent of the entire population aged 65 and over were found to be suffering from mental disorder. In half of the cases due to dementia, the mental deterioration had progressed to a severity that was equal to those found in demented hospital patients, yet fewer than one-fifth were in hospital; and of the cases of depressive illness, the majority were not receiving any form of psychiatric treatment. Other studies have indicated that elderly patients seem particularly reluctant to seek medical attention; Parsons (1965) in a domiciliary survey of the elderly found about half the mental disorders in this age group were unknown to their general practitioners, and in a study among

149

their own patients by Stokoe and his colleagues (Stokoe 1965) the figure was higher: 84 per cent. Apart from the absence of appropriate medical treatment, many of these patients had pronounced social needs that could have been helped by the community social services.

2 *Types of mental disorder among the aged*

The mental disorders that occur in old age are comprised of the organic dementias and the functional disorders, of which depression is the commonest. Paranoid disorders form only one per cent of domiciliary psychogeriatric conditions.

On the basis of community surveys, it has been estimated (Bergmann, 1972) that in a hypothetical practice of 10,000 patients, of whom one would expect 1,200 (12 per cent) to be aged 65 and over, the psychiatric morbidity would be distributed as follows:

Dementia	6·7 per cent	=	81 patients
Early cerebrovascular involvement without dementia	2·9 per cent	=	35 patients
Patients with suspected mild or early dementia	2·8 per cent	=	34 patients
Patients with moderately severe functional disorder (mainly depression)	10 per cent	=	120 patients
Total 'Morbidity Pool' within practice		=	270 patients

(This represents 22·5 per cent of all patients over 65 within the practice).

Dementia. Two types of dementia are described: arteriosclerotic and senile, each of which has distinctive pathological features. In practice, there may be overlap which makes it difficult to distinguish clinically between them, but the general practitioner need not be too concerned with the differentiation. Both involve damage to cerebral tissue, both are progressive, and each shares an equivalent bad prognosis; in a follow-up study of hospitalised cases 70 per cent were found to have died two years after admission to hospital (Slater and Roth, 1969). An alteration in personality and a deterioration of intellectual faculties are the two ultimate main consequences of both conditions. The most important intellectual decline is manifest by a disorder of memory, particularly in the capacity for remembering *recent* events. While dementing patients can often recall accurately early events in their lives, the capacity to remember recent events may show marked impairment. As both conditions progress, however, earlier personal memories also become affected. It is the deterioration in these abilities that forms the basis for the clinical detection of dementia.

The diagnosis of arteriosclerotic dementia would be suggested by a previous history of cerebrovascular accidents. Hypertension is present in about half the cases (Slater & Roth, 1969) and neurological abnormalities like aphasia, visual field defects, or occasionally signs of Parkinson's disease may be present. There may be also a history of fleeting episodes of vertigo or loss of consciousness, or even generalised epileptiform seizures. Initially, judgment and basic personality tends to be better preserved than in senile dementia; the patient retains insight, and with the realisation of his general decline may become depressed. Characteristically, the course of the illness fluctuates, and acute confusional episodes, in which the patient is disorientated, and may wander about at night, can be brought about by further cerebral episodes or concurrent physical disorders such as cardiac failure, or infections of the chest and urinary tract.

In senile dementia, which is probably hereditary in origin and slightly more common than the arteriosclerotic form, the development is slower and in the early stages is indistinguishable from the more benign memory difficulties experienced as part of the ageing pattern of normal subjects. It is in the *progressive decline* that the differences between benign senescence and senile dementia emerge. As the memory of a senile dementing patient deteriorates, the patient tends increasingly to mislay possessions in the home, leave on cookers, electric fires, etc. Whatever the type, the ends of both arteriosclerotic and senile dementia merge into a common clinical picture of personality decline and memory failure. The patients are easily provoked into bouts of fatuous laughter or outbursts of explosive rages, speech may be incoherent, general physical debility with incontinence of bowels and bladder occurs, and they become generally incapable of looking after themselves. The degree of disorientation may be such that they are unaware of the current day, month or year.

Depression. There is little point in the practitioner attempting to distinguish between 'endogenous' and 'reactive' forms of depression in the aged. The form most likely to be encountered is reactive (Roth, 1964) which has been brought about by social vicissitudes, such as bereavement, and family worries, or as a result of the social and physical restrictions imposed by physical illness. The practitioner's suspicions of depression, as also dementia, may be aroused from points in the history and subsequently confirmed at interview by observations of the patient's demeanour and symptom complaints.

It is unusual for some degree of anxiety not to co-exist, and vague bodily sensations are also common. Hypochondriasis, fear or conviction of the presence of underlying physical disease, which in its more severe forms can reach delusional intensity, is a common presenting feature of depression and is the diagnosis most easily missed if the underlying mood state is not ascertained. Insomnia, either in the form of early morning wakening or difficulty in getting off to sleep, is often present.

Paranoid states. Paranoid symptoms are sometimes seen as part of a severe depressive picture, but usually the illness is a specific syndrome, which in its fully-developed picture is characterised by ideas of persecution and auditory hallucinations. The previous personalities of the patients in which it develops are frequently characterised by suspiciousness, cantankerousness and eccentricity. Often they are bachelors and spinsters who in their declining years have become isolated and withdrawn from society. Sensory defects such as blindness and deafness which contribute to their social isolation are common among paranoid patients (Post, 1962).

Scope for treatment. Until a few decades ago, it used to be assumed that all mental disorders in old age were variants of an irreversible destruction of cerebral tissue. Such is now known not to be the case, and the group of functional disorders, such as depression and paranoia, have no underlying equivalent organic cerebral pathology. Although there is no known remedy which will either arrest or reverse the organic process of dementia, the outlook and susceptibility to treatment in depressive disorders is strikingly different. Advances in psychopharmacology have made available effective drugs that can considerably alleviate the distressing symptoms of depressive illness and reduce the risk of suicide which is particularly prominent in elderly patients with this disorder. Similarly, appropriate drug treatment can control the symptoms of paranoid illness, and has made it possible for elderly patients with this disorder to live a reasonable life in the community. While drugs form an important part in the treatment for depression, there has been an increasing awareness that a system of management to be comprehensive and effective must also take into account that these disorders often arise in the setting of social adversity, such as bereavement, loneliness and isolation, or physical ill-helath. These patients need help in the form of emotional support, and, in the case of a physical handicap, advice and practical measures to help deal with the handicaps arising from physical illness.

Hitherto, the course of dementias has always been held to be uninfluenced by drugs, but in recent years there have been a number of favourable reports drawing attention to the benefit of pharmacological agents in this condition. While such reports hold hope for future therapy, at present the main justification for the recognition of dementia must rest on two counts. First, because the stress on other members of the family looking after demented patients can be considerable (Grad and Sainsbury, 1965), and although many relatives are prepared to care for dementing patients at home, they may suffer penalties in the form of emotional distress, restriction of leisure, and in some cases, financial deprivation. It is clearly important that in such circumstances all possible assistance is given by the community health and social services. Secondly, the condition of elderly patients with dementia may not come to light until social stress or the development of a physical illness provokes a crisis. Such situations are invariably accompanied by a considerable degree of social disruption, which does not lend itself to the making of calm decisions about management. Previous assessment and supervision would enable plans to be drawn up to meet such contingencies, so that they can be dealt with more easily should they arise.

Evaluation of screening

While the substantial evidence from research programmes relating to the extent of undisclosed mental illness in the community highlights the scope for psychogeriatric screening clinics, there has to date been little evaluative research that has concentrated on the outcome of mental disorders detected by such measures. The methods of operation of a number of screening clinics have been described; most of these have included an assessment of mental state, which has usually been undertaken by a psychiatrist. While the published overall results relating to outcome are favourable, the extent of subsequent change in the mental disorders discovered by screening has not been described in the reports.

The work of Anderson and Cowan (1955) who described the pioneer screening clinics at Rutherglen, indicates that early detection of illness avoids hospitalisation. The follow-up by Lowther and his colleagues (1970), who looked principally at a high-risk group of elderly patients such as the bereaved, those living alone, and patients recently discharged from hospital found that of those whose mental health was already known to be impaired, comprising two-thirds of all patients examined, 70 per cent were improved or unchanged, but in those whose condition had been detected by the initial screen at an early stage, only 23 per cent had improved. While they question whether such a low figure of improvement can justify the operation of such clinics, they, nevertheless, point out that early detection is humane, reduces the period of suffering and, as in the Rutherglen project, avoids admission to hospitals. Fourteen to sixteen per cent of their patients were found initially to be suffering from depression, but how much the overall figures of improvement relate to this group is not clear. Although the lack of detailed evaluative research indicates that psychogeriatric screening must be considered to be still in the experimental phase, on ethical grounds alone, the amount of potentially treatable morbidity is sufficient justification for such screening.

Practical procedures in screening

Reports from some of the screening clinics to which reference has already been made indicate the feasibility of incorporating a psychiatric assessment into a geriatric screening programme, and apart from practical convenience it is also desirable that physical and psychiatric assessment should not be made separate procedures, as mental disorder in old age is frequently accompanied by physical illness (Anderson, 1971).

Use of ancillary personnel. In the reports of experimental ventures, physical examinations have taken place in the surgery. The patients previously received a visit from ancillary staff such as a health visitor, who organised the practical arrangements, including appointments and transport, if needed, to the surgery. A key feature of this method of approach is that it enables these personnel both to observe the patients in their home circumstances and to make specific enquiry into social functioning, which is essential to any geriatric investigation. Thus, details of such items as housing difficulties, financial and family worries, restrictions in leisure, social contacts, and recent bereavement can be incorporated in a preliminary medical and psychiatric history. The latter would need to include enquiry into such features as memory failure, oddities of behaviour, and depression. This information can help the general practitioner to focus on relevant features, when the time comes for assessment at the surgery.

It has been suggested by official authorities that ancillary medical personnel such as health visitors and nurses could be used specifically to identify psychiatric disorder among the elderly (HMSO, 1970) and there are reports of surveys which have given support to this idea. A Scottish pilot survey of elderly people reported that health visitors successfully identified all the cases of moderately severe psychogeriatric illness. but failed to recognise mild cases (Player *et al.*, 1971). In a general practice survey in which a group of district nurses were asked to assess the mental state of elderly patients with physical illness living at home, a substantial majority of the patients subsequently confirmed by the author as suffering from a mental disorder, were successfully identified by the nurses (Harwin, 1973). Few severe cases were missed; such results are certainly encouraging for paramedical staff to be deployed in this way, but suggest that in order to increase their efficiency in identification they should receive more specialised training in this field.

Assessment of the mental state. Two possible approaches are available and used by psychiatrists in screening programmes for mental disorder: one is by a questionnaire which is completed by the patient, the other is by actual interview. Self-administered questionnaires have not been used for elderly patients and are unlikely to be of value, as the presence of dementia would preclude reliable answers by patients with this condition. The approach, therefore, must be by direct interview.

Although to date there is no psychogeriatric screening interview that has been designed and tested specifically for use by general practitioners, the doctor should not be discouraged by this from carrying out such procedures. A suggested interview which is not lengthy and would be suitable for screening purposes in the setting of general practice is outlined in Appendices A and B (pp. 157–158). Its two basic aims are to establish the presence or absence of dementia and depression. The assessment of dementia is based on a modification of the Tooting Bec questionnaire (Doust et al., 1953) which has been found to be useful in identifying dementia in community studies of the elderly (Goldberg et al., 1970). The interview comprises a series of questions to test the patient's memory and orientation, as indicated in Appendix A. All questions must be put to the patient and the answers scored as indicated; a total score is obtained by the addition of the individual scores of each question answered correctly.

The assessment of depression and anxiety by interview is outlined in Appendix B. This approach has been found by the author to be useful in eliciting such symptoms in general practice psychogeriatric screening, and the questions have the additional advantage of being quite acceptable to patients. The format is a series of mandatory questions followed by optional probes, if indicated. It is advisable to record some of the replies verbatim, and although in practice the doctor's technique will need to be flexible as patients may often choose to steer their own courses through the interview, each manadatory question must be asked. If these are answered in the affirmative, the subsequent questions serve as probes for further exploration. The practitioner should not fight shy of asking patients about intimate thoughts of suicide and hopelessness. Apart from the need to identify such a risk, such patients never resent it and are often relieved to be able to divulge such ideas. Nevertheless, there will always be a few who will find it difficult or painful at first to acknowledge they are depressed. When this is suggested by points in the history of the patient's demeanour, tact, understanding and perseverence can usually succeed in bringing to light any hidden distress.

Evaluation of the interview. The score on the cognitive tests (Appendix A) serves as a guide for the presence of dementia but it is sometimes difficult to distinguish between this condition and depression. As a consequence of apathy, uninterest in life and its events, or lack of concentration, depressed patients can sometimes perform poorly on the memory and orientation tests. Conversely, dementing patients can be depressed. A score of eight or below in these tests would strongly *suggest* the presence of a dementing process, but there is no known psychological test which indicates unequivocally its presence or absence, particularly in border-line cases. Other evidence from the history or behaviour, as outlined in the account in a previous section, needs to be taken into consideration. However, the practitioner need not be disconcerted by not always reaching a precise diagnosis. It is valuable and sufficient in the circumstances to have identified the patient as a 'case', and appropriate action can then be taken to seek a specialist psychiatric opinion. In assessing the severity of the depression the practitioner must draw upon his clinical judgment, supplementing his own observations of the patient's manner, and replies given to his questions, with evidence available in the history. At one extreme will be the patient who is tearful and agitated, with perhaps suicidal pre-occupations; at the other is the patient whose depressive symptoms are mild, and although intrusive into his thoughts and outlook, do not conspicuously interfere with his life. In between lies a whole range of moderately severe conditions which cause the patient subjective distress and significantly impair his functioning.

It is suggested that enquiry about the possible presence of hallucinations or persecutory ideas be left to the discretion of the doctor, and made when there is a severe degree of depression evident at interview, or where reports of disturbed behaviour have been provided in the history.

At the end of the interview, the practitioner should preface his final evaluation of the case with brief comments about the patient's demeanour at interview.

Some case examples are described in Appendix C (p. 158).

APPENDIX A. The Assessment of Dementia

Question	*Patient's reply*	*Score*
1 What is your name?		
2 How old are you?		
3 Are you married?		
4 What was your (husband's) work?		
5 What year is it?		
6 How long have you lived here?		
7 What is the name of this street? (I am going to tell you an address, and I want you to try to remember it:- 74 Columbia Road).		
8 When did the Second World War start?		
9 When did the Second World War finish?		
10 Who was Prime Minister at the beginning of the War?		
11 Who was Prime Minister at the end of that War?		
12 Who is the Prime Minister now?		
13 Who is on the throne of England?		
14 (Some question relating to recent world events).		
15 What is the name of the Queen's eldest son (Prince of Wales)?		
16 (Another question relating to recent world events).		
17 What was that address I told you a few minutes ago?		
	TOTAL	

Score 1 point for each correct answer, except for Question 17 which should be scored 2 points.

MAXIMUM SCORE = 18

APPENDIX B. *The Assessment of Depression and Anxiety*

Questions   *Patient's reply*

How do you keep in your spirits nowadays?
   — are there periods when you feel low or sad?

If the replies suggest depression, carry on:
How often does this happen?
   — is this most of the time or just occasionally?
Do you know what brings it on?
   — is it connected with anything that happens?
Do you feel like crying sometimes?
Do you sometimes feel you don't want to go on?
Have you ever felt like making an end to it all?
Do you worry a lot about things?
   — what sort of things worry you at present?
Is your physical health a worry to you?
Do you ever worry about developing physical illness?
   (e.g. heart or bowel trouble, stroke, cancer)
How do you sleep at night?
   — do you have trouble getting off?
   — do you wake early?

If YES,

   — have you any idea why you can't sleep?
   — how often do you have bad nights?

APPENDIX C. *Case examples found by screening*

Case 1
Severe bereavement masquerading as hypochondriasis

The medical records of a 74-year-old widow showed that she had been radiologically investigated six months previously for dysphagia. The patient at the time had voiced a pronounced fear of underlying carcinoma, from which her husband had died a year before. At interview the patient, a thin, careworn and agitated figure, revealed that she still had not overcome the grief following her husband's death. She was convinced the sensation in her throat derived from underlying cancer and when asked about her spirits, wept and said she was seldom free from thoughts of her dead husband, and would only be happy when she ultimately joined him. She had little interest in living and lay awake at night, sometimes hearing his voice. The marriage had been a particularly happy one, and each partner was devoted to the other. The true nature of her husband's condition had not been disclosed to her until shortly before his death and had come as a profound shock. Social isolation added to her distress; they had only moved into the area shortly before the busband's death and had not had an opportunity to make new friends. A married son and a daughter lived a long distance away and were precluded from visiting her frequently. The patient was considered a suicidal risk and referred for psychiatric supervision.

Case 2
Depressive reaction to family difficulties and physical disabilities

Since the onset of rheumatoid arthritis, a 72-year-old bachelor had lived with his sister and her family. The arthritis had limited the patient's physical mobility and considerably restricted his leisure and social outlets. Haemoglobin estimation confirmed the anaemia that his pallor suggested. He seemed a pleasant, quiet, pensive, unhappy man at interview, who initially denied any depression. With patience and understanding, it was suggested that perhaps he was covering up his feelings, and he went on to admit this was true and revealed how dispirited he was. He found little pleasure and interest in living at present, and on occasion had felt like weeping, but had 'not reached the stage of wanting to make an end of it'. His presence in the household had created tensions, which centred principally on the resentment by his sister's husband. The sister's difficulties had been further aggravated by worries over the behaviour problems of one of her two children.

Arrangements were made to investigate further the patient's anaemia and for a social worker to make contact with the family to see what advice and practical help could be given in the situation.

Case 3
Concealed dementia

A 75-year-old married woman had a history of being taken to the casualty department of the local hospital five months previously, following a fall. Only a mild injury to the ankle had been sustained, and the patient had been returned home by ambulance. The husband, who suffered from recurrent bronchitis and was in poor physical health, reported that his wife had become rather forgetful in the house and neglectful in her appearance and hygiene, and had on several occasions in recent times left on cooker taps. When interviewed, the patient seemed content, cheerful and superficially mentally well preserved. However, formal testing revealed marked deficiencies of cognitive functioning. Although she correctly gave her age and date of birth, and knew the day and month, she was ten years out with the current year and believed George III to be the ruling monarch. She was quite unable to recall the address given to her in testing, and incorrectly maintained that she had seen the interviewer the previous day. Physical examination revealed hypertension, slight one-sided weakness and an extensor plantar reflex. On this evidence it seemed likely that the patient's previous fall had been due to a mild cerebrovascular accident.

Arrangements were made for a health visitor to call in regularly and for the domiciliary 'Meals-on-Wheels' service to be provided.

REFERENCES

Anderson, W. F. & Cowan, N. R. (1955). Prevention of illness in the elderly—the Rutherglen experiment. *Lancet*, 2, 239.

Anderson, W. F. (1971). The inter-relationship between physical and mental disease in the elderly. In *Recent Developments in Psychogeriatrics*. Kent: Headley.

Bergmann, K. (1971). *Proceedings of VIth World Congress of Psychiatry*. In the press.

Bergmann, K. (1972). Psychogeriatrics. *Medicine*, 9, 647.

Brooke, E. M. (1965). The psychogeriatric patient: some statistical considerations. In *Psychiatric Disorders in the Aged*. Manchester: Giegy.

Doust, J. W. L., Schneider, R. A., Talland, G. A., Walsh, M. A. & Barker, G. B. (1953). The correlation between intelligence and anorexia in senile dementia. *Journal of Neurology and Mental Diseases*, 117, 383.

Goldberg, E. M., Mortimer, A. & Williams, B. T. (1970). *Helping the Aged*. London: Allen & Unwin.

Grad, J. & Sainsbury, P. (1965). An evaluation of the effects of caring for the aged at home. In *Psychiatric Disorders in the Aged*. Manchester: Geigy.

Harwin, B. G. (1973). Psychiatric morbidity among the physically impaired elderly in the community. In *Roots of Evaluation: the Epidemiological Basis for planning Psychiatric Services*. Oxford University Press.

HMSO (1970). *Services for the Elderly with Mental Disorder*. Scottish Health Services Council.

Kay, D. W. K., Beamish, P. & Roth, M. (1964). Old age mental disorders in Newcastle-upon-Tyne. *British Journal of Psychiatry*. 110, 146.

Lowther, C. P., MacLeod, R. D. M. & Williamson, J. (1970). Evaluation of early diagnostic services for the elderly. *British Medical Journal*, 3, 275.

Parsons, P. L. (1965). The mental health of Swansea's old folk. *British Journal of Preventive and Social Medicine*, 19, 43.

PEP (1966). Trends in psychogeriatric care. *Political and Economic Planning*, XXXII, No. 497.

Player, D. A. Irving, G. & Robinson, R. A. (1971). Psychiatric, psychological and social findings in a pilot community health survey. *Health Bulletin*, XXIX, 2.

Post, F. (1962). The significance of affective symptoms in old age. In *Maudsley Monograph*, 10, Oxford University Press.

Roth, M. (1964). Prophylaxis and early diagnosis and treatment of mental illness in late life. In *Current Achievements in Geriatrics*. London: Cassell.

Shepherd, M., Cooper, B., Brown, A. C. & Kalton, G. W. (1966). *Psychiatric Illness in General Practice*. Oxford University Press.

Slater, E. & Roth, M. (1969). Mental diseases of the aged. In *Clinical Psychiatry*. London: Baillière, Trindal & Cassell.

Stokoe, I. M. (1965). Physical and mental care of the elderly at home. In *Psychiatric Disorders in the Aged*. Manchester: Geigy.

Watts, C. A. M., Cawte, E. C. & von Kuenssberg, E. (1964). Survey of mental illness in general practice. *British Medical Journal*, 2, 1351.

III Screening for Specific Diseases

16 Urinary Infection

P.J. Constable

'In principle a normal urinary tract remains sterile'.

H. G. Hanley, 1965.

After respiratory disease, urinary tract infection is the commonest infectious illness that the general practitioner has to deal with. A survey conducted by London and Greenhalgh (1962) showed that a general practitioner can expect to see 12 cases of acute urinary infection per year, per 1,000 patients on his list, the greatest incidence being in young women between the ages of 20 and 30.

But this is only part of the problem. Kass (1956) has described a technique for identifying urinary infections in clean catch specimens of urine, based on quantitative estimation of bacteria, thereby avoiding the need for catheterisation. When infection is present the organisms multiply rapidly in the bladder urine until they reach concentrations greater than 100,000 per ml, this level being termed 'significant bacteriuria'. In contrast, contaminated urine shows bacterial counts generally less than 1,000 organisms per ml, and thus it has become possible to differentiate infection from contamination in clean catch specimens of urine.

With this tool it rapidly became apparent that symptomless urinary infection, or asymptomatic bacteriuria, was more prevalent than had been realised. During the past fifteen years countless studies have attempted to throw light on the significance of this finding and to determine the natural history of urinary tract infection in man. Sadly, our knowledge remains patchy and incomplete; while a greater understanding exists of the particular problems of urinary infection in infancy and pregnancy, any relationship that exists between asymptomatic bacteriuria, acute frank urinary infection and end-state renal failure in adults remains in doubt.

163

As a result of this increased interest in urinary infection, a variety of screening tests have been developed which offer the general practitioner an opportunity to extend his diagnostic ability by confirming or excluding the presence of infection without complete reliance upon the hospital laboratory and its associated delays.

The need for bacteriological screening tests arises partly from the poor correlation that exists between the presence of urinary infection, the exhibition of symptoms and abnormal physical signs. As was so well demonstrated by Mond *et al.* (1965), nearly half the patients with symptoms of dysuria and frequency in fact have no bacteriological evidence of urinary infection. While the classical sign of loin tenderness in the presence of renal infection was found helpful by Manners *et al.* (1972), this is in contrast to the findings of many others. In a study from an Australian general practice, Fairley *et al.* (1971), though observing loin tenderness in renal infection, pointed out that often dysuria and frequency were the only symptoms occurring in patients with proven renal infection. With such fallibility in the symptoms and physical findings, the importance of bacteriological assessment of urine becomes apparent. Renal tract infection in infancy and childhood, when diagnosis is more difficult, is more sinister. It has been demonstrated conclusively that the growing kidney is extremely sensitive to infection and if this is allowed to proceed unchecked, it rapidly results in pyelonephritic scarring of the renal parenchyma. The relationship of asymptomatic bacteriuria in infancy to frank infection is a matter for further study to determine. It has been demonstrated by Abbott (1972) that it is possible for bacteriuria in infancy to clear spontaneously, presumably as a result of the same host defence mechanisms that are present in adults, namely the mechanical clearing of organisms by voiding and the antibacterial activity of the bladder wall (Norden, Green and Kass, 1968). As childhood advances the incidence of urinary infection in the sexes shows a marked change. By school age there is an incidence of significant bacteriuria of 1·2 per cent in girls and 0·03 per cent in boys, a reversal of the incidence at birth. Continuous study of this population shows that the incidence in schoolgirls rises steadily with age though the prevalence of bacteriuria remains at about the same level (Kunin, Zacha and Paquin, 1962; Asscher *et al.*, 1973). This apparently innocuous observation is of particular importance because it indicates that to identify these children any screening procedure would have to be repeated at intervals throughout their school life and, having identified and treated their bacteriuria, Kunin has shown that 75 per cent of infections had recurred within two years.

In the adult, epidemiological studies have revealed some three to four per cent of healthy women to have asymptomatic bacteriuria

(Kass, Savage and Santamarina, 1965; Freedman *et al.*, 1963; Asscher, Chick and Waters, 1971). The turnover of bacteriuria in the population is substantial. Each year a quarter of adult bacteriurics clear spontaneously, only for a similar number to develop bacteriuria. The prevalence of bacteriuria appears to increase with age but its relation to frank infection and the value of treatment has not been established.

There has been intensive study of asymptomatic bacteriuria in pregnancy and here the incidence has been shown to be similar to that in non-pregnant women, namely four per cent (Kass, 1958; Kincaid-Smith and Bullen, 1965). In contrast, however, is the fact that in pregnancy some 40 per cent of the asymptomatic bacteriurics develop frank pyelonephritis and by eradication of the bacteriuria it is possible virtually to abolish pyelonephritis of pregnancy.

The long term effects of significant bacteriuria in adult women are unknown. Prospective studies are currently under way and may confirm the findings of Freedman and Andriole (1969) who in a series of 250 women with urinary infection found no deterioration in renal function over a period of 12 years.

It is with this rather patchy background of the natural history of urinary infection that the practitioner must judge when screening is justified and interpret his findings in the light of these observations.

SCREENING TESTS FOR URINARY INFECTION

The recognition of urinary tract infection is now dependent upon the statistical concept of 'significant bacteriuria' which may be defined as the presence of more than 100,000 organisms per ml in two or more clean catch specimens of bladder urine. The accuracy of all screening tests depends upon their ability to differentiate between contamination and infection. For this, they must be compared with standard quantitative bacteriological techniques such as pour plate colony counts or surface viable counts. There are a wide variety of methods available to practitioners, ranging from simple microscopy, through indirect chemical tests to semiquantitative bacteriological methods. Whilst, in practice, it is commonplace to regard a single positive test as presumptive evidence of infection it is important to remember that Kass (1956) showed that the accuracy of examination increases from about 80 per cent on a single specimen to greater than 95 per cent following examination of two specimens. The three groups of techniques that are available for use as screening tests for urinary tract infection may be considered in greater detail.

Microscopical methods

1 *Detection of infection by the presence of pyuria*
The urine may be examined microscopically for the presence of

white cells. An increased number of white cells is evidence of inflammatory change somewhere in the urinary tract, but not necessarily of infective origin.

Semiquantitative method: The standard method of assessing the excretion of pus cells is to examine the unstained film of fresh urine and record the number seen per high power field. By using a Fuchs-Rosenthal counting chamber it is possible to standardise the count and figures varying from 10 to 50 white cells per cu. mm of urine have been regarded as the upper limit of normal. Gadeholt (1964) observed many variables in the cellular counting of urinary sediment and felt that centrifugation causes an unpredictable cellular loss, this inaccuracy having been observed earlier by Little (1962). The accuracy of the test is a little suspect. Brumfitt and Percival (1964) found a good correlation with quantitative bacteriological tests in a group of 43 symptomatic infected patients from general practice. In contrast, in their observations on 163 patients with bacteriuria of pregnancy only 57 per cent had an excess of white cells. In the surveillance of infants and children, simple microscopy of the urine has repeatedly been advocated as an aid to diagnosis. Providing the incidence of false negative tests is realised it is well suited for use in general practice, requiring little time to perform the test and obtain an immediate result (Dunn, Hine and MacGregor, 1964; O'Doherty, 1968).

Quantitative method: The most satisfactory way to detect small increases in urinary white cell excretion is by collecting a timed sample, measuring the total volume, counting the white cells in the pooled specimen and calculating the rate of white cell excretion per hour. Little (1962) showed this to be far more accurate than examining films of urine, but sebsequently Fairley and Barraclough (1967) showed that though it is a good screening test for urinary tract disease it gives a high rate of false positive results in uninfected urine.

2 Staining of urinary sediment

Gram stain of urinary deposit: For many years it has been recognized that one of the simplest screening tests for bacteriuria is a gram stain of the unspun urinary sediment. This offers only a moderately good correlation, however, being positive in 80 per cent of specimens with significant bacteriuria. In many cases it offers an immediate method of distinguishing infection from contamination. The method is ideally suited to the conditions of general practice and has been rather attractively described as the poor man's colony count (Finnerty et al., 1961). All reports have not been so enthusiastic; for example, Deutch and Jespersen (1964) found that in their hands the method was unsatisfactory.

Methylene blue stain of urinary deposit: Schamadan (1964) assessed the accuracy of staining slides of unspun urinary deposit with Methylene Blue. While he reported an agreement with quantitative methods in over 95 per cent of samples, this work remains to be confirmed and the method appears to have little to recommend it compared with the more usual Gram stain.

Indirect biochemical screening tests

1 *Greiss-Ilosvay nitrite test*

This test depends upon the reduction in urine of nitrates to nitrites by actively respiring bacteria. The nitrites in the urine may then be identified by means of a chemical spot test, giving an obvious colour change. The test was originally adopted by Greiss (1879) as a means of assessing bacterial contamination of water. Subsequently Cruickshank and Moyes (1914) showed that nitrites could be detected in urine by using this reaction. In recent years, application of this test to the detection of bacteriuria of pregnancy has produced indifferent results when compared with standard quantitative bacteriological studies, though it has been marketed commercially both in Europe and North America (Smith and Schmidt, 1962; Verhoef, 1973).

Sleigh (1965) modified the original test by incubating the urine at 37°C for four hours with potassium nitrate, before adding the reagent and testing for nitrites. He found this refinement to be more accurate than other chemical screening tests. Kincaid-Smith and her associates (1964), however, found this modified nitrite test gave only 35 per cent positive results in a series of infected urines and that this degree of accuracy compared unfavourably with alternative chemical screening tests.

2 *The triphenyl tetrazolium chloride test (TTC)*

This substance has the advantage of being one of the comparatively few organic compounds that is coloured in the reduced state, colourless triphenyl tetrazolium chloride being reduced to red insoluble triphenylformazan.

Interest in this substance as an indicator of bacterial growth was initiated by Wundt (1950) who, while investigating factors inhibiting bacterial growth, observed the colour change of TTC to red formazan by bacterial cultures. Using Seitz filtration he established that this colour change was due to the organisms themselves and not to their metabolites. Simmons and Williams (1962) developed these observations into a practical test for the recognition of significant bacteriuria.

In this, a solution of the salt is incubated with an aliquot of urine for four hours at 37°C. At the end of this time the mixture is examined by the naked eye, a red precipitate indicating the presence of significant bacteriuria and a negative result being shown by the absence of any colour change. The authors found a high degree of correlation existing between the TTC test and quantitative bacterial urinary counts.

Interest was aroused in using this technique as a screening test for antenatal patients (Pinkerton, 1964; Kincaid-Smith et al., 1964) and in children (Neter, 1964), these authors finding that the method was a reliable screening test when more complex bacteriological techniques were not available. Other studies have criticized various aspects of the method. Bulger and Kirby (1963) found, in their series, a poor correlation between the TTC test and quantitative bacterial urinary counts. Its use in general practice is handicapped by the rather unstable character of the solution and the four hour incubation period (Constable, 1966). In a study of the remote Scottish island community of Tiree (Calvert et al., 1972) the authors felt that while the test might be sufficiently accurate for survey purposes, it could miss up to 40 per cent of infected urines and this was unacceptable as a diagnostic agent. The technique has proved sufficiently popular in North America to be marketed commercially as 'Uroscreen' and this has been reviewed favourably (Hnatko, 1966). In an informed and thorough review on screening procedures for urinary infection, Brumfitt and Reeves (1968) considered the TTC and the modified nitrite test to be the best of the chemical procedures then available.

3 Detection of urinary catalase

The enzyme catalase occurs in most bacteria that attack the urinary tract. It is also present in high concentrations in kidney tissue and its cell free extract. Catalase may be detected by observing the release of oxygen resulting from its action upon hydrogen peroxide.

Gagnon, Hunting and Esselen (1959) developed a rapid technique of catalase determination by impregnating a paper disc with a solution of the substance under test and observing its flotation in a column of hydrogen peroxide. Oxygen bubbles, realised by the catalase acting on the hydrogen peroxide, cause the paper disc to rise in the column. This technique was used in investigating urinary tract infection by Braude and Berkowitz (1961). False positive results were disappointingly frequent; this finding was confirmed by other studies and led to the technique falling rapidly into disuse.

4 *Subnormal levels of urinary glucose as an indicator of bacteriuria*

Since the mid-nineteenth century it has been realised that normal urine contains very small amounts of glucose. Scherstén and Fritz (1967) used a hexokinase-glucose-6-phosphate method to determine the range of fasting urinary glucose levels in a large group of persons. They found 96 per cent of this group to fall in the range between 2 mg and 20 mg per cent. In a pilot study those who had less than 2 mg per cent of urinary glucose were found to have significant bacteriuria. They postulated that this decrease in urinary glucose level was a result of the bacteria in the bladder metabolising the glucose. By using a glucose specific test paper together with a colour reagent they developed a practical screening test which has been marketed commercially under the name 'Uriglox' (Scherstén *et al.*, 1968).

Emmerson (1972) used this technique in screening for pregnancy bacteriuria. He found it a simple, rapid and accurate test to perform. There are, however, certain disadvantages. A fasting specimen of early morning urine is needed and this requires testing within three hours of collection. Furthermore, some bacterial species, notably *Proteus mirabilis* and *Pseudomonas aeruginosa*, utilise glucose too slowly to give a positive result. Moreover, in a small study screening neonates, Dosa and Houston (1972) found too high a proportion of false negative results to justify its continued use; whilst Cahalane and Kelly (1972) found the somewhat rigid requirements of specimen collection, together with its high cost, rendered it unsuitable as a mass screening test for children. Emmerson and Mond (1973) were encouraged by a trial of this technique in general practice, but their careful study showed a disappointingly high proportion of false negative results. This finding was confirmed in a Scottish study (Hendry, 1973), where it was felt that the conditions required for the test were too strict for general use in family practice.

Semiquantitative bacteriological methods

1 *Standard loop*

This technique, long proved useful in dairy bacteriology, entails inoculating surface media with a 2, 3 or 5 mm loopful of uncentrifuged urine and subsequently counting the number of colonies grown. Although Randolph and Greenfield (1964) recommended the adoption of this technique as a practical method for use in the North American consulting room, I fear that contemporary general practitioners in Great Britain would not regard it in the same light. Indeed only a fair correlation has been found with this technique when compared with pour plate methods (Liggins and Whittington, 1966).

2 *Filter paper strips*

Ryan, Hoody and Luby (1962) developed a technique using strips of filter paper whereby small aliquots of urine could be uniformly distributed upon the surface of an agar plate. A standard curve may thus be plotted relating the number of bacteria per ml to the number of colonies per filter strip area. This is prepared by contrasting standard plate counts of dilutions of pure cultures of various organisms with the filter strip readings.

This method was assessed by Brumfitt and Percival (1964), who found it to be a rapid, economical and suitably accurate method of screening for significant bacteriuria. A slight variant of this technique was introduced by Leigh and Williams (1964) using a measured area of blotting paper of particular absorbancy, and this has been shown to be a reliable and practical method in the hands of enthusiastic general practitioners.

3 *Dip slide inoculum*

Mackey and Sandys (1965) conceived the idea of the dip inoculum transport medium with the particular needs of general practitioners in mind. They designed a readily transportable screw topped bottle containing a metal spoon, holding a suitable culture medium. A standard inoculum of urine is obtained by dipping the medium coated spoon into a freshly passed mid stream specimen of urine. They demonstrated that the spoon colony counts showed a direct proportional relationship to the standard quantitative methods. Two years later, Guttmann and Naylor (1967) developed this method by using a microscope slide coated with nutrient media, instead of a spoon. Laboratory and clinical testing showed it to give consistent quantitative results, comparing well with pour plate colony counts. Finding no false negative results in 385 specimens, they recommended this technique both for routine use by general practitioners and where large scale screening was required. The equipment is simple both to use and read and the dip slide can, if necessary, be sent through the post. The reliability and value of this method in communities remote from laboratory services has been well demonstrated by Calvert *et al.* (1972).

The earlier studies were confirmed rapidly (Cohen and Kass, 1967) and the technique has been found to be reliable and effective, prompting world-wide commercial marketing. Further encouragement to its widespread acceptance in general practice was given by Arneil, McAlister and Kay (1970) who demonstrated that the method was reliable not only when the specimen is incubated at 37°C but also when cultivated at room temperature for 18 hours.

However, in studies from general practice (Maclean, McCallum and Davies, 1971; Dove *et al.*, 1972) it was shown that the accuracy of positive results rises from 80 per cent to 95 per cent when incubation is either at 37°C for 24 hours or at room temperature for 48 hours. The method has now become widely accepted for use in general practice because of its convenience and the lack of special equipment or skill needed in the interpretation of the result.

4 *Suprapubic bladder aspiration (SPA)*

Suprapubic aspiration of urine from the bladder provides a means of obtaining uncontaminated urine, any bacterial growth from a single specimen obtained by this method being strongly indicative of urinary infection. Beard *et al.* (1965) employed this technique as part of a screening programme in puerperal patients at Queen Charlotte's Hospital and found it an easy method to perform, without complications. Using a combination of this technique with dip slide culture of the aspirate, Dove *et al.* (1972) were able to identify 93 per cent of cases of urinary infection on a single specimen, compared with only 72 per cent on dip slide culture of a single mid stream specimen of urine. In this study, from general practice, they found no false negative results even though in order to facilitate the technique a diuresis was produced in some patients.

O'Doherty (1968) recommends the use of this technique in neonates and infants, describing it as an easy, reliable and safe diagnostic test. The technique of SPA is not new (Monzon *et al.*, 1958; Stamey, Govan and Palmer, 1965). The procedure is simple and, for the patient, comparable to a venepuncture. The bladder should be readily palpable and, after skin cleansing, punctured about two inches above the symphisis pubis, using a 1½ inch 23 gauge needle; the urine may then be aspirated. Despite the merits of this technique and the enthusiasm of its protagonists, its use in general practice has been criticised because of the need for careful sterility techniques, its time consuming nature and the small increase in accuracy compared with other less onerous methods.

THE USE OF SCREENING TESTS FOR URINARY INFECTION IN GENERAL PRACTICE

The existence of so many screening tests for bacteriuria indicates that the ideal test for this condition has yet to be developed. This is particularly so in relation to the requirements for use in general practice. Yet the wide variety of fairly satisfactory methods may be matched by the diversity that exists in the character of practices throughout the country, and it should be possible for most practitioners to select a technique that is suitable for their particular circumstances. So many excellent studies demonstrating the value of various screening tests in general practice have been published in recent years that it is salutory to read Professor Arneil's comment (1971) that even now many practitioners work under the misapprehension that the presence of proteinuria is an adequate indication of urinary infection.

The role of screening tests for urinary infection in general practice is still uncertain. There are two differing requirements. Firstly the general practitioner is in a particularly favourable position to participate in observations on the natural history of urinary tract infection in different sections of the community. For these large scale surveys the chemical screening tests such as the TTC or Greiss test appear to be suitable methods, though recently Asscher et al. (1973) have demonstrated the value of dip slides in large scale community surveys. The second requirement is in screening the individual patient, either for suspected urinary infection or in supervision following treatment. For many practitioners, faced with this situation, the dip inoculum semiquantitative bacteriological methods have proved invaluable.

Perhaps the most important function of these techniques in general practice lies in establishing the diagnosis of urinary infection in patients presenting with symptoms referable to the urinary tract. Mond et al. (1965) showed that lower urinary tract symptoms occurred just as commonly in patients with normal urine as in those with infected urine. It is the identification of patients with true recurrent urinary infection that leads to the selection of those who warrant thorough urological investigation, and in whom identification of unsuspected renal tract abnormality is more likely. Furthermore, the general practitioner is ideally placed to follow up the patient who has been treated for urinary infection. By the use of screening tests he may establish that the infection has been eradicated and, where both doctor and patient are suitably motivated, ensure by surveillance that infection has not recurred.

In antenatal care, the value of identifying those four per cent of women with asymptomatic bacteriuria has been established. Eradication of the bacteriuria in this group of patients has been shown to reduce greatly the incidence of pyelonephritis of pregnancy. Although the claims that link asymptomatic bacteriuria with toxaemia and prematurity remain in doubt, there is no doubt that here is an aspect of antenatal care where the general practitioner has an opportunity to extend his supervision of the patient.

Any of the screening tests that have been described would, if used routinely, add to the value of the consultation. Indeed, some are sufficiently simple that they can be used by the midwife with only minimum supervision. In contrast, renal tract infection in infancy and childhood appears to have attracted rather less interest from general practice than its importance warrants. Perhaps this is due, in part, to the time consuming difficulties in obtaining suitable urine specimens for examination. When medical resources are being focussed on the management of chronic renal failure, it is relevant to recall that urinary infection in this age group may result, in a proportion of cases, in chronic and progressive disease. It is incumbent upon those engaged in primary medical care to identify those children at risk by the early recognition of the presence of urinary infection.

The problem of screening for urinary tract infection in the aged is a complex one, hampered by the rather limited published information. Although there is an increased prevalence of urinary tract infection with age (Kass, 1972) it would seem to run a more benign course in this group of the population, while the suggestion that vascular disease is a contributing factor to renal infection has still to be established (Dontas et al., 1966). The picture is further complicated by the fact that the symptomatology of urinary infection in the aged is often atypical or even frankly bizarre.

In conclusion, while it can be argued that the value and purpose of screening tests for urinary tract infection remains to be established, there is little doubt that they already offer the general practitioner an opportunity to extend his interest in this common infective process. Whether he uses them in a population survey or, more likely, in the monitoring of an individual patient's health, the screening tests that are already available can add to the quality of care in general practice.

REFERENCES

Abbott, G. D. (1972). Neonatal bacteriuria—a prospective study in 1,460 infants. *British Medical Journal*, 1, 267-269.

Arneil, G. C. (1971). Urinary tract infection in childhood. Supplement to the *Postgraduate Medical Journal*, 47, 35-37.

Arneil, G. C., McAllister, T. A. & Kay, P. (1970). Detection of bacteriuria at room temperature. *Lancet*, 1, 119-121.

Asscher, A. W., Chick, S. & Waters, W. E. (1971). Clinical aspects of urinary tract infection: The need for treatment. Supplement to the *Postgraduate Medical Journal*, 47, 28-30.

Asscher, A. W., McLachlan, M., Verrier Jones, R., Meller, S., Sussman, M., Harrison, S., Johnston, H., Sleight, G. & Fletcher E. (1973). Screening for asymptomatic urinary tract infection in schoolgirls. *Lancet*, 2, 1-4.

Beard, R. W., McCoy, D. R., Newton, M. R. & Clayton, S. G. (1965). Diagnosis of urinary infection by suprapubic bladder puncture. Lancet, 2, 610-611.

Braude, A. I. & Berkowitz, H. (1961). Detection of urinary catalase by disc flotation. *Journal of Laboratory and Clinical Medicine*, 57, 491-493.

Brumfitt, W. & Percival, A. (1964). Pathogenesis and laboratory diagnosis of nontuberculous urinary infection: a review. *Journal of Clinical Pathology*, 17, 482-490.

Brumfitt, W. & Reeves, D. S. (1968). Screening procedures for urinary infection. In *Presymptomatic Detection and Early Diagnosis*, Chap. 8. Ed. C. L. E. H. Sharp & H. Keen. Pitman Medical.

Bulger, R. J. & Kirby, W. M. M. (1963). Simple tests for significant bacteriuria. *Archives of Internal Medicine* 112, 742-746.

Cahalane, S. F. & Kelly, D. G. (1972). Evaluation of the 'Uriglox' method in screening for bacteriuria. *Journal of the Irish Medical Association,* 65, 339-341.

Cohen, S. N. & Kass, E. H. (1967). A simple method of quantitative urine culture. *New England Journal of Medicine,* 277, 176-178.

Constable, P. J. (1966). The triphenyl tetrazolium chloride test in general practitioner antenatal care. *Lancet,* 2, 195-196.

Cruickshank, J. & Moyes, J. M. (1914). The presence and significance of nitrites in urine. *British Medical Journal,* 2, 712-714.

Calvert, F. R., Hawthorne, V. M., Mann, P. G., & Sandys, G. H. (1972) Bacteriuria in a Scottish Island community. A comparison of chemical and cultural tests for bacteriuria applied in remote surroundings. *Journal of Hygiene,* 70, 105-112.

Deutch, M., & Jespersen, H. G. (1964). The detection of significant bacteriuria. *Acta Medica Scandinavica,* 2, 191-193.

Dontas, A. S., Papanayiotou, P., Papanicolaou, N., Marketos, S., & Economou, P. (1966). Bacteriuria in old age. *Lancet,* 2, 305-306.

Dosa, S., & Houston, I. B. (1972). Neonatal bacteriuria and 'Uriglox'. *Archives of Diseases of Childhood,* 47, 674-676.

Dove, G. A., Bailey, A. J., Gower, P. E., Roberts, A. P. & de Wardener, H. E. (1972). Diagnosis of urinary tract infection in general practice. *Lancet,* 2, 1281-1283.

Dunn, P. M., Hine, L. C., & MacGregor, M. E. (1964). Search by clinical methods for persistent urinary infection in childbirth. *British Medical Journal,* 2, 1081-1084.

Emmerson, A. M. (1972). The use of a simple test for hypoglycosuria (Uriglox) in the diagnosis of bacteriuria of pregnancy. *Journal of Obstetrics and Gynaecology of the British Commonwealth,* 79, 828-830.

Emmerson A. M & Mond. N. C. (1973). A simple strip test for the diagnosis of urinary tract infection in general practice. *Journal of the Royal College of General Practitioners,* 23, 592.

Fairley, K. F. & Barraclough, M. (1967). Leucocyte excretion rate as a screening test for bacteriuria. *Lancet,* 1, 420-422.

Fairley, K. F., Carson, N. E., Gutch, R. C., Leighton, P., Grounds, A. D., Laird, E. C., McCallum, P., Sleeman, R. L. & O'Keefe, C. M. (1971). Site of infection in acute urinary tract infection in general practice. *Lancet,* 2, 615-618.

Finnerty, F. A., Massaro, G. D., Kakaviatos, N., & Chupkovich, V. (1961). Incidence of unsuspected urinary tract infection in normal pregnant and toxaemic patients. *New England Journal of Medicine,* 265, 534-537.

Freedman, L. R. & Andriole, V. T. (1969). *Abstracts of the IVth International Congress of Nephrology.* Stockholm. Vol. 1, 386-389.

Freedman, L. R., Phair, J. P., Seki, M., Hamilton, H. B., & Nefzger, M. D., (1963). The epidemiology of urinary tract infection in Japan. Second International Congress of Nephrology. *Excerpta Medica,* 67, 53-59.

Gadeholt, H. (1964). Qualitative estimation of urinary sediment, with special regard to sources of error. *British Medical Journal,* 1, 1547-1549.

Gagnon, M., Hunting, W. M., & Esselen, W. B. (1959). New method for catalase determination. *Analytical Chemist,* 31, 144.

Greiss, P. (1879). Bemerkungen zu der Abhandlung der HH. Weselsky und Benedikt. Ueber einige Azoverbindungen. *Bericht. deutsch. chem. gesslach.,* 12, 426-427.

Guttmann, D. & Naylor, G. R. E. (1967). Dip-Slide: an aid to quantitative urine culture in general practice. *British Medical Journal,* 3, 343-344.

Hanley, H. G. (1965). The urethral syndrome and pyelonephritis. *Proceedings of the Royal Society of Medicine,* 58, 1035-1038.

Hendry, D. W. W. (1973). The assessment of two consulting room tests for bacteriuria. *Journal of the Royal College of General Practitioners,* 23, 365.

Hnatko, S. I. (1966). The triphenyl tetrazolium chloride test alone and in combination with the gram smear as a screening procedure for significant bacteriuria in hospital patients. *Canadian Medical Association Journal,* 95, 103-105.

Kass, E. H. (1956). Asymptomatic infections of the urinary tract. *Transactions of the Association of American Physicians,* 69, 56.

Kass, E. H. (1958). Asymptomatic bacteriuria and pyelonephritis of pregnancy. *Journal of Clinical Investigation,* 37, 906-909.

Kass, E. H. (1962). Pyelonephritis and bacteriuria. A major problem in preventive medicine. *Annals of Internal Medicine,* 56, 46-50.

Kass, E. H., Savage, W. & Santamaria, B. A. G. (1965). The significance of bacteriuria in preventive medicine. In *Progress in Pyelonephritis,* ed. E. H. Kass, Philadelphia; F. Davis & Co.

Kincaid-Smith, P., Bullen, M., Mills, J., Fussell, U., & Huston, N. (1964). The reliability of screening tests for bacteriuria of pregnancy. *Lancet,* 2, 61-63.

Kincaid-Smith, P. & Bullen, M. (1965). Bacteriuria in pregnancy. *Lancet,* 1, 395-396.

Kunin, C. M., Zacha, E., & Paquin, A. (1962). Urinary tract infection in schoolchildren. *New England Journal of Medicine,* 266, 1287.

Leigh, D. A. & Williams, J. D. (1964). Methods for the detection of significant bacteriuria in large groups of patients. *Journal of Clinical Pathology,* 17, 498-504.

Liggins, G. C. & Whittington, E. (1966). A routine procedure for the detection of bacteriuria in pregnancy. *Journal of Obstetrics and Gynaecology of the British Commonwealth,* 73, 244-248.

Little, P. J. (1962). Urinary white cell excretion *Lancet,* 1, 1149-50.

Loudon, I. S. L. & Greenhalgh, G. P. (1962). Urinary tract infection in general practice. *Lancet,* 2, 1246-1247.

Mackey, J.P. & Sandys, G. H. (1965). Laboratory diagnosis of infection of the urinary tract in general practice by means of a dip-inoculum transport medium. *British Medical Journal,* 2, 1268-1270.

Maclean, D. W., McCallum, F. M., & Davies, B. I. (1971) Dip-slide urine cultures in general practice. *Journal of the Royal College of General Practitioners,* 21, 710.

Manners, B. T. B., Grob, P. R., Dulate & Grieve, N. W. P. (1972). The interrelationships of asymptomatic bacteriuria, acute bacterial pyelonephritis and bacterial cystitis in women. Paper read at Second National Symposium of Urinary Infection, London. Publication pending.

Mond, N. C., Percival, A., Williams, J. D. & Brumfitt, W. (1965). Presentation, diagnosis and treatment of urinary tract infection in general practice. *Lancet,* 1, 514.

Monzon, O. T., Ory, E. M., Dobson, H. L., Carter, E. & Yow E. M. (1958). A comparison of bacterial counts of the urine obtained by needle aspiration of the bladder, catheterisation and mid-stream voided methods. *New England Journal of Medicine,* 259, 764.

Neter, E. (1964). Bacteriology and the immune response in urinary tract infections. *The Pediatric Clinics of North America,* 11, 3517.

Norden, C. W., Green, G. M. & Kass, E. H. (1968). Antibacterial mechanisms of the urinary bladder. *Journal of Clinical Investigation,* 47, 2689.

O'Doherty, N. (1968). Urinary tract infection in the neonatal period and later infancy. In *Urinary Tract Infection: Proceedings of the First National Symposium on Urinary Infection,* Ed. F.O'Grady & W. Brumfitt,. Oxford Medical Publications.

Pinkerton, J. H. M., Gibson, G. L. & Houston, J. K. (1964). Screening tests for bacteriuria *Lancet,* 2, 313.

Randolph, M. F. & Greenfield, M. (1964). The incidence of asymptomatic bacteriuria and pyuria in infancy. *Journal of Pediatrics,* 65, 57.

Ryan, W. L., Hoody, S. & Luby, R. (1962). A simple quantitative test for bacteriuria. *Journal of Urology,* 88, 6, 838-840.

Schamadan, W. E. (1964). Bacteriuria during pregnancy. *American Journal of Obstetrics and Gynaecology,* 89, 10.

Schersten, B. & Fritz, H. (1967). Subnormal levels of glucose in urine—a sign of urinary tract infection. *Journal of the American Medical Association,* 201, 949-952.

Schersten, B., Dahlqvist, A., Fritz, H., Kohler, L. & Westlund, L. (1968). Screening for bacteria with a test paper for glucose. *Journal of the American Medical Association,* 204, 205-208.

Simmons, N. A. & Williams, J. D. (1962). A simple test for significant bacteriuria. *Lancet,* 1, 1377.

Sleigh, J. D. (1965). Detection of bacteriuria by a modification of the nitrite test. *British Medical Journal,* 1, 765.

Smith, L. G. & Schmidt, J. (1962). Evaluation of three screening tests for patients with significant bacteriuria. *Journal of the American Medical Association,* 181, 431.

Stamey, T. A., Govan, D. E. & Palmer, J. M. (1965). The localisation and treatment of urinary tract infection. *Medicine (Baltimore),* 44, 1-36.

Verhoef, J. (1973). Detection of bacteriuria. *Lancet,* 1, 1066-1067.

Wundt, W. (1950). Untersuchungen uber die radktionswirkung von baktenen auf Triphenyltetrazolium chlorid. *Deutische Medizinische Wochenschrift,* 75, 1471.

17 Diabetes Mellitus
I.H. Redhead

'The protean spectre of diabetes mellitus haunts the consulting room of every practising physician. It lurks behind the folliculitis, furunculosis and pruritus ani in the office of the dermatologist. It peers out from retinal microaneurysms, pigmentation, haemorrhages and retinitis proliferans at the ophthalmologist's. It hides behind the altered sensation and reflexes in the clinic of the neurologist, and leers through an albuminous cloud in the test tube of the urologist. It troubles the sleep of the surgeon concerned about wound healing; and of the obstetrician vacillating between forceps and caesarean. It hides behind the cough of the phthisical and the elevated T-wave on the cardiogram. It complicates the life of the general practitioner and specialist alike . . .'

Milton Weed.

The hypothesis that if a disease is diagnosed in its early stages the results of treatment will be better seems logical. In the early days of screening for diabetes this was the spur that drove on workers in this field. Blotner and Marble (1951), two leading American workers, wrote 'early diagnosis of the disease prolongs life, increases efficiency and decreases disability; it prevents or postpones the onset of complications.' This opinion was shared by many experts, some of whom, for example, Joslin (1946), suggested the occurrence of a period of reversibility after the onset of the disease during which, with adequate treatment, a recurrence might be prevented. This opinion was controversial when first expressed and today it remains so. This controversy and the question as to whether or not early treatment really does modify the disease makes it doubly difficult to assess the value of screening.

The incidence

The first systematic attempt to estimate the true incidence of diabetes in a community was made by Wilkerson and Krall (1947) in the USA. Other workers followed, notably Kenny (1951). These investigations were accompanied by a series of diabetes detection drives which were heralded by much publicity in an effort to gain public support.

The introduction of the glucose oxidase strip test for glycosuria facilitated the search for diabetes and in 1960 a survey from a large general practice in Newcastle was reported (Redhead, 1960). A constructed sample of 20 per cent of the 9,940 patients in the practice was tested. Walker (1961) tested 87 per cent of the total population of Ibstock, Leicestershire. The Working Party of the Royal College of General Practitioners (1962) investigated the patients on the lists of members taking part. After strenuous efforts no less than 95·50 per cent of the total of 19,412 were tested. The results of these and other whole population surveys is shown in Table 13.

Table 13. Results of some whole population surveys for diabetes.

	Population at risk	Percentage tested	Percentage of those tested with glycosuria	Percentage of those tested found to be diabetic	
				Known	New Cases
Wilkerson & Krall (1947)	4,983	70·6	4·7	0·8	0·6
Kenny, Chute & Best (1951)	3,502*	81·0	1·7	0·75	0·5
Redhead (1960)	1,991†	100·0	5·27	0·45	0·5
Walter & Kerridge (1961)	5,406	81·0	4·8	0·8	0·6
College of Gen. Pract.(1962)	19,412	95·5	2·66	0·64	0·69
Harkness (1962)	5,843	95·3	2·66	0·62	0·57

* Over 6 years old.
† Constructed sample

Varying methods and criteria of diagnosis were adopted by the different workers. The most usual method was to obtain a sample of urine passed an hour after a large meal, the urine being tested with the glucose oxidase strip. In several of the surveys (College of General Practitioners, Redhead) all cases of glycosuria were given an oral glucose tolerance test. Wilkerson and Krall (1947) collected both urine and venous blood samples. 'Dextrostix,' an exzyme test for blood sugar, was first utilised in a survey in 1965 by Kent and Leonards. This test, so it was claimed, reduced to some extent the use of the autoanalyser.

Malins (1968), in an analysis of whole population surveys, pointed out that whatever the method used for detection and whatever diagnostic criteria were set up (and certainly both these features varied considerably from survey to survey), the proportion of newly diagnosed diabetics was much the same as and always approximate to the number of known cases in the community. Malins went on to state that the diagnosis of most new cases of diabetes depended upon the finding of a small deviation in the glucose tolerance test or a minor elevation in the blood sugar without the clinical features of the disease: 'All the variations of initial screening, of laboratory techniques and interpretation of results fail to produce any wide variation in the proportion of cases finally labelled diabetic.' This surely is an extraordinary fact.

From the available evidence it seems that the incidence of diabetes is 1—1·5 per cent of the population. This estimate is based on abnormality of glucose tolerance and not on the incidence of symptomatic disease. Work performed subsequent to their initial screen by the Working Party of the Royal College of General Practitioners (1963, 1970) indicates that the incidence could be in excess of this figure.

The value of early detection and screening

There is now such a large body of knowledge about diabetes in whole populations that probably no more such surveys are required. These surveys have indicated those groups of the population in which most diabetics are to be found. To spend time screening outside these groups is wasteful and unrewarding.

Selected group screening. An analysis of whole population surveys indicates that screening for diabetes should be limited by age, concentrating in those over fifty. Other groups who are considered to be at high risk are those with a family history of diabetes, women who have had a baby of over 10 lb (4·5kg) birth weight, women who have had six or more children, and women who have had two or more unexplained stillbirths or excessive weight gain in pregnancy.

Diagnostic classification of diabetes

The diagnosis of diabetes does not necessarily depend on the presence of symptoms. The fundamental diagnostic criterion remains an abnormal glucose tolerance test. The interpretation of that which is normal or abnormal is still a matter for debate. A classification of the test was formulated and accepted by the medical and scientific section of the British Diabetic Association and reported by Fitzgerald and Keen in 1964. This is still accepted by many experts.

Classification recommended by the British Diabetic Association

1 **Potential.** These persons have a normal glucose tolerance test (GTT, defined below) but have a potential risk of developing diabetes:

(a) an identical twin, the other twin being diabetic.

(b) a person with both parents diabetic.

(c) a person with one diabetic parent whose other (non-diabetic) parent has, or had, either a diabetic parent, sibling or offspring, or a sibling having a diabetic child.

(d) a woman who has given birth to a live or stillborn child weighing 10 lb (4·5 kg) or more at birth, or a stillborn child showing hyperplasia of the pancreatic islets not due to rhesus incompatibility.

2 **Latent.** (a) a person with a normal GTT who is known to have had a diabetic GTT at some time during pregnancy, infection, or other stress or when obese.

(b) a person who has abnormal blood glucose responses (similar to those found in diabetes mellitus) to provocative tests, such as the cortisone augmented GTT or the intravenous sodium tolbutamide test.

3 **Asymptomatic.** (sometimes referred to as subclinical or chemical):

(a) a person with a diabetic response to the GTT whose fasting blood sugar is below 130 mg per 100 ml (capillary) or 125 mg per 100 ml (venous).

(b) as above, but with fasting blood sugars above the stated values.

4 **Clinical.** A person with an abnormal GTT with the symptoms or complications of diabetes.

The term 'prediabetic' is reserved for the period in the life of a diabetic before the diagnosis is made.

Oral glucose tolerance test

Conditions. Unrestricted diet and physical activity for at least three days, 12 hours of fasting, and 30 minutes sitting quietly before the test. Subject to remain seated and non-smoking during the test.

Method. After withdrawing the fasting blood sample, 50 g glucose in 200-500 ml of flavoured water to be drunk in five minutes. Zero time to be taken as the beginning of the drink and samples to be withdrawn at 30-minute intervals for two hours.

Standard of abnormality. Capillary blood glucose level of 120 mg per 100 ml or more at two hours and of 180 mg per 100 ml or over at some other time point in the test. (Corresponding venous blood glucose values 110 mg and 160 mg per 100 ml respectively.) The blood glucose values above refer to measurements by either the glucose oxidase method or ferricyanide method after dialysis using the autoanalyser.

The Working Party of the Royal College of General Practitioners (1970) has suggested in a follow up report of their original survey that the criteria for diagnosis should be modified so that the two-hour level capillary blood glucose should be raised to 135 mg per cent. The figure suggested by the British Diabetic Association in 1964 was 120 mg per cent.

The problem of the asymptomatic diabetic

In screening for diabetes some cases will come to light who already have symptoms but who have not complained. These obviously need treatment. Problems arise from the fact that the diagnosis of diabetes is a biochemical one and it is vital that the 'patient' should not be left in a state of uncertainty and puzzlement. The management of the asymptomatic diabetic is yet another subject for controversy. Stowers (1967, 1970) believes that if after treatment by diet the chemical abnormality persists, chlorpropamide should be used in small dosage. He claims that in those under 35 years of age the diabetes is reversed in the majority of cases and in some this reversal has been maintained for as long as eight years (Stowers, 1973). This would confirm the hypothesis that there is a period of reversibility and if treatment is instituted during this time the disease can be cured. The opposite view is taken by Malins (1968) who believes that there is no evidence that early treatment modifies the disease.

Method of detection in screening programmes

The fundamental criterion for the diagnosis of diabetes remains an abnormal GTT. Using this test as a screening method will probably uncover about twice as many diabetics as any other testing technique. Screening with this method, however, is not a practical proposition. One must therefore accept less efficient methods. The choice lies between spot blood and urine specimens. The former will probably uncover a higher proportion of latent disease, especially in the elderly who frequently have a high renal threshold for glucose. Specimens could be taken two hours post prandially and sent to the hospital for autoanalysis. A patient with a reading of 130 mg per cent or higher should be referred for an oral GTT.

Alternatively dextrostix could be used. This would avoid the laboratory being involved in a large number of autoanalyser tests, but dextrostix has its limitations in practice, mainly to do with the varying degree of readout error involved in the ocular assessment of the colour changes on the test strip with reference to the colour scale (Schersten, 1971). Malins (1973) considers the dextrostix has not made any fundamental difference to the screening for diabetes and does not think it suitable for survey work. However, Stowers (1973) believes that dextrostix is of considerable value if used in association with the Ames reflectance meter. This device at the present time costs almost £200 and unless screening is being performed in a group practice in which diabetes is being managed under clinic circumstances this method would seem to be unacceptable in view of the cost of the instrument. A new reflectance meter, called the Eyetone, has recently been described, but this is not yet widely available in Britain (Schersten *et al.*, 1974).

There remains the enzyme strip test for glycosuria, which will reveal a considerable proportion of the latent cases of diabetes if a two hour post prandial specimen is tested. All cases of glycosuria should be subjected to a two hour post prandial blood sugar estimation. If the capillary blood specimen shows a reading of 130 mg per cent or higher, then an oral GTT should be performed.

A screening programme for diabetes in general practice

As in all screening programmes it is of fundamental importance that a practice should have an age-sex register. A morbidity register is of almost equal value so that relatives of a case of diabetes can be traced with ease.

Screening should be confined to selected peak risk groups. These can be listed as follows:

1 Those of fifty years of age and over.
2 Those with a family history of diabetes.
3 Women who have had a baby of 10 lb (4·5 kg) birth weight or over.
4 Women who have had six or more children.
5 Women who have had six or more unexplained stillbirths.
6 Women who show excessive weight gain during pregnancy.

Investigations of these groups depends upon practice circumstances. If the practice runs its own diabetic clinic it might consider it worthwhile to own an Ames reflectance meter. In these circumstances the following procedure is suggested: A capillary blood glucose reading of 130 mg per cent two hours after a meal should be referred for a full oral GTT. Without a reflectance meter the use of dextrostix as a screening method is not recommended, and it is probably preferable to use in those under fifty years of age the enzyme glucose oxidase test for glycosuria If a two hour post prandial urine specimen contains glucose then a two hour post prandial capillary blood sugar should be performed. In those over fifty years of age it is preferable to screen by performing a two hour post-prandial capillary blood sugar. If the reading is greater than 130 mg per cent an oral GTT should be performed. The interpretation of the GTT should be based on the criteria laid down by the British Diabetic Association detailed previously.

Follow-up

All cases showing a diabetic glucose tolerance curve present no problems regarding future management; their diabetes requires treatment. Borderline cases, and other non-diabetic abnormalities of glucose tolerance require firm reassurance and prolonged follow-up. Full explanations must be provided to help the puzzled and bewildered. It is just as important to reassure the patients with non-diabetic glycosuria as it is to treat the diabetic.

REFERENCES

Blotner, H. & Marble, A. (1951). Diabetes control: detection, public education and community aspects. *New England Journal of Medicine*, 245, 567-574.
Fitzgerald, M. G. & Keen, H. (1964). Correspondence. *Lancet*, 1, 1325.
Harkness, J. (1962). Prevalence of glycosuria and diabetes mellitus. A comprehensive survey in an urban community. *British Medical Journal*, 1, 1503-1507.
Joslin, E. P., Root, H. F., White, P., Marble, A. and Bailey C. L. (1946). In *Treatment of Diabetes Mellitus*. Philadelphia: Lea and Febiger.
Kenny, A. J., Chute, A. L. & Best, C. H. (1951). A study of the prevalence of diabetes in an Ontario community. *Canadian Medical Association Journal*, 65, 233-241.
Kent, G. T. & Leonards, J. R. (1965). Mass screening for diabetes in a metropolitan area using finger blood glucose after a carbohydrate load. *Diabetes*, 14, 295-299.
Malins, J. (1968). *Clinical Diabetes Mellitus*. London: Eyre and Spottiswoode.
Malins, J. (1973). Personal communication.
Redhead, I. H. (1960). Incidence of glycosuria and diabetes mellitus in a general practice. *British Medical Journal*, 1, 695-699.
Schersten, B. (1971). The dextrostix Reflectance Meter. *Lakartidningen*, 68, 4,001-4,004.
Schersten, B., Kuhl, C., Hollender, A. & Ekman, R. (1974). Blood glucose measurement with Dextrostix and a new reflectance meter. *British Medical Journal*, 3, 384-387.
Stowers, J. (1967). Prevention of diabetes. Clinical results. International Congress Series No. 172. *Proceedings of the Sixth Congress of the International Diabetes Federation.* 743-746. Amsterdam: Excerpta Medica Foundation.
Stowers, J. (1970). Treatment of subclinical diabetes. *Early Diabetes*, 449-454. New York: Academic Press.
Stowers, J. (1973). Personal communication.
Walker, J. B. & Kerridge, D. (1961). *Diabetes in an English Community*. Leicester University Press.
Wilkerson, H. L. C. & Krall. L. P. (1947). Diabetes in a New England town. *Journal of the American Medical Association*, 135, 4, 209-216
Working Party of the Royal College of General Practitioners (1962). A diabetes survey. *British Medical Journal*, 1, 1497-1503.
Working Party of the Royal College of General Practitioners (1963). Glucose tolerance and glycosuria in the general population. *British Medical Journal*, 2, 655-659.
Working Party of the Royal College of General Practitioners (1970). Five year follow-up report on the Birmingham Diabetes Survey of 1962. *British Medical Journal*, 3, 301-305.

18 Obesity

D. Craddock

Obesity occupies a special place among conditions for which screening should be considered, as screening for obesity gives a greater yield than any other specific condition.

Definition of obesity

To determine the prevalence of obesity in any population group, obesity must first be defined. Many authorities regard a weight that is 10 per cent above an individual's fit lean weight as indicative of obesity. Those who would accept only 15 or 20 per cent above the fit lean weight as abnormal should ponder the fact that even the 10 per cent definition allows a 12 stone (76 kg) man to put on 16 lbs (7 kg) of fat without being considered obese. To obtain the base line of a person's fit lean weight is easy if their weight was known in their twenties and if they were then slim and fit. Recourse must otherwise be made to tables of some sort.

Tables of normal weight for height

Tables which show increasing weight with age are based on averages and are useless. Fit adults maintain the same weight throughout their life except for a slight decline after the age of 60 (Slome *et al.*, 1960; Gastineau, 1972).

It is now generally accepted that the tables produced in 1959 by the New York Metropolitan Life Insurance Society are the most reliable. They give desirable ('ideal' or 'best') weights for each height which are the weights giving the lowest mortality rates. Individuals are grouped into those with small, medium and large frames, thus rationalising the considerable differences in weight between individuals of the same height. (See Table 14). How are you to decide to which group a person belongs? Those who put on weight often look broader than they really are and an attempt must therefore be made to estimate the basic build by judging shoulder and hip width. (Accurate somatotyping requires 17 measurements, at least three

Table 14. Chart showing desirable weights in indoor clothing related to height and build. After Statistical Bulletin Metropolitan Life Insurance Company No. 40, Nov-Dec. 1959.

MEN AGED 25 AND OVER

Height ft in	Small frame lb	kg	Medium frame lb	kg	Large frame lb	kg
5 2	112-120	50·5-54·5	118-129	53·5-58·5	126-141	57·0-64·0
3	115-123	52·0-56·0	121-133	55·0-61·0	129-144	58·5-65·0
4	118-126	53·5-57·0	124-136	56·0-62·0	132-148	60·0-67·0
5	121-129	55·0-58·5	127-139	57·5-63·0	135-152	61·0-69·0
6	124-133	56·0-60·0	130-143	58·5-65·0	138-156	62·5-71·0
7	128-137	58·0-62·0	134-147	60·0-66·5	142-161	64·5-73·0
8	132-141	60·0-64·0	138-152	62·5-69·0	147-166	66·5-75·0
9	136-145	62·0-66·0	142-156	64·5-71·0	151-169	68·5-77·0
10	140-150	63·5-68·0	146-160	66·0-72·5	155-174	70·0-79·0
11	144-154	65·0-70·0	150-165	68·0-75·0	159-179	72·0-81·0
6 0	148-158	67·0-71·5	154-170	70·0-77·0	164-184	74·0-83·5
1	152-162	69·0-73·5	156-175	71·5-79·0	168-189	76·0-85·5
2	156-167	71·0-76·0	162-180	73·5-81·5	173-194	78·5-88·0
3	160-171	72·5-77·5	167-185	76·0-79·0	178-199	80·5-90·5
4	164-175	74·0-79·0	172-190	78·0-86·0	182-204	82·5-92·5

WOMEN AGED 25 AND OVER

Height ft in	Small frame lb	kg	Medium frame lb	kg	Large frame lb	kg
4 10	92-98	42·0-44·5	96-107	43·5-48·5	104-119	47·0-54·0
11	94-101	42·5-46·0	98-110	44·5-50·0	106-122	48·0-55·0
5 0	96-104	43·5-47·0	101-113	46·0-51·0	109-125	49·5-56·5
1	99-107	45·0-48·5	104-116	47·0-52·5	112-128	51·0-58·0
2	102-110	46·5-50·0	107-119	48·5-54·0	115-131	52·0-59·5
3	105-113	47·5-51·0	110-122	50·0-55·0	118-134	53·5-61·0
4	108-116	49·0-52·5	113-126	51·0-57·0	121-138	55·0-62·0
5	111-119	50·5-54·0	116-130	52·5-58·5	125-142	57·0-64·5
6	114-123	52·0-56·0	120-135	54·5-61·0	129-146	58·5-66·0
7	118-127	53·5-57·5	124-139	56·0-63·0	133-150	60·0-68·0
8	122-131	55·0-59·5	128-143	58·0-65·0	137-154	62·0-70·0
9	126-135	57·0-61·0	132-147	60·0-66·5	141-158	64·0-71·5
10	130-140	58·5-63·5	136-151	62·0-68·5	145-163	66·0-74·0
11	134-144	61·0-65·0	140-155	63·5-70·0	149-168	67·5-76·0
6 0	139-148	63·0-67·0	144-159	65·0-72·0	153-173	69·5-78·5

photographs and years of practice!) Fortunately, most obese individuals are obviously so and over the years I have found clinical estimation fails only with borderline cases which are of minimal importance to health.

Clinical assessment of obesity

Skin fold calipers are necessary only for research. If thick rolls of fat can be picked up between finger and thumb in the mid triceps area or below the scapulae then obesity is present. Rolls of fat are also commonly found around the waist, the hip girdle and upper thigh. Some men accumulate fat mainly in the greater omentum and the main evidence of obesity may be an expanding waistline, although there is invariably some excessive subcutaneous fat in addition.

What is the likely yield of screening?

The prevalence of obesity in this country has not yet been accurately determined, but is likely to be at least 30-50 per cent of women over the age of thirty and 20-40 per cent of men (Craddock, 1973a).

Screening for obesity in general practice in this country has been carried out mainly during multiphasic screening of whole adult population of specific groups (Table 15). The table shows that about half of the available population are usually screened and 30-60 per cent of these have been found to be overweight, which is in keeping with the estimated prevalence in the general population. In an average practice population of 2,500 individuals this means that somewhere between 600 and 1,000 are likely to be obese and between 300 and 500 may be picked up as a result of multiphasic screening. One can see why only the grossly obese were offered treatment! This is certainly understandable when screening for obesity was merely incidental to the main purpose of the exercise.

Monophasic Screening for obesity

Few practices are well enough organised or have sufficient enthusiasm for large scale multiphasic screening, but screening for obesity gives such a high yield that it should be undertaken by every practice which is geared towards the prevention of the disease. The prevention and control of obesity are the most important measures for preventing diabetes, hypertension and coronary artery disease, all of which shorten life. Obesity directly or indirectly is now one of the major killing diseases of western civilisation. Middle aged individuals

Table 15. General Practice Obesity Surveys

Name	Date	Age-Group	Number Screened	Percentage of Practice Population	Obese Number	Obese Percentage	Grossly Obese Number	Grossly Obese Percentage
Evans, Wilkes & Dalrymple-Smith	1969	15+	355 males 436 females	25			14 30	4 7
Cope & Smith	1972	15+	1,836	52·5	442 males 622 females	54 61		
Taylor	1970	35-64 ($\frac{1}{3}$ sample)	436	68·5	84 males 74 females	33·5 30		
Bernstein & Dolan	1969	Women 35-45	170	42·3	94	55·3		
Pike	1972	Men 35-45	140	45·3	44	31		
Pike	1969	68+	150 males 136 females	72 30			10 8	6·6 5·9

in the USA who are 30 per cent over their best weight have a mortality rate about 40 per cent above average (New York Metropolitan Life Insurance Society). *The prevention, detection and treatment of obesity if carried out systematically are likely to be productive of greater benefit to the community than any other single health measure.* For the effects on health of the unbalanced diet enjoyed in the affluent society the reader should consult Cleave *et al.* (1969) and the writings of Denis Burkitt. Apart from diabetes, hypertension and coronary artery disease, other conditions which are probably due in the main to our unbalanced, unnatural diet in the affluent countries include peptic ulcer, haemorrhoids, varicose veins, diverticulitis, carcinoma of the colon and even carcinoma of the body of the uterus.

Practical aspects of screening—a pilot scheme

Screening for obesity could well become part of each normal consultant session. A start might be made during a slack time of the year with a pilot scheme involving, for example, men between 35 and 45 or 35 and 55, as they are most likely to be co-operative in weight reduction and to benefit most in terms of increased longevity. The average practice with 2,500 patients will have about 150 men in each decade, of whom about 10 or 15 are likely to attend each week. This type of pilot screening could be done initially by one of the reception staff or by a health visitor or practice nurse. It should take only two or three minutes to record the weight and height of each individual and this could be done immediately after leaving the reception area. The weighing and measuring could be carried out on the way back to the waiting area in a room set aside for the purpose such as a spare consulting room or examination room.

Developing the screen

If a pilot scheme proves successful and it is decided to commence a scheme involving the whole practice population, more detailed planning will be required.

First of all it is essential to decide what action should be taken about those who are found to be over-weight. It is worthwhile pondering why it is that only a small proportion of obese individuals approach their doctor about their weight problem. The main reason appears to be that many people feel that this is not purely a medical problem, and they are diffident about approaching a busy doctor. These are the ones in particular who can be helped if their weight problem is brought to notice as the result of a survey. Other individuals enjoy their food so much that they are willing to put up with an expanding waistline rather than deny themselves the pleasures of the table, while yet others eat to compensate for something missing in their lives and accept moderate obesity as a fair price to pay for the satisfaction they need and get from eating.

It may well be therefore that about half of all those who are overweight will be glad to accept treatment. Should pressure be brought to bear on the other overweight people to accept treatment or not? If people are only one or two stones overweight it may well do them harm to try to upset their compromise with their life situation. I feel that those on whom pressure ought to be brought to bear include the following:

1 *Children.* Here one must be careful to obtain the child's co-operation and to persuade the mother that the family should sacrifice themselves to some extent by altering their own eating habits for the benefit of the child. It is especially important with children to make sure that they are not unhappy or feel unloved in any way as, if they are eating for compensation, any attempt to reduce the pleasure they get from eating may make them feel even more insecure.

2 *Young adults.*

3 *Men between 35 and 55.*

4 *Any other people who are considerably overweight.* Here one can take an arbitary figure of 25 to 30 per cent over fit lean weight as a minimum. In many of these people a considerable shortening of life can occur if obesity is allowed to persist.

Having considered all these facts a choice should now be made between the following courses of action:

1 *A continuation of the pilot scheme for men between 35 and 55 with the aim of eventually screening all men in these age groups.* When screening during normal consulting sessions has been carried on for one or two years a list can be made from the practice age-sex register of those who have not yet been screened. These can be contacted by letter or telephone and invited to come to a few special evening sessions at which screening for obesity could be combined with screening for hypertension to make the project worthwhile both for staff and patients. It could be pointed out perhaps that abnormalities of weight or blood pressure are those which are regarded as of the utmost importance by all life insurance companies, as an increase above the normal range in either is associated with a decreased expectation of life.

2 *A survey of the whole practice population.* This could possibly arise out of the pilot scheme and in some practices could be organised as a continuous survey during normal consulting sessions if

the pilot scheme has gone smoothly. In most practices volunteers can be found to carry out the task of weighing, measuring and recording, or extra part time staff from outside the practice can be employed at a small extra cost. The height and weight could be recorded on the patient's record card by the receptionist.

To deal with the hundreds of individuals who would eventually be offered treatment as the result of this sort of survey would necessitate the setting up of an obesity clinic, and I have detailed suggestions concerning this elsewhere (Craddock, 1973b). Does the phrase 'hundreds' seem to be fanciful? Even if only half the adult population were surveyed and only half of these wished to accept treatment this could in fact involve up to 10 per cent of the total practice population in treatment. Once an obesity clinic is in existence each individual doctor would note the height and weight recorded by the receptionist on the patient's record card, would assess the patient for build, make a clinical assessment as to whether true obesity was present and offer treatment at the clinic, applying pressure if necessary to the special groups outlined above.

Many practices will feel that this is too big a load to bear, even though it will mean eventually reducing the incidence of coronary artery disease, hypertension and diabetes. The alternative here is to refer only those patients who would normally justify pressurising, which would cut the number by about half.

Obesity is a slow killer and its importance as one of the major killing diseases of western civilisation is only just receiving recognition. The pursuit of positive health demands a change of attitude from us all, from the concept of a national *ill health* service to that of a national *health* service. Screening for obesity need not be a complicated and specific exercise. Providing a practice runs an obesity clinic, perhaps the best method of screening is for the individual general practitioner to have the problem continually in mind and to offer treatment at the clinic to any patient seen during normal consulting sessions who is clinically obese.

REFERENCES

Burkitt, D. (1970). Relation as a clue to causation. *Lancet*, 2, 1237.
Burkitt, D. (1972). Varicose veins, deep vein thrombosis and haemorrhoids: epidemiology and suggested aetiology. *British Medical Journal*, 2, 556.
Bernstein, J. M. & Dolan, L. J. (1969). Multiphasic screening as part of family doctoring. *Practitioner*, 203, 798-805.
Cleave, T. L., Campbell, G. G. & Painter, N. S. (1969). *Diabetes, coronary thrombosis and the saccharine disease*. 2nd edn. Bristol: Wright.
Cope, J. T. & Smith, D. H. (1972). A second multiple screening clinic in a rural general practice. *Journal of the Royal College of General Practitioners*, 22, 113.
Craddock, D. (1973a). *Obesity and Its Management*, 2nd edn. London and Edinburgh: Churchill, Livingstone.
Craddock, D. (1973b). Special Clinics: Obesity. *Update*, 7, 1309.

Evans, S. M., Wilkes, E. & Dalrymple-Smith, D. (1969). Presymptomatic diagnosis. *Journal of the Royal College of General Practitioners,* 17, 237-240.

Gastineau, C. F. (1972). Obesity. Risks, causes, and treatments. *Medical Clinics of North America,* 56, 1021-1028.

Pike, L. A. (1969). A screening programme for the elderly in a general practice. *Practitioner,* 203, 805-812.

Pike, L. A. (1972). Screening middle-aged men in a general practice. *Practitioner,* 209, 692-695.

Slome, C., Gampel, B., Abramson, J. H. & Scotch, N. (1960). Weight, height and skin fold thickness in Zulu adults in Durban. *South African Medical Journal,* 34, 505.

Taylor, M. P. (1970). Periodic health examination combined with multiple screening tests in general practice. *Journal of the Royal College of General Practitioners,* 19, 146-157.

19 Hypertension

Robert G. Sinclair

'It is clear that mortality rises steadily and markedly with increasing elevation of both systolic and diastolic blood pressure. The excessive mortality of individuals with hypertension is primarily due to cardiovascular and renal diseases. In the group with the highest blood pressures, and those are not regarded as seriously high by many clinicians, the mortality from cardiovascular and renal disease was nearly four and a half times the average for all standard risks.'

Dublin, Lotka and Spiegelman, 1949.

High blood pressure is not, in its own right, a common cause of death or of admission to hospital. It is, however, a major factor associated with atherosclerosis and its complications. Effective treatment of hypertension requires early detection and regular surveillance of patients even if treatment is not considered to be justified initially. A clear understanding of those groups of people who could be considered a being at high risk is very desirable.

It is now accepted that the prevention of atherosclerotic disorders depends in part on finding means to prevent high blood pressure. The problem is one of definition and measurement. At present, hypertensives are not sought out and treated on a systematic basis. There are wide variations in the action that different doctors take in similar cases. Many general practitioners seem to prefer not to treat asymptomatic hypertensives as a matter of routine unless their pressures are very high. It is important therefore to determine the merits of seeking out and treating people with raised blood pressure in the general population as a matter of routine, and to determine also what level of blood pressure should be taken as the dividing line between hypertension and the normal.

Definition of hypertension

A person can be considered hypertensive only if his blood pressure is consistently raised in the absence of any stimulus that may cause a temporary rise in pressure. For this reason it is important to measure the individual patient's blood pressure more than once under standard conditions before making the decision to regard the reading as falling outside the accepted range of normality.

There is controversy whether hypertension per se can be considered as a diseased state. Studies of blood pressure levels in the population at large have shown that levels are distributed continuously throughout the population. Even life insurance information does not provide a clear line of division between the normal and the abnormal (Society of Actuaries, 1959; Dublin, Lotka and Spiegelman, 1949). It indicates, however, that the risk to health and life increases without doubt as the systolic or diastolic blood pressure rises.

Pickering (1968) classified hypertension in two ways, by kind and by degree. In the classification by kind, the condition is divided into essential hypertension, which is the commonest, where there is no apparent cause, and secondary hypertension. The latter occurs as a manifestation of a known condition such as disease of the kidney, narrowing of the aorta, Cushing's syndrome, toxaemia of pregnancy and various conditions affecting the nervous system. He also wrote (1968) that if we choose to call essential hypertension a disease, it is a disease of a kind hitherto unrecognised by medicine, a disease characterised by a quantitative, not a qualitative deviation from the norm. However, what matters is that the higher the blood pressure the greater is the risk of illness or death.

In deciding on the level of blood pressure which I regard as the upper limit of normal, I take as my guide the comments of the World Health Organisation's Expert Committee on Cardiovascular Disease and Hypertension. Their suggestion that blood pressure below 140/90 mm Hg can be regarded as normal seems reasonable. There are many who would disagree with this figure and in the final analysis each doctor must make up his own mind on the upper level of normality he is going to accept.

Taking the blood pressure

It is generally accepted that the cuff method of measuring blood pressure can on occasion be liable to error, but it remains the only practical method of recording the blood pressure in clinical medicine, where an easy, painless and repeatable method is of greater importance than absolute accuracy in a single measurement.

I feel that is is important that the details of the examination must be correctly carried out to ensure as accurate a reading as possible. A test not correctly performed can hardly be considered worth doing.

If possible the same sphygmomanometer and cuff should be used at all times. The cuff should be placed firmly and evenly round the arm about three inches above the elbow, which should be quite free to move, so that the bell of the stethoscope can be easily placed over the brachial artery in the antecubital fossa.

The cuff is inflated to a pressure well over that necessary to obliterate the pulsation of the peripheral artery. As the cuff is deflated and the column of mercury drops, the first characteristic tapping sound is heard. This begins at the systolic blood pressure level and is due to the return of the pulse wave to the previously collapsed artery. A murmur develops at phase two, but disappears at phase three when the initial pulse sound becomes louder. At the fourth phase the sound muffles. In Britain this is usually taken as the diastolic level, the level of pressure where blood flow can take place through the artery through the entire cardiac cycle. The sound then disappears altogether and this is called the fifth phase; in which there is no obstruction at all to the blood flow in diastole. This is the point which is taken to represent the diastolic pressure in the United States of America and some other countries.

In interpreting studies of blood pressure the technical problems must be realised. Blood pressure is higher in cold weather and often higher when taken by the opposite sex. The orienteering reflex is the name given to the phenomenon in which blood pressure readings tend to fall on successive occasions when taken by the same person under the same conditions. It has been shown in hospital clinics that blood pressure falls from the first to the second and from the second to the third visit but not thereafter, and this with no treatment. The blood pressure is higher in people with fat arms, unless a large cuff is used.

Assessment of screening programmes

There is no doubt that the cost of a screening programme deliberately carried out would be large in terms of increased work load on doctors and ancillary staff. There would also be an increase in cost to the National Health Service caused by the therapy. In 1969, hypertensive disease cost the National Health Service £20·6 million, or 1·6 per cent of those sections of the National Health Service where costs could be broken down by disease groups. Over half of this was spent on hypotensive drugs. This accounts for about six per cent of the total cost of the pharmaceutical service, a proportion which has doubled over 10 years. It may well be true that for every case of hypertension attending a general practitioner or a hospital clinic, there are two or three others of the general population unaware that their blood pressure is raised. In fact, recent

American sources suggest that there may be as many as 5,000,000 undiagnosed cases in the United States. This could mean that there might be as many as 1,000,000 undiagnosed in the United Kingdom. If treatment were to be extended to a considerable proportion of people in this group, the cost to the National Health Service would be considerable. Added to this many people, though diagnosed, are not being treated (at present) for many reasons; if treatment were to be started on this group the outlook would become financially alarming. Clearly, expenditure of this magnitude would entail the postponement of many other projects within the National Health Service and could only be justified by very convincing evidence of the benefits to be derived from detection and treatment.

It must also be remembered that many present day drugs used to treat hypertension still have unpleasant and sometimes potentially dangerous side effects which are clearly apparent to patients. A person who is placed on antihypertensive therapy is likely to remain so for life; and if doctors deliberately set out to detect the condition in younger age groups, we are going to have increasing numbers of people on such drugs for increasing number of years. The risk of long term treatment with certain drugs is still an important unknown factor which demands that close supervision of those on treatment must be maintained.

However, there is no doubt that there is much to be gained from detection and treatment of hypertension. It is difficult to measure the personal hardship and disability to the victim of complications related to hypertension. In 1969 the economic cost in Great Britain of absence from work attributed to strokes was £16 million. In 1968/69 a total of 7·5 million days of certified absence from work were attributed to hypertension. If the primary objective of the health services is the extension of life which is both healthy and socially active, then the prevention of some of this long term incapacity, which is disastrous for the individual and his family in both personal and financial terms, is much to be desired. Another aspect of the personal cost to a family is the premature death of the husband. Reference to insurance data of the Metropolitan Life Insurance Company of New York (1961) shows that a man of 45 years with a blood pressure of 150/100 mm Hg could expect to live for only 20½ years, compared with the 32 years of life expectancy of a similar man with a blood pressure of 120/80 mm Hg or below. This means 11½ years more of widowhood for the wife, with the added effects on the family of being deprived of their father. The consequences in some families could well be disastrous.

The important question is the extent to which benefits of detection and treatment for various levels of asymptomatic hypertension have been demonstrated in both sexes and at various levels of blood pressure (Stuart *et al.*, 1974).

Several useful points have arisen from the trials done so far. No clear benefits have been shown to arise from the treatment of women without severe symptoms. The trial of Hamilton, Thomson and Wisniewski (1964) has been the only one to include women under 60 years of age. All of them were asymptomatic and all had diastolic pressures over 110 mm Hg. The treated group did not fare better than the untreated group.

Controlled trials to measure the effectiveness of treatment and blood pressure control on women of various ages, symptoms and levels of blood pressure are urgently required.

For middle aged men on the other hand two controlled trials, Veterans' Administration (1967) and Hamilton, Thomson and Wisniewski (1964) have shown significant benefits from treatment when diastolic pressures are over 110 mm Hg. Such evidence suggests that it is the level of pressure per se and not the associated signs and symptoms which is the main factor in prediction of excess mortality or morbidity from a stroke. There is therefore very strong (though not yet conclusive) evidence that successful lowering of the blood pressure amongst men discovered by screening for hypertension would confer benefits far exceeding those to be obtained by haphazard treatment of persons who consult their doctor with signs and symptoms that prompt him to take their blood pressure. A screening programme to detect hypertension in middle aged men and to offer treatment to those with diastolic blood pressures over 110 to 115 mm Hg would almost certainly be justified (Coope, 1974). This is the group of the population which is so important both to industry and the professions and to family life. It would place no extra burden on general practitioners to take the blood pressure of this group of patients at every available opportunity and the benefits to these patients and their wives and families could be immense.

For those with a diastolic pressure below 115 mm Hg there has been reported only one controlled trial upon which one can base conclusions. Again, it was a Veterans' Administration (1970) trial of middle aged men with diastolic pressures above 90 and below 115 mm Hg. Benefits were shown but most were concentrated within the upper portion of the range.

The immediate problem therefore is not pressing if general practitioners develop a habit of screening all middle aged men to pick out those with diastolic pressures in the 110 to 115 mm Hg range and above. This is not a difficult task as the average general practitioner sees 60 per cent of his middle aged male patients in the course of a year (HMSO 1958).

To treat or not to treat

Normally the general practitioner decides what is best to be done for his patient according to his own judgement and knowledge. In the case of high blood pressure detected through screening, the patient is likely to be symptomless. Also, the doctor is not able to tell the patient that he is suffering from a disease per se. All the doctor can do is to assess the risks associated with the patient's level of blood pressure and explain them precisely and quantitatively to the patient, together with the benefits and possible side effects of treatment. The patient could then come to a rational decision of his own whether to accept treatment. He could furthermore try treatment to decide whether the side effects were acceptable. It would be important to indicate to the patient that the treatment, if accepted, must be at an effective level and that ineffective treatment would be quite unacceptable to the doctor.

This suggestion obviously poses problems both for doctor and patient, and would require a good deal of educational effort on the part of the doctor to provide himself and his patient with a clear and reliable summary of the present state of knowledge of the condition. Clearly also, doctors must be selective in deciding who should or should not be given the facts, and I can think of no better person to have this position of responsibility than the conscientious general practitioner who knows his patient personally as well as the family's social, work and recreational background.

Here is a condition that is a fascinating challenge to those of us who are in general practice. It is possible to study it in all its manifestations and effects in a large number of our own patients. By doing so we will not only know a great deal about hypertension in our practice, but we will learn even more about our patients. All in all, a most satisfying experience.

REFERENCES

Coope, J. (1974). A screening clinic for hypertension in general practice. *Journal of the Royal College of General Practitioners,* 24, 161.
Dublin, L. I., Lotka, A. J. and Spiegelman, M. (1949). *Length of Life: a study of the Life Table.* 2nd edn. New York.
Hamilton, M., Thomson, E. N. & Wisniewski, T. K. M. (1964). *Lancet,* 1, 235.
HMSO (1958). *Morbidity Statistics from General Practice,* Vol. 1. W.P.D. Logan & W.W. Cushion, London: HMSO.
Metropolitan Life Insurance Company, New York (1961). *Blood Pressure: Insurance experience and its implications.*
Pickering, G. (1968). *Hypertension.* London: Churchill.
Society of Actuaries (1959). *Build and Blood Pressure Study,* Vol. 1, Chicago, Illinois.
Stuart, K. L., Desai, P. & Lalsingh, A. (1974). Approach to assessment of risk factors in mild hypertension. *British Medical Journal,* 2, 195.
Veterans' Administration (1967). Co-operative study group on antihypertensive agents. *Journal of the American Medical Association,* 202, 1028.
Veterans' Administration (1970). Co-operative study group on antihypertensive agents. *Journal of the American Medical Association,* 213, 1143.

20 Ischaemic Heart Disease *Julian Tudor Hart*

'. . . how we can and ought to serve our neighbour, to his advantage and not to his hurt.'

Paracelsus.

Ischaemic heart disease is the greatest single cause of premature male death in fully industrialised countries. It causes about a quarter of all male deaths at ages 35-44 in Britain, and about one third at ages 45-54. Mortality is increasing annually at a higher rate in the young than in the middle-aged. There is some evidence that in the United States mortality may have reached its peak in younger men and is now levelling off about 30 per cent higher than ours (WHO, 1967), so that may be where we are going. The problem in pre-menopausal women is very much smaller, and is not discussed further in this chapter. The annual cost in Social Security benefits and lost years of working life has been estimated at £300 million, about one per cent of the gross national product (Morris and Gardner, 1968).

It is on these grounds that screening for IHD has been proposed, despite much doubt in relation to other criteria for screening. Valid specific preventive treatment for high-risk groups found is doubtful, and discrimination between high and low-risk groups is poor. However, the techniques for measuring risk factors for IHD are well known and fairly simple, can be integrated into normal primary care procedures, are acceptable to patients and not very costly.

There is good evidence that angina due to coronary insufficiency is historically independent from myocardial infarction/sudden cardiac death, and failure to realise this may have led to confusion. Angina alone, in the absence of ECG changes, carries a fair prognosis, with an annual male mortality of about 5 per cent (Seim, 1960). Use of the WHO chest pain questionnaire certainly leads to the diagnosis of many cases not previously known to the doctor, but it has never been convincingly validated (how can it be?) (Meade and Gardner, 1968), and probably misses about 17 per cent of cases (Rose, 1962). The value of early diagnosis of angina seems to me doubtful, except perhaps to reinforce advice on smoking. However, these remarks refer to stable, classical angina. Unstable angina and the prodromal symptoms of infarction are a very different problem.

Risk factors

The classical epidemiological studies at Framingham (Dawber *et al.*, 1962) defined five major risk factors for ischaemic heart disease: high blood pressure, high serum cholesterol, cigarette smoking, diabetes and abnormal ECG. Numerous studies in many countries have confirmed these and they must be included in any screening programme.

Many other minor risk factors have been less certainly established. **Obesity** is probably not an independent causal factor; multivariate analysis of 5 years' prospective data for 11,400 men in the USA and Northern and Southern Europe, aged 40-59, showed that neither weight-for-height nor skinfold thickness made a significant contribution to mortality, once age, blood pressure, cholesterol and smoking were standardised (Keys *et al.*, 1972). However, those grossly overweight are probably more likely to die from their infarct, even if they are no more likely to get one, and there are many other good reasons for reducing excess weight. **Physical inactivity** probably has the same sort of association; the unfit are less likely to survive their infarcts, but it is not yet firmly established that exercise really reduces the infarction rate as opposed to mortality. Even if it does, the exercise must certainly be vigorous, sustained, and habitual (Morris *et al.*, 1973). **Aggressive personality and behaviour** has been strongly incriminated by research in San Francisco (Freidman and Rosenman, 1959) which initially was of doubtful quality; there has ensued a flood of papers from the same school (Rosenman *et al.*, 1966; Freidman *et al.*, 1968) confirming this prospectively. There is more convincing evidence of an association with **social and/or geographical mobility** (Syme, Hyman and Enterline, 1964; Werkö, 1971). Raised serum uric acid is probably a minor risk factor, male sex is a huge factor but unalterable, and the same might be said for family history. Concordance in twin studies is not high (Harvald and Hange, 1965), and probably most of the heritable effect is mediated through blood pressure. Myxoedema exerts its effect through hypercholesterolaemia, and some cases may be accounted for by states of subclinical hypothyroidism; this matter is very much *sub* *judice* at present. A rapid resting pulse is an interesting and rather neglected risk factor, though well established (Paul *et al.*, 1963).

Despite this wealth of causes and associations, the plain fact is that 20 years of prospective data from the Framingham study have shown that two thirds of the sudden coronary deaths occur in people without previous clinical or electrocardiographic evidence of coronary artery disease (Gordon and Kannel, 1970), and even when all known risk variables are taken into account by the most sophisticated methods of multivariate analysis, half of those who develop overt IHD have risk factors within the range of those who do not (Cotton, *et al.*, 1972). American data show that for the highest risk groups with raised blood pressure and cholesterol, only about one third of men will develop IHD over a 10 year period in the age group 30-39, and one fifth in the age group 40-59 (Epstein, 1967). British data suggest a risk of about one in seven over a five year period for the same age and risk groups (Morris, *et al.*, 1966).

There are huge gaps in our knowledge of IHD/sudden cardiac death. We know from large international post-mortem studies (Kagan, *et al.*, 1968) that about 25 per cent of 'coronary' deaths with obvious fresh infarctions show coronary arteries completely free from thrombotic or other occlusion, though a smaller British study demonstrated only 10 per cent (Harland and Holburn, 1966). There is much evidence that the epidemic of ischaemic heart disease has developed quite independently of changes (if any) in mural atheroma (Morris, 1951), and that mortality from cerebrovascular accidents has remained stationary and roughly equal between the sexes, while male mortality from IHD has risen dramatically. No doubt atheroma is a necessary precursor of IHD, and microscopically obvious coronary arteriosclerosis is present in more than three-quarters of fit American men of 22 (Enos, Holmes and Beyer, 1953); but something else must be added, and this is probably neither high serum cholesterol nor raised blood pressure. There is no evidence that the mean blood pressure of male populations is rising. The important and possibly causal association of soft water supplies with IHD and sudden death is entirely unexplained, there is evidence to support a myocardial, perhaps myopathic co-factor (Anderson, 1970, 1973), and differences in fibrinolytic activity, and other factors involved in the thrombotic process may account for a good deal of the missing variance (Chakrabarti *et al.*, 1968; Meade, 1973). When these new fields are fully explored, we may be able to forecast IHD with some precision. For the present, screening for IHD will identify three groups: those without risk factors or evidence of current IHD; those with risk factors, without evidence of current IHD; and those with evidence of current IHD. The size of each of these groups will depend on definitions. Customary (but arbitrary) cutting points are systolic pressure 160, diastolic pressure 95, cholesterol 260 mg/100 ml.

The first group can be reassured that they are unlikely to develop IHD, but are not immune from it. If we evaluate only three major factors (blood pressure, smoking, serum cholesterol), American data suggest that about 17 per cent of men aged 40-59 will have no risk factors, of whom less than 1 per cent will get clinical IHD in the next five years; 33 per cent will have any one risk factor, of whom 2 per cent will get IHD: 32 per cent will have any two risk factors, of whom 2·5 per cent will get IHD: and 18 per cent will have all three risk factors, of whom 9 per cent will get IHD (Stamler, 1967). While the progression in risks is striking, so is the very poor discrimination in prognosis and the large size of the high risk group obtained. An average primary care list of 2,500 patients of all ages will yield about 440 men aged 35-64 (17·6 per cent), of whom about 90 might be expected to fall in the high risk group. A further small group, perhaps 2 or 3 per cent, will have ECG's classifiable as abnormal on the Minnesota code, without symptoms (Dick and Stone, 1973), giving us about 100 in all.

What is to be done with these people? A number of reputable enthusiasts have for many years advocated energetic programmes for informed self-help by modifications of diet, exercise, body weight, the treatment of hypertension and stopping smoking. In most cases, for instance the Anti-coronary Club of New York (Lancet, 1967), these are volunteer populations, so controlled studies, and therefore definite conclusions, are impossible. Some large-scale controlled studies have been done, mostly on those who have already had infarcts, or on captive populations where both methodology and acceptability of diet to the general population have been questioned (Meittinen et al., 1972). In my opinion this evidence is still inconclusive, and does not justify the very great effort required of both doctor and patients in managing such a shift in diet for such a large number of people; anyone who attempts it will certainly have to develop collective methods with mutual support, along the line of 'Weight Watchers'. The alternative for hypercholesterolaemia is the use of cholesterol-lowering agents. The evidence of the Edinburgh and Newcastle secondary prevention trials of clofibrate, (i.e. prevention of second infarcts in those who have survived a first) (Newcastle, 1971; Scottish Society of Physicians, 1971) I find unconvincing, and I think this opinion is now widely held. Even if some drug were fully effective in wholly abolishing raised cholesterol as a risk factor, there are good theoretical reasons to anticipate that this would only reduce the number of new IHD events from 14 per cent to 11 per cent in a male cohort over a period of 10 years (Epstein, 1968).

Blood pressure

The greatest single risk factor for IHD, hypertension, is now fairly easy to treat, and the reduction in mortality from stroke, renal failure and cardiac failure is dramatic: but so far there is little evidence of any reduction in the incidence or mortality of myocardial infarction (Aurell and Hood, 1964; Veterans Administration, 1967; Mathisen *et al.*, 1969; Breckenridge, Dollery and Parry, 1970; Veterans Administration, 1970). This may be because most cases are not being treated early enough (younger and at lower levels of pressure), or because treatment is frequently so inefficient (Werkö, 1971). In his prospective study of 834 randomly sampled men aged 50 in Göteborg, Werkö maintained careful treatment of all ascertained hypertensive, including those supposed to be already under treatment but actually out of control. He concluded that 'early recognition of high blood pressure and its adequate treatment is still the most promising single preventive measure. In our population elevated blood pressure did not appear as a risk factor, for which we would like to credit active treatment.' The hope that treatment of hypertension by beta-adrenergic blocking drugs would kill two birds with one stone by reducing the incidence of arrhythmia at the onset of infarction has not been borne out in practice (Fitzgerald, 1972; Multicentre Trial, 1966), and it may be that increased deaths from pump failure are balancing gains from suppressed arrhythmia.

ECG

Identification of ECG abnormalities certainly defines a high-risk group. The Framingham study showed a threefold higher incidence of attacks, a higher mortality in those who had them, and in those with initial electrocardiographic left-ventricular hypertrophy (Kannel *et al.*, 1970). Criteria were the presence of several or all the following ECG features: increased R amplitudes with ST depression and flat or inverted T waves in leads I, II, aVL and V4-6; deep S waves over right precordial leads; left axis deviation exceeding—30 degrees, and a ventricular activation time of at least 0·05 seconds. All these features relate closely to blood pressure, but make an independent contribution to mortality, and certainly add to the significance of single casual BP readings. Non-specific T wave inversion also seems to be a predictor of raised mortality and is associated with all the main risk factors (Ostrander, 1970). Frequent (more than 10 per cent) ventricular ectopics in a resting ECG are probably an additional risk factor, and left-bundle-branch block certainly is.

Gross observer variability in ECG interpretation, even between very experienced consultants, is now well recognised, and the use of a standard convention is essential. The obvious one is the Minnesota Code, which also provides convenient standard interpretation procedure even for novices. It is given in full in Rose and Blackburn's book, together with other standard questionnaires and procedures mentioned in this chapter, and this is really an essential possession for anyone doing any kind of cardiovascular screening (Rose and Blackburn, 1968). Even this does not eliminate inter- or even intra-observer error (Meade and Gardner, 1968). Use of nutmeg-grater electrodes for the limb leads is a practical advantage in ECG screening (Lewes, 1970). Exercise tests may add to the usefulness of ECG screening (Godfrey, 1970), but they greatly increase the staff time required; I have no experience of them.

There may be a good case for limb leads only on ECG screening. Not only do these give about 80 per cent of the information on a standard 12-lead ECG, but they give us the only true comparability between successive records in the same patient, because of the siting errors inherent in the precordial leads. In my opinion the main justification for screening ECGs is the building up of a complete ECG baseline for the entire population at substantial risk, that is, men over 35 and post-menopausal women. In this way the primary doctor can always have a previous tracing to compare with a new one, after the onset of possible IHD symptoms; there should be no substantial difference in any of the limb leads, and minor changes can be spotted easily, which in association with symptoms may be highly significant. These changes can be small (Short, 1968), and are easily missed without a baseline record.

Smoking

Smoking history should be taken and defines a high-risk group for all cardiorespiratory disease. The value of this must lie in the opportunity to concentrate advice at a vulnerable time, in conjunction with other evidence. There is no doubt that smoking is a causal factor in IHD, and that stopping smoking rapidly reduces liability to that of non-smokers (Hammond and Horn, 1958). The harmful effect seems to be maximal in those under 55 (Doll and Hill, 1956). The proportion of doctors who smoke fell from 43 per cent in 1951 to 21 per cent in 1966 (Action on Smoking and Health, 1971), so there is no doubt that people can react rationally in this matter. However, even the most intelligently planned personal medical advice to patients, given in the presence of respiratory symptoms, has so far been quite ineffective in a controlled trial in general practice (Porter, 1972).

Practical aspects of screening for IHD

My experience of screening for IHD in primary care is based on a survey of all the men aged 30-64 in my village (a total of 350, with a refusal rate of 1·4 per cent, response rate of 93·7 per cent, the rest of the non-respondents having moved away or died during the survey). The work was carried out by myself and my partner, Dr Reg Saxton, with the help of our wives and one secretary-receptionist, at a special weekly evening session at the Health Centre, and has not yet been published. All the men were recruited for the survey by home visits. This procedure was carried out as part of a research project, so we were aiming at very high response rates, and this imposed a more arduous protocol than that required for service purposes only. The parts of the procedure that would normally be included in IHD screening took about 40 minutes for each subject, of which about 10 minutes was doctor-time and 30 minutes ancillary-staff-time. All the work except the venepunctures can be undertaken by lay staff if they are trained, including ECGs and sphygmomanometry. We had no help from attached nursing or health visiting staff, but this would normally be available and should lighten the load a good deal. We were also helped by the fact that the whole male and female population over 20 had already been screened 3 years earlier for hypertension.

The variables that can be measured in such a procedure are as follows:

Minimum programme	*Maximum programme*
Identification data, age, etc.	Occupational history
Smoking questionnaire (current and previous)	Family history
Chest pain and claudication questionnaire	
ECG limb leads	Chest leads
BP after 15 minutes' rest, seated, same arm	ECG after standard exercise
Pulse rate	
Examination of chest for valvular disease and left ventricular hypertrophy	
Corneal arcus, palmar and orbital xanthelasma under 50 years	
Weight for height	Skinfold thickness
Venous blood for serum cholestcrol	Serum uric acid
	Serum triglycerides
Femoral and ankle pulses	Postprandial urine, modified glucose tolerance test

Estimation of cholesterol is now cheap and well standardised by nearly all regional laboratories, though values have been very unreliable until quite recently. It is not usually feasible or necessary to obtain fasting cholesterols, but very high values should be repeated. Estimation of triglycerides is expensive and very unreliable, unless your regional laboratory has a special interest in the procedure. As Kannel says: 'Any particular lipid can be used for assessing vulnerability to coronary heart disease, but none would appear superior to the simple total cholesterol for this purpose' (Kannel, 1970). It is not generally recognised, despite a wealth of evidence from many sources, that 'only in younger persons is the diastolic pressure superior to systolic in discriminating potential IHD cases. There appears to be a declining influence of diastolic pressure and a corresponding increase in the contribution of the systolic component of the blood pressure with advancing age' (*ibid*). There is no diagnostic advantage in estimating pressures in different postures. Lay staff (and doctors) usually find diastolic phase 5 (disappearance) easier to define than phase 4 (muffling), and trained lay or nursing staff usually record BP more consistently and with less bias than doctors. Use of an electronic sphygmomanometer may be an advantage. Pulse rate should be recorded just before estimation of BP, and venous blood taken well afterwards. Examination of peripheral pulses is reproducible (Meade and Gardner, 1968) despite some published assertions to the contrary.

Conclusions

I am not convinced that screening for IHD is yet a moral obligation in primary care, though I am quite sure that screening for hypertension has been for some time. Addition of ECG to measurement of BP is useful, mainly to provide a baseline for future care. For the present, only enthusiasts will undertake more than this, and gains, if any, will be marginal.

The work of these pioneers, providing they do it seriously and aim at worthwhile response rates, will be valuable. Preventive care is undoubtedly going to become very important in IHD, far more so than any surgical circus-tricks. We are probably on the eve of great things, and the techniques and attitudes of mind evolved for the barely justified screening procedures of today, will be needed urgently when those great things arrive.

For the time being we must beware of dogmatic advice to patients not fully justified by the evidence; we have said a great many silly things in the past, and should not burden the lives of patients with transient medical fashion. We must also beware of encouraging them to have excessive faith in IHD screening, particularly electrocardio-graphy, nor should we frighten them with the results, especially those relating to blood lipids.

It seems likely that IHD screening will develop in two opposite directions. There is a lot of evidence that most fatal acute myocardial infarctions are preceded by minor symptoms for several weeks or months (Kinlen, 1973; Short and Stowers, 1972). With baseline data from previous screening, we may be able to identify those with impending infarction, and do something effective to avoid it. The group with unstable angina is of special importance here (Fulton *et al.*, 1972). On the other hand, if we are to deal with causes, screening may have to be extended to a much younger group, possibly before school-leaving. We are at the very beginning, with only a candle in the darkness; haste will only blow it out.

REFERENCES

Anderson, T. W. (1970). Role of myocardium in the modern epidemic of ischaemic heart disease. *Lancet,* 2, 753.

Anderson, T. W. (1973). Nutritional muscular dystrophy and human myocardial infarction. *Lancet,* 2, 298.

Aurell, M. and Hood, B. (1964). Cerebral haemorrhage in a population after a decade of active antihypertensive treatment. *Acta Medica Scandinavia,* 176, 377.

Action on Smoking and Health, (1971). *Smoking and health now.* London: Royal College of Physicians.

Breckenridge, A., Dollery, C. T. & Parry, E. H. O. (1970). Prognosis of treated hypertension: changes in life expectancy and causes of death between 1952 and 1967. *Quarterly Journal of Medicine,* 39, 411.

Chakrabarti, R., Hocking, E. D., Fearnley, G. R., Mann, R. D., Attwell, T. N. & Jackson, D. (1968). Fibrinolytic activity and coronary artery disease. *Lancet,* 1, 987.

Cotton, S. G., Nixon, J. M., Carpenter, R. G. & Evans, D. W. (1972). Factors discriminating men with coronary heart disease from healthy controls. *British Heart Journal,* 34, 485.

Dawber, T. R., Kannel, W. B., Revotskie, N. & Kagan, A., (1962). The epidemiology of coronary heart disease—the Framingham enquiry. *Proceedings of the Royal Society of Medicine,* 55, 265.

Dick, T. B. S., & Stone, M. C., (1973). Prevalence of three cardinal risk factors in a random sample of men and in patients with ischaemic heart disease. *British Heart Journal,* 35, 381.

Doll, W. R. & Hill, A. B., (1956). Lung cancer and other causes of death in relation to smoking: a second report on the mortality of British doctors. *British Medical Journal,* 2, 1071.

Enos, W. F., Holmes R.H. & Beyer, J. (1953). Coronary disease among United States soldiers killed in action in Korea. *Journal of the American Medical Association* 152, 1090.

Epstein, F. H. (1967). Risk factors in coronary heart disease—environmental and hereditary influences. *Israeli Journal of Medical Science,* 3, 504.

Epstein, F. H. (1968). Multiple risk factors and the prediction of coronary heart disease. *Bulletin of the New York Academy of Medicine,* 14, 916.

Fitzgerald, J. D., (1972). The role of beta-adrenergic blockers in acute myocardial ischaemia, in *Effect of Acute Ischaemia on Myocardial Function,* ed. M. F. Oliver, D. G. Julian and K. W. Donald. London and Edinburgh: Churchill Livingstone.

Friedman, M. & Rosenman, R. H., (1959). Association of specific overt behaviour pattern with blood and cardiovascular findings. *Journal of the American Medical Association,* 169, 1286.

Freidman, M., Rosenman R. H., Straus, R., Wurm, M. & Kositchek, R. (1968). The relationship of behaviour pattern A to the state of the coronary vasculature: a study of 51 autopsy subjects. *American Journal of Medicine,* 44, 525.

Godfrey, S. (1970). Role of exercise tests in diagnosis of fitness in suspected heart or lung disease. *Lancet*, 2, 973.

Gordon, T. & Kannel, W. B. (1970). *The Community as an Epidemiological Laboratory*, p.123, Ed. P.I. Kessler and M.L. Levin, Baltimore: John Hopkins Press.

Hamilton, M. (1968). The need for early reduction in blood pressure illustrated by the long term results of treatment of hypertension. *New Zealand Medical Journal*, 67, 275.

Hammond, E. C. & Horn, D. (1958). Smoking and death rates: report on 44 months of follow-up of 187,783 men. *Journal of the American Medical Association*, 166, 1159 and 1294.

Harland, W. A. & Holburn, A. M. (1966). Coronary thrombosis and myocardial infarction. *Lancet*, 2, 1158.

Harvald, B. & Hange M. (1965). *Genetics and the Epidemiology of Chronic Diseases*. Ed. J. V. Neel, M. W. Shaw and W. J. Schull. Public Health Service Publication No.1163, Washington, D.C.

Kagan, A., Livsic, A. M., Sternby, N. & Vihert, A. M. (1968). Coronary artery thrombosis and the acute attack of coronary heart-disease. *Lancet*, 2, 1199.

Kannel, W. B., Gordon, T., Castelli, W. P. & Margolis, J. R. (1970). Electrocardiographic left ventricular hypertrophy and risk of coronary heart disease. *Annals of Internal Medicine*, 72, 813.

Kannel, W. B. (1970). Results of the epidemiologic investigation of ischaemic heart disease, illustrated by the Framingham study. In *Ischaemic Heart Disease*, ed. J. H. De Haas, H. C. Hemker, and H. A. Snellen, Holland: Leiden University Press, p.285.

Keys, A., Aravanis, C., Blackburn, H., Van Buchem, F. S. P., Buzina, R., Djordjevak, R., Fidauza, F., Karvonen, M., J. Menotti, A., Punnd, V. & Taylor, H. L. (1972). Coronary heart disease: overweight and obesity as risk factors. *Annals of Internal Medicine*, 77, 15.

Kinlen, L J. (1973). Incidence and presentation of myocardial infarction in an English community. *British Heart Journal*, 35, 616.

Lancet, (1967). Annotation: The Anti-Coronary Club, *Lancet*, 1, 148.

Lewes, D. (1970). Techniques of ECG recording. *British Journal of Hospital Medicine*, 721.

Mathisen, S., Loken, H., Brox, D. & Stenbach, O. (1969). The prognosis in long-term treated and untreated essential hypertension. *Acta Medica Scandinavica*, 185, 253.

Meade, T. W. & Gardner, M. J. (1968). Observer variability in cardiology. *Proceedings of the Royal Society of Medicine*, 61, 451.

Meade, T. W. (1973). In *Portfolio for Health 2: The developing programme of the DHSS in health services research*. ed. G. McLachlan, p.204. Oxford University Press.

Meittinen, M., Turpeinen, O., Karvonen, M., Elosuo, R. & Paavilainen, E. (1972). Effect of cholesterol-lowering diet on mortality from coronary heart disease and other causes. *Lancet*, 2, 836.

Morris, J. N. (1951). Recent history of ischaemic heart disease. *Lancet* 1, 1 & 69.

Morris, J. N., Healey, J. A., Raffle, P. A. B. Roberts, C. G. & Parks, J. W. (1953). Coronary heart disease and physical activity of work. *Lancet*, 2, 1053.

Morris, J. N., Chave, S. P. W., Adarn, C., Sirey, C., Epstein, L. & Sheehan, D. J. (1973). Vigorous exercise in leisure time and the incidence of coronary heart disease. *Lancet*, 1, 333.

Morris, J. N., Kagan, A., Pattison, D. C., Gardner, M. J. & Raffle, P. A. B. (1966). Incidence and prediction of ischaemic heart diseases in London busmen. *Lancet*, 2, 553.

Multicentre trial (1966). Propranolol in acute myocardial infarction. *Lancet*, 2, 1435.

Newcastle (1971). Trial of Clofibrate in the treatment of ischaemic heart disease. *British Medical Journal*, 4, 767.

Ostrander, L. D. (1970). The relation of silent T wave inversion to cardiovascular disease in an epidemiologic study. *American Journal of Cardiology*, 25, 325.

Paul, O., Lepper, M. H., Phelan, W. H., Dupertius, G. W., Macmillan, A., MacKean, H. & Park, H. (1963). A longitudinal study of coronary heart disease. *Circulation*, 28, 20.

Porter, A. M. W. & McCullough, D. M. (1972). Counselling against cigarette smoking. *Practitioner*, 209, 686.

Rose, G. A. & Blackburn, H. (1968). *Cardiovascular survey methods*. WHO Monograph Series, No. 56.

Rose, G. A. (1962).*Bulletin of the World Health Organisation*, 27, 645.

Rosenman, R. H., Freidman, M. Jenkins, C. D., Strauss R., Wurm, M. & Kositchek, R. (1966). The prediction of immunity to coronary heart disease. *Journal of the American Medical Association*, 198, 1159.

Scottish Society of Physicians (1971). Ischaemic heart disease: a secondary prevention trial using Clofibrate. *British Medical Journal*, 4, 775.

Seim, S. (1960). Angina pectoris: a prognosis study. *Acta Medica Scandinavica*, 166, fasc.4,225.

Short, D. (1968). Value and limitations of electrocardiogram in diagnosis of slight and subacute coronary attacks. *British Medical Journal*, 4, 673.

Short, D. & Stowers, M. (1972). Earliest symptoms of coronary heart disease and their recognition. *British Medical Journal*, 2, 387.

Stamler, J. (1967). *Lectures on Preventive Cardiology*. New York: Grime and Stratton.

Syme, S. L., Hyman, M. M. & Enterline, P. E. (1964). Some social and cultural factors associated with the occurrence of coronary heart disease. *Journal of Chronic Diseases*, 17, 277.

Veterans Administration Cooperative study group (1967). Effects of treatment on morbidity in hypertension. *Journal of the American Medical Association*, 202, 1028.

Veterans Administration Cooperative study group (1970). Effects of treatment on morbidity in hypertension: results in patients with diastolic blood pressure averaging 90 through 114. *Journal of the American Medical Association*, 213, 1143.

Werkö, L. (1971). Can we prevent heart disease? *Annals of Internal Medicine*, 74, 278.

WHO (1967). *Epidemiological and Vital Statistics Report*, 20, Cardiovascular diseases supplement.

21 Glaucoma

J.T. Cope and D.H. Smith

'And that one talent which is death to hide
Lodged with me is useless.'

Milton. On his blindness.

Chronic glaucoma appears at first sight to be a condition ideally suited to early diagnosis and treatment. It is a major source of blindness, ranking high in the figures for blind registration in the elderly (1,400 out of 11,500 new cases registered in 1962), and because the visual loss does not involve central vision until a late stage, signs of the disease may be present for a long time before the patient notes any symptoms (Graham, 1967).

In essence chronic glaucoma is an insidious disease developing over many years, and in its natural state it will progress to channel vision or complete blindness. Frequently its presence is demonstrated by chance examination, as for example in the course of a heavy goods vehicle licence examination, or during routine ophthalmoscopy. Regretably screening for glaucoma is not simple or straightforward, and it is bedevilled by the fact that there is no one test by which all cases of glaucoma can be recognised at an early stage. Indeed, as yet no-one is certain of the natural history of chronic glaucoma, and there is not even complete agreement on its aetiology.

Definition

Opthalmologists define chronic simple glaucoma as an eye disease in which the complete clinical picture is characterised by increased intra-ocular pressure, excavation and degeneration of the optic disc, and typical nerve fibre damage producing defects in the field of vision. Any or all of these signs may be present at a given examination

211

(Becker and Burd, 1970). So basically, to make a diagnosis of chronic simple glaucoma it is necessary to have evidence of raised intra-ocular pressure and damage to the optic nerve, and this damage is shown either by cupping of the optic disc or field defects. The normal intra-ocular pressure is less than 21 mm Hg. A pressure that is greater than 21 mm Hg on repeated examination occurs only in 2·5 per cent of the normal population. Glaucoma may be defined for the individual eye as that intra-ocular pressure which produces damage to that particular optic nerve. Consequently, it is true to say that glaucoma develops when intra-ocular pressure rises, and that chronic glaucoma is the result of imbalance between inflow of fluid into the eye and its drainage out of the eye. Fluid enters the eye through the ciliary bodies and drains out through the trabecular channels in the anterior chamber of the eye, probably via the Canal of Schlemm. It can be shown that there is both a daily and a diurnal variation in intra-ocular pressure, and some people believe that raised intra-ocular pressure is not the sole cause of simple chronic glaucoma.

For the purposes of screening, chronic glaucoma can be divided into four types:

1 *Chronic simple glaucoma*
This is the commonest form of glaucoma, and is the one with which we are most concerned in screening. It exists when one or both eyes have an intra-ocular pressure in excess of 21 mm Hg, when there are visual field defects, and when glaucomatous cupping of the disc is present. In addition there must not be evidence of angle closure on examination of the anterior chamber of the eye.

2 *Ocular hypertension*
This is present when tonometry reveals intra-ocular pressure greater than 21 mm Hg in one or both eyes, but when other signs of glaucoma are absent.

3 *Low tension glaucoma*
In this type of glaucoma there are visual field defects and cupping of the optic discs, but the intra-ocular pressure is persistently less than 21 mm Hg.

4 *Congestive or Closed Angle Glaucoma*
In this condition there may be a history of haloes (which are caused by corneal oedema), and there is a narrow angle on examining the anterior chamber of the eye. Alternatively, there may just be an intra-ocular pressure greater than 21 mm Hg associated with a narrow angle.

The Bedford Glaucoma Survey (1968) gives some idea of the relative frequency of these various types of glaucoma. In this survey 5,941 people over the age of 40 years living in Bedford were screened for glaucoma, and they eventually found 55 new cases of primary glaucoma. Of these, 42 were cases of chronic simple glaucoma, 3 were low tension glaucoma and 10 people had closed angle glaucoma. At our local ophthalmic department two thirds of all new cases of glaucoma are chronic simple in type.

From the above definitions it is obvious that there is no single test available to general practitioners which can with accuracy detect most of the incipient cases of glaucoma. For example, a screener who relies on tonometry alone will completely miss all the people with low tension glaucoma. In addition, he may create a lot of unnecessary work and cause much needless apprehension by throwing up a lot of false positives in patients with ocular hypertension. If visual field examination alone is used, then there is the risk that the glaucoma may be considerably advanced before detection, as it is notoriously difficult to detect early visual field changes. Statistically, at this early stage in the development of glaucoma there is very little difference between the effectiveness of tonometry and visual field screening in the picking up of new cases, or for that matter, in the throwing up of false positives.

Tonometry

Intra-ocular pressure is measured by means of a tonometer, of which there are several different types available but the easiest for use in the surgery is the Schiøtz tonometer (fig. 6). This measures intra-ocular pressure by recording the depth of indentation of the cornea when the foot of the instrument is placed carefully on the eye. Local anaesthetic is first instilled into both eyes, and the patient lies in a recumbent position. A given weight is placed on the tonometer and the amount of indentation is read off a scale. By using a set of tables supplied with the instrument it is then possible to read off the instruments using the Schiøtz tonometer foot are available. The Schiøtz tonometer is easily portable and relatively cheap, but it is important that a properly calibrated instrument is used whenever tonometry is carried out.

A refined method of measuring intra-ocular pressure is by an applanation tonometer. This instrument fits onto a slit lamp and measures the pressure needed to flatten a given area of cornea. It does not indent the eye and has the advantage that its measurement is independent of ocular rigidity. It is the standard method of measuring intra-ocular pressure in cases referred for glaucoma investigation, but if used for screening would require ophthalmic trained personnel. The reason for introducing applanation tonometry in this chapter is that it is the standard method by which

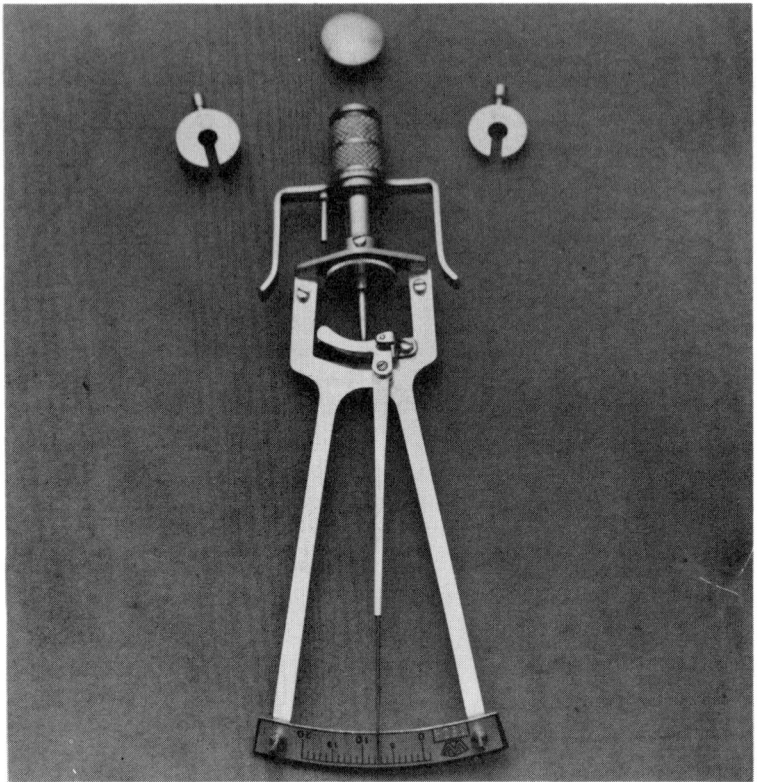

Figure 6. Schiøtz tonometer.

ophthalmologists measure intra-ocular pressure, and they express this pressure as so many mm Hg applanation.

A new electronic tonometer called the Mackay Marg which gives automatic recordings on a tape has not yet received universal acceptance, but holds out great promise of being a simple accurate instrument.

All people found with pressures greater than 21 mm Hg in one or both eyes should be regarded with great suspicion, and will need to be referred to an ophthalmic clinic for further investigation.

Assessment of visual fields

The reason that the visual fields are affected in glaucoma is that the raised intra-ocular pressure produces ischaemic changes in the optic nerve fibres by pressure effects on the small blood vessels round the optic nerve. Good central vision is retained until late in the disease simple because these central fibres are by their position most resistant to damage.

Normal methods of investigating visual fields are unsuitable for use in screening because they are too tedious and require considerable personnel training. It is essential that any method used to screen for early visual defects in glaucoma must be accurate and detect as many visual field defects as possible; in addition it must not throw up too many false positives. The examination must be quick, not too demanding on the patient, and it must be possible to reproduce the same findings easily. There are two types of machine available. Instruments such as the Friedmann Visual Field Analyser give an assessment quickly and accurately of central visual field defects and are quite satisfactory for screening purposes. However, recent work suggests that the Goldmann Perimeter has a higher sensitivity (Rock, Drance and Morgan, 1971). This instrument plots the blind spot and 72 points in the central field. It takes approximately 5 minutes to examine each eye and trials show that the perimeter is capable of great accuracy and that it picks up a high percentage of field defects without creating too many false positives.

The first indication of a defect in the visual field is a scotoma leading from the nasal side of the blind spot. Later other scotomata develop, become confluent, and join with the blind spot. Enlargement of the blind spot itself is a late sign. In early glaucoma there is difficulty in finding these blind spots at all, and many opticians who have had experience with visual field screeners have abandoned them for this reason. Visual field examination requires a fair degree of patient co-operation and this is not always forthcoming in the old and in those patients who are most at risk.

Ophthalmoscopy

This is the oldest method of screening and of course is a regular part of an eye examination by an ophthalmologist or optician. Its use is limited by the fact that a glaucomatous cupped disc is not easy to detect in its early stages, and frequently is not diagnostic till late changes are present. Clinically the disc first enlarges, then shows a sharply defined central depression, with a tendency for the vessels to move towards the nasal side. Even in expert hands it is not easy to detect cupping until field defects are present. Ophthalmoscopy is an excellent method of following up suspected cases of glaucoma, since there appears to be a quantitative relationship between the deterioration of the visual field and progressive changes seen in the optic disc.

Selection of patients for screening

1 **Age.** The incidence of glaucoma increases with age. It is rare

below the age of 40 years. In the Bedford Glaucoma Survey nearly 80 per cent of the people detected were aged over 60 years, and in a large scale population survey in the Rhondda Valley, 90 per cent of the patients with chronic glaucoma were 55 years of age and over (Hollows and Graham, 1966). In this survey no cases of glaucoma were detected in people under 50 years of age. Thus it would seem logical that the GP should direct his screening efforts at people over 55 to 60 years of age.

2 **Family history.** Chronic simple glaucoma is much more common in first degree relations (siblings, parents, or children) of known cases. It is therefore most productive to screen members of known glaucoma families. Tonometry, followed by a full glaucoma investigation in those discovered to have a pressure greater than 21 mm Hg in either eye, is probably as good a screening method as any in these cases. Such relations should have glaucoxa testing at regular intervals after the age of 40 years. Once suspicion has been aroused these people should have regular ophthalmoscopic examinations, preferably using retinal photography. In a survey carried out in our practice, 2 cases of chronic glaucoma were found in one family; subsequent checking of brothers and sisters revealed 5 more cases in this large family (Cope and Smith, 1967).

Results of screening

The incidence of glaucoma discovered by tonometry in the general population varies from 0·93 per cent in the Bedford Survey to 0·43 per cent in the Rhondda Valley Population Study (Hollows and Graham, 1966). Both these surveys discovered a high rate of ocular hypertension, 3 per cent and 8·6 per cent respectively. Now the main stumbling block is that it is not known how many cases of raised ocular tension will proceed to glaucoma with field defects, let alone complete blindness. In a long term follow up of 141 people found to have ocular hypertension at the Bedford Survey, only 5 (3·54 per cent) developed glaucoma over 5-7 years (Perkins, 1973). Two out of the 25 cases of ocular hypertension from our own study in 1967 have so far developed glaucoma.

Glaucoma is far more likely to arise in those cases of ocular hypertension that have readings greater than 25 mm Hg. Conversely, it would seem that in patients with pressures between 21 and 25 mm Hg on first examination, the natural history is for the intra ocular pressure to revert to its normally accepted levels with the passage of time. It must be said that ocular hypertension is the curse of screening, in that its follow-up creates a vast amount of work in ophthalmological departments; yet it is likely that the long term follow-up of ocular hypertension holds the key as to whether screening for chronic glaucoma is or is not of worthwhile benefit. Professor Goldman (1972) said 'I am convinced that it is necessary to keep under observation those whose tension is found after repeated examination to be 22 to 25 mm Hg applanation without a visual field defect, and to begin medical treatment in cases with a persistently higher pressure even in the absence of any field defect.'

What then should the GP do? The possibilities are:

1 Screening of all people 40 years of age and over

Using tonometry, this method has enjoyed a considerable vogue over the past decade, but analysis has shown it to be wasteful of time and energy in respect of the large number of false positives discovered.

2 Selective screening

Given that there is a familial incidence of 38 per cent in cases of fully developed chronic simple glaucoma, then it would appear that the most productive line of attack for the GP screener would be to concentrate his efforts on the first degree relations of known cases of chronic simple glaucoma. The obvious snag is that someone by some means has to pick up the first case.

Conclusion

Tonometry is not infallible and it will fail to detect a significant number who suffer from glaucoma. It creates a lot of work in following up cases of ocular hypertension. Nevertheless, in early glaucoma (as opposed to glaucoma with established field defects) it is probably as accurate as visual field screening and consequently the Schiøtz tonometer should still remain the main weapon of the GP screener. The one certainty that exists amid all the uncertainty that surrounds the subject, is that further research is urgently needed to improve our ability to detect glaucoma at an early stage.

REFERENCES

Becker, B. & Burd, R. M. (1970). *Shaffer's Diagnosis & Treatment of the Glaucomas*. 3rd Ed. Mosby, USA.

Bedford Glaucoma Survey (1968). *British Medical Journal*, 1, 791.

Cope, J. T. & Smith, D. H. (1967). A health week in rural general practice. *British Medical Journal*, 2, 756.

Goldman, H. (1972). *British Journal of Ophthalmology*, 56, 307.

Graham, P. A. (1967). *The Early Diagnosis of Field Defects*, Paper No. 2. Office of Health Economics.

Hollows, F. C. & Graham, P. A. (1966). Intra-ocular pressure glaucoma and glaucoma suspects in a defined population. *British Journal of Ophthalmology*, 50, 570.

Perkins, E. S. (1973). *British Journal of Ophthalmology*. 57, 179.

Rock, W. J., Drance, S. M., & Morgan, R. W. (1971). An evaluation of the Armaly technique for screening glaucomatous fields. *Canadian Journal of Ophthalmology*, 6, 283.

22 Anaemia

R.M.A. Moore

'Before recommending countrywide facilities for haemoglobin testing, one should perhaps pause a little to ask whether "screening" in general is not liable to produce a certain amount of smugness because one is "doing something for the community", and one should also ask whether it is not a little too easy to do compared with the difficult, boring, prolonged, all-too-often not statistically significant though certainly more rewarding, task of carrying out properly randomised controlled clinical trials.'

G. S. Kilpatrick, 1966.

The criteria for diagnosis of anaemia

It is a simple matter to obtain a sample of venous or capillary blood, from which values for haemoglobin, white cell count and red cell absolute indices can be calculated, and in cases where values are abnormal a film can be examined under the microscope. In view of the frequent occurrence of low haemoglobin and other abnormal indices, it would seem that screening procedures could easily be used for the detection and early diagnosis of anaemia. However, 'anaemia' is not a single disease entity, but rather a clinical sign which is present in many diseases and which may require considerable investigation to diagnose fully. Furthermore, haemoglobin levels at or below the lower range of normal may be found in persons who are apparently very fit and active, so that the specificity of screening for low haemoglobin may be very poor in terms of significant diseases detected by the screening procedure.

Numerous population surveys have been carried out to establish normal values for haematological indices, to delineate criteria for the diagnosis of anaemia, and to estimate the incidence of anaemia in the population screened. Table 16 shows the normal values determined by Wintrobe and accepted as standard, and it may be noted that there is

Table 16. Normal values for haemoglobin at various ages
(after Wintrobe)

Age	Haemoglobin (g/100 ml)
First day	19.5 ± 5.0
2—3 days	19.0
4—8 days	18.3 ± 4.0
9—13 days	16.5
14—60 days	14.0 ± 3.3
3—5 months	12.2 ± 2.3
6—11 months	11.8
1 year	11.2
2 years	11.5
3 years	12.5
4 years	12.6
5 years	12.6
6—10 years	12.9
11—15 years	13.4
Adults: Females	14.0 ± 2.0
Males	16.0 ± 2.0

a marked fall in haemoglobin from birth to one year, followed by a continuous rise to adult levels. But these figures are mean, and as the distribution of haematological indices in the population is Gaussian, difficulty arises in determining a point below which anaemia can be said to be present. Choosing that point at too high a level will include many people who are healthy but have relatively low values, and choosing too low a level will exclude many who are, in fact, anaemic.

For a screening procedure to be worthwhile the condition being sought must be amenable to correction, or at least must be one in which early diagnosis offers an improved prospect of cure or benefit. In the case of anaemias the great majority of positive findings in screening programmes have been due to deficiencies of iron, vitamin B_{12} or folate, or to blood loss. The more serious causes of anaemia such as aplastic anaemia, leukaemias, Hodgkin's disease and myeloma and those secondary to renal failure and other chronic diseases, form a much smaller proportion. Nevertheless, they cause a large number of deaths every year and if and when a curative treatment becomes available it will become as important to diagnose these diseases at an early stage as it now is, for instance, for carcinoma. Table 17 compares death rates from blood dyscrasias with some other diseases detectable by screening.

Table 17. Comparison of death rates from some kinds of anaemia and some other diseases detectable by screening procedures (Registrar General's Statistics for England and Wales, 1971).

Cause		Total Numbers	Rate per Million Population
ICD No.			
204	Lymphatic Leukaemia	1,146	23
205	Myeloid Leukaemia	1,480	30
206	Monocytic Leukaemia	118	2
280	Iron Deficiency Anaemia	171	(3)
281	Other Deficiency Anaemias	349	(7)
281·0	Pernicious Anaemia	344	(7)
282	Hereditary Haemolytic Anaemias	63	(1)
284	Aplastic Anaemia	291	6
011	Pulmonary Tuberculosis	850	17
174	Carcinoma of Breast (female only)	11,182	446
180	Carcinoma of Cervix	2,315	92
162	Carcinoma of Trachea, Bronchus and Lung	30,744	634
400–404	Hypertensive Disease	9,302	191
250	Diabetes Mellitus	4,893	100

Figures in brackets are approximate calculations from total numbers.

Some screening surveys (Table 18)

In two comparable surveys in the Rhondda Fach (Kilpatrick and Hardisty, 1961) and Wensleydale (Kilpatrick, 1961) the incidence of low haemoglobins in these populations was examined. Subjects found to have haemoglobin levels below 12·5 g/100 ml in men and 12·0 g in women were considered to be anaemic. In the Rhondda 3·3per cent of the men and 13·9 per cent of women (aged 55-64 only) fell below these criteria, and in Wensleydale the proportion was higher—7·7 per cent of men and 20·9 per cent of women (of all ages). Women in the menstruating years in the Wensleydale survey, and both sexes over the age of 60 in both surveys provided the majority of positive findings. In the Rhondda survey the causes of anaemias were investigated and the majority were found to be due to menstrual blood loss of deficient diets, but peptic ulcer, gastrectomy, chronic lymphatic leukaemia, carcinoma of stomach, and larynx, and pernicious anaemia were also diagnosed. Another study (Parsons, Withey and Kilpatrick, 1965) was concerned with the population over 65 years of age in Swansea. Two hundred and eight subjects were examined, and 10·8 per cent of men and 15·7 per cent of women were found to be anaemic, and in the 75 years-olds and over

Table 18. Comparison of the findings of some surveys investigating the incidence of low haemoglobins (Hb g/100 ml)

Authors	Place	Population	Criterion (Hb g/100ml) Male	Female	Number examined Male	Female	Total	% below criterion Male	Female
Kilpatrick & Hardisty	The Rhondda	Men 35-64 yrs Women 55-64 yrs	12·5	12·0	543	180	723	3·3	13·9
Kilpatrick	Wensleydale	Men & Women 15-75 +	12·5	12·0	182	230	412	7·7	20·9
Kilpatrick et al.	Swansea	Men & Women over-65	12·5	12·0	93	115	208	10·5	15·7
Lovric	Sydney	Children attending Baby Clinics	10·0	10·0	—	—	1,000	3·1 per cent of total	
Anyon & Clarkson	Rural New Zealand	Children under 1 year	9·5	9·5	—	—	82	10 per cent of total	
Natvig et al.	Norway	Children 7-20 yrs	Varied		777	734	1,511	1·7	2·5
Natvig et al.	Norway	Adults 15-60 +	14·0	12·5	1,117	322	1,439	3·1	5·3
Macfarlane et al.	Glasgow	Women in General Practice	—	12·0	—	500	500	Patients 9·7 Controls 2·0	
Rees, Moore & Wycherley	Shrewsbury	1 in 4 sample of General Practice. Children 1-3 yrs	12·0	11·0	—	—	504	13 overall	
			11·0	11·0					
Kaufman, Grant & Moorhouse	Manitoba, Canada	Whole Population Screen	10·0	10·0	7,415	9,336	16,751	13 overall 0·1	2·4

the figures were even higher (20·8 per cent and 23·3 per cent respectively). One case each of pernicious anaemia and of carcinoma of colon were diagnosed.

Unsuspected anaemia will be found in children, also, if a screening procedure is undertaken, as studies in Australia and New Zealand show. Lovric (1970) examined 1,000 children attending baby health clinics in Sydney and found 31 (3·1 per cent) to have iron deficiency anaemia with haemoglobin below 10 g/100 ml. There was no correlation between incidence of low haemoglobin and family income; indeed there were more children with haemoglobin below the mean in the higher income group than the lower. Nor was there any correlation with prematurity in this study, although another group of 458 children admitted to hospitals was found to have mean haemoglobins of 10·6 g/100 ml (mean for the health clinic group was 12·0 g/100 ml) and of these 458 hospital children one third had been premature. Another interesting finding was that 60 per cent of children of mothers aged less than 19 years had haemoglobins below the mean. This study shows that babies who are not under surveillance at baby clinics, and especially those of very young mothers, are more likely to suffer from iron deficiency anaemia; and that those who are iron deficient are more likely to suffer illness requiring admission to hospital than those who are not. Anyon and Clarkson (1971) studied 82 apparently healthy babies in a rural community in New Zealand. Ten children under one year of age were found to have haemoglobin values below 9·5 g/100 ml and eight of these had occult blood in the stools. It is postulated that cows milk can cause excessive desquamation of intestinal mucosal cells, thereby producing loss of 'free' iron sufficiently great to lead to anaemia.

In Norway a survey of 1,511 school children aged between seven and 20 years (Natvig, Vellar and Anderson, 1967) revealed 13 boys and 18 girls who were anaemic with signs of iron deficiency, and improved to normal on iron therapy. A study of adults by the same authors revealed evidence of iron deficiency in 3·1 per cent of men and 5·3 per cent of women in all ages over 15 years (Natvig and Vellar, 1967).

An interesting study in Glasgow (Macfarlane, Pinkerton, Dagg and Goldberg, 1967) examined 500 women attending at a general practice. Of these 402 attended as patients, and 98 came without complaint or were accompanying a patient, being described in the study as 'Subjects'. The overall incidence of iron deficiency anaemia, defined in this survey as haemoglobin less than 12·0 g/100 ml, was 8·2 per cent (9·7 per cent in patients and two per cent in 'subjects'). In addition there were 105 women (20 per cent) who were not anaemic but were considered to be iron deficient in that they showed less than 16 per cent saturation of the total iron binding capacity. There were 17 cases of anaemia due to other or uncertain causes, including pernicious anaemia (five cases) chronic lymphatic leukemia (one case) and suspected monocytic leukaemia (one case).

The finding of iron deficiency without anaemia is becoming recognised more frequently and indicates a depletion of iron reserves to the point where blood loss, pregnancy or infection could produce overt anaemia. If iron deficiency anaemia is to be prevented attention should also be paid to iron stores, because therapy sufficient to return haemoglobin and red cell values to normal in circulating blood may be insufficient to restore depleted iron stores, which should be not less than 1·0 to 1·5 g and perhaps as much as 4·0 g. This is sufficient iron for two to three litres of blood, and at an average absorption of 1·0 mg/day is equivalent to three or four years dietary supply. In a study of college women in Dallas, Scott and Pritchard (1967) demonstrated that two thirds of apparently healthy young women, who had never had a haemorrhage or other cause of iron depletion, were unable to mobilise more than 350 mg of iron in response to haemorrhage, only enough for one quarter to one half litre of blood, and some of them much less.

A screening procedure to detect the incidence of known and unsuspected anaemia was undertaken in a randomly selected sample of a general practice in Shrewsbury (Rees, Moore and Wycherley, 1969). A one-in-four sample of a country town practice was invited, by letter, to submit to a blood test. 584 people of all ages (73 per cent of those approached) agreed to co-operate. 76 people were found to have haemoglobin levels below those defined as anaemic in this study, that is males 12 g/100 ml, females 11 g/100 ml, and children one to three years 11 g/100 ml. These included 15 children (ten girls and five boys) with iron deficiency, one case of Vitamin B_{12} deficiency, six folate deficiencies (three children, one woman of 37 and two over 70 years) and 16 cases of secondary anaemia, mainly in children with recurrent infections. There were 17 cases of blood loss, of whom three were men and three were children, including gastro intestinal bleeding due to aspirin and butazolidin, haemorrhoids and ulcers, as well as the anticipated cases of menstrual loss.

Perhaps the largest screening procedure carried out for anaemia was that done by Kaufman, Grant and Moorhouse (1969a, 1969b) in rural Manitoba, in conjunction with a survey to detect tuberculosis, diabetes and raised blood urea. The haemoglobin levels of 16,751 persons were examined, and the screen test was said to be positive when below the arbitrarily chosen figure of 10 g/100 ml, which is rather lower than in other surveys quoted. Positive screen tests were found in 194 women (2·1 per cent of women screened) and eight men (0·1 per cent). 24 were false positives, and after allowing for this and previously known cases 65 women and only three men were left who were not previously known to be anaemic. The causes of anaemia in these cases is not specified as follow-up was done after referral to the patients' own physicians. It is therefore difficult to draw conclusions from the women, but the yield of three cases in over 7,000 men examined is very small. The cost of the survey was $19,000 but the urea and haemoglobin analysis accounts for only $800 so that in this context, as one item in a multiphasic screening programme the cost of detecting the previously unknown cases does not add greatly to the overall cost.

The interpretation of findings in screening programmes

The surveys described above have shown that screening, either of volunteers, randomly selected samples, or groups selected for particular reasons will reveal a high proportion of cases of 'anaemia'. If anaemia is defined as a haemoglobin level of below 12·0 g/100 ml, many people who feel perfectly well will be diagnosed as 'anaemic'; if the level of 10 g/100 ml is taken there may be many who are truly anaemic but symptomless, not included in the 'positive' group. The question must therefore be asked 'How important is the finding of a haemoglobin level of between 10·0 and 12·0 g/100 ml?' There is no clear answer to this but the evidence suggests that to have haemoglobin levels in that range is not harmful in itself and does not cause symptoms, as was shown in a very carefully studied survey of 880 women (Elwood et al., 1969). An attempt was made to correlate the level of haemoglobin with six symptoms commonly regarded as those of anaemia, namely irritability, palpitation, dizziness, breathlessness, fatigue and headaches, and also to correlate these symptoms with a neurotic grading of the subjects. The presence of symptoms and the degree of neurosis was examined by means of standard questionnaires. Those women with haemoglobin levels between 8·0 and 12·0 g/100 ml were admitted to a trial, one half taking oral iron and the other a placebo. A group of women with high neurotic grade but haemoglobin levels of 13·5 g or higher were also given iron or placebo in the same way. It was found that there was no significant correlation between the symptoms specified and the haemoglobin levels, except in the case of palpitations, and here the symptom was commoner with higher levels than lower. However, there was positive and significant correlation between the specified symptoms and neurotic grading. Those with low haemoglobins who were given iron improved their haemoglobin levels, but there was no greater improvement in symptoms in this group, of whom 53 per cent noticed general improvement in well-being, than the placebo group, of whom 58 per cent improved though their haemoglobin levels did not rise. Of those with high haemoglobins 43 per cent reported a general improvement in wellbeing after iron and 61 per cent after the placebo. The conclusion drawn from this study is that there is no clear evidence that iron deficiency is a disease which causes symptoms unless the deficiency is severe. This conclusion is supported by Simpson and Gourley (1971) who investigated the prevalence of anaemia in 316 women working in jute factories. Although 11·7 per cent overall had haemoglobin of 12·0 g/100 ml or less, the study failed to show a relationship between low haemoglobin and poor work performance.

Screening as a diagnostic aid

As far as the commonest cause of anaemia, iron deficiency, is concerned we have evidence of its widespread occurrence but no evidence that in its less severe degrees it causes any symptoms. It is probable that it does not cause any interference with function unless the haemoglobin falls well below 8·0 g/100 ml and the surveys quoted above have rarely detected previously unknown cases of anaemia of this degree. Indeed Elwood *et al.* (1969) found only 18 cases in 3,000 women screened and most of these were already known to their doctors. Furthermore, anaemia of this degree due to other causes, such as leukaemia or agranulocytosis is likely to be advanced beyond the hope of cure; or there will already be symptoms or signs of the underlying disease in many cases sufficient to draw the patient's or the physician's attention to the anaemia. Mass population screening for anaemia as a single entity therefore cannot be expected to make a big impact in terms of reducing morbidity or improving well being, nor in reducing mortality from serious disease. But there can be little doubt that taken in conjunction with other diagnostic procedures, including screening programmes, a continuous awareness of the possibility of anaemia in certain groups will lead to earlier and more accurate diagnosis and there is a good case for selective screening in those groups.

For this to be effective it is important that laboratory investigation should be accurate, and that therapy should be avoided until a firm diagnosis has been made to avoid interfering with subsequent investigations. Automation of laboratory techniques, such as the use of the Coulter 'S' counter, produces quick accurate results that are comparable between laboratories. The laboratories working within the National Health Service regularly compare their results with each other and therefore maintain standards which are comparable not only between different people at the same time, but also between the same person at different times. It is doubtful if a physician not constantly using a haemoglobinometer can come near the degree of accuracy achieved in haematology laboratories, which are now readily accessible to general practitioners in the Health Service. Furthermore a trained observer can obtain vital information in a few minutes from the microscopic study of a blood smear, which is not feasible for the clinician to do in a screening programme. One unexpected disadvantage of automated techniques, however, is that reliance can not now be placed on the mean corpuscular haemoglobin content (MCHC) as an indicator of iron deficiency because it is calculated in a way different from the original method and must be interpreted differently (Rose, 1971; England, Walford and Waters, 1971). However, the mean corpuscular haemoglobin and the mean cell volume, both calculated by automated processes, are reliable indicators of iron deficiency. Haemoglobin estimation, therefore, can be used as a screening procedure in two ways: either as one phase of a multiphasic screening programme, or as one criterion in the examination of patients suspected of having diseases involving anaemia.

Selection of 'at risk' groups

What groups then should be regarded as being vulnerable to anaemia and therefore selected for screening? It is suggested that the following should be included:-
1 Those liable to iron deficiency.
2 Those liable to dietary deficiency of other substances essential for haemopoiesis.
3 Those with evidence of blood loss or in whom occult blood loss may occur.
4 Those with recurrent infections.
5 Women during and after pregnancy.
6 The elderly.
7 Those being investigated for diseases of which anaemia may be a complication.
8 Those undergoing health checks.
9 Those in whom sickle cell trait or other congenital diseases of the blood are possible.

Iron deficiency. Much has been said in this chapter about the prevalence of iron deficiency so it will suffice to say that the following, amongst others, are prone to this condition:-

(a) Infants with dysmaturity and or low birth weight; those who are weaned late without supplementary iron; infants of very young mothers and those with poor appetites.

(b) Children of any age in periods of fast growth where the red cell mass may be expanding faster than dietary resources can supply the necessary iron.

(c) Those at any age who have previously had known or suspected depletion of iron stores with or without anaemia.

Dietary deficiency. This may cause inadequate absorption of iron, Vitamin B_{12}, folic acid and proteins, all of which are necessary for haemopoiesis. The causes of the deficiency may be external or internal. External factors include poverty, ignorance, emotional disorders and alcoholism; and internal factors include oral or alimentary disease, gastrectomy, malabsorption syndrome and anorexia due to diseases of other systems, especially infections and neoplasms. The follow up of those suffering from malabsorption and postgastrectomy anaemia is important as it is easy to forget these long term conditions; especially so with post-gastrectomy anaemia as this is iatrogenic. Ideally a screening programme in which long term disease of this nature is found should cause the positive cases to enter a scheme of periodical re-examination. One group at risk for dietary deficiency has recently been described, namely immigrants in poor social circumstances. Britt, Harper and Spray (1971) describe 17 cases of anaemia due to dietary deficiency among Indian immigrants, an incidence in Indians three times greater than in the white population of the area in which they lived. In 15 of these cases the anaemia was profound—less than 7·0 g/100 ml.

Pregnancy must also be considered as possibly leading to both iron and folic acid deficiency, and all pregnant women should have haemoglobin estimations throughout pregnancy—especially unmarried mothers who are more prone to anaemia than the married (Barwin, 1970).

There is some evidence that recurrent abortions may be associated with folic acid deficiency (Martin, Harper and Kelso, 1965). Such cases should be examined with this in mind.

Blood loss. Overt blood loss from such causes as epistaxis, haematemesis, melaena and haemorrhoids, and of course menorrhagia, requires a blood count if at all heavy or prolonged. In this context the blood loss of childbirth must be remembered and the post natal examination should include haemoglobin estimation. Occult blood loss is easily overlooked, and especially that from salicylates and other anti-rheumatic preparations. Sufferers from rheumatism and recurrent painful conditions, whether under medical treatment or self-medicated should be suspected and tested. Patients with hiatal hernia, peptic ulcers, colitis, diverticulitis and alimentary malignant conditions may all bleed without knowing it.

Infectious diseases. Recurrent infections, especially of the respiratory tract in children, may depress haemopoiesis and diminish appetite, thereby producing normo- or hypochromic anaemia. Such cases should be screened selectively and anaemia corrected when present.

Women in and after Pregnancy. Screening for anaemia in this group is discussed in Chapter 11.

The elderly. There is probably a case for multiphasic screening of people over 70 years of age and detection of anaemia should certainly be included. The elderly are prone to many causes of anaemia, and more than one cause may be present simultaneously.

Investigation for other diseases. Clearly a haemoglobin and full blood count must form part of the investigation of all serious disease. If a specific disease is suspected it will be part of the routine investigation to examine the blood picture. In the approach from general practice however, the discovery of anaemia in a patient with no clear physical signs on which to base a diagnosis will help to confirm the presence of organic disease. This is an important function of the primary physician, who is often confronted by a patient with symptoms but little other evidence of organic disorder. Similarly health checks would be incomplete without screening for anaemia which may be a pointer to other, otherwise asymptomatic disease not detectable by the methods employed in such checks.

Haemoglobinopathy. Detection of the sickle cell trait is important for two reasons. First, the presence of the disease can cause severe complications such as nephropathy, splenic and renal infarction and sudden death under anaesthesia involving hypoxia. The latter are preventable if the presence of the disease is known before anaesthesia is undertaken. Second, if the presence of the trait is known genetic counselling can be employed with the intention of reducing the incidence of the disease in future generations. The screening test for sickle trait costs only a few pence, and is easily performed. In one study 1,000 consecutive U.S. Army Negro recruits were screened, with 7·5 per cent being positive (Binder and Jones, 1970), and in another the Kaiser Multiphasic Screening Clinic in San Francisco detected 8·7 per cent of 4,028 people of all ages (Petrakis *et al.*, 1970). Sickle cell trait is less common in this country than in USA but only because of the smaller Negro population, and is common enough to be sought. In 1972 two hundred and twelve screening tests were carried out at the Royal Salop Infirmary, Shrewsbury, and 15 (7·7 per cent) were positive (Wycherley, 1973). This suggests that a screening programme carried out through general practice or by Area Health Authorities, before the patients need to go to hospital, would yield worthwhile results, both in reducing anaesthetic hazards and in enabling genetic counselling to be offered.

In conclusion, it is argued that, at the present time, there is little value in mass population screening for anaemia, but that screening of selected cases and high risk groups is an important contribution to health care. The difficulties lie not in the screening procedure, but in the interpretation of results and the investigation of positive cases.

REFERENCES

Anyon, C. P. & Clarkson, K. G. (1971). Cow's milk: A cause of iron-deficiency anaemia in infants. *New Zealand Medical Journal*, 74, 24.

Barwin, B. N. (1970). Pregnancy in the unmarried mother. *Ulster Medical Journal*, 39, 143.

Binder, R. A. and Jones, S. R. (1970). Prevalence and awareness of Sickle Cell haemoglobin in a military population. *Journal of the American Medical Association*, 214, 910.

Britt, R. P., Christine Harper, and Spray, G. H. (1971). Megaloblastic anaemia among Indians in Britain. *Quarterly Journal of Medicine*, New Series XL, 160, 499.

Elwood, P. C., Waters, W. E., Greene, W. J. W., Sweetnam, P. & Wood, M. M. (1969). Symptoms and circulating haemoglobin level. *Journal of Chronic Diseases*, 21, 615-628.

England, J. M., Walford, D. M. and Waters, D. A. W. (1971). Epitaph for the MCHC. *British Medical Journal*, 4, 232.

Kaufman, B. J., Grant, D. R., and Moorhouse, J. A. (1969a). An analysis of blood glucose in a population screened for diabetes mellitus. *Canadian Medical Association Journal*, 100, 692-698.

Kaufman, B. J., Grant, D. R. and Moorhouse, J. A. (1969b). An analysis of blood urea nitrogen and haemoglobin values in a population screened for diabetes mellitus. *Canadian Medical Association Journal*, 100, 744-747.

Kilpatrick, G. S. (1961). Prevalence of anaemia in the general population: a rural and an industrial area compared. *British Medical Journal*, 2, 1736.

Kilpatrick, G. S. (1966). The presymptomatic diagnosis of anaemia. *Proceedings of the Royal Society of Medicine*, 59, 122.

Kilpatrick, G. S. & Hardisty, R. M. (1961). The prevalence of anaemia in the community: a survey of a random sample of the population. *British Medical Journal*, 1, 778.

Lovric, V. A. (1970). Normal haematological values in children aged 6-36 months and socio-medical implications. *Medical Journal of Australia*, 2, 366.

Martin, R. H., Harper, T. A. & Kelso, W. (1965). Serum folic acid in recurrent abortions. *Lancet*, 1, 670.

McFarlane, D. B., Pinkerton, P. H., Dagg, J. H. & Goldberg, A. (1967). Incidence of iron deficiency, with and without anaemia, in women in general practice. *British Journal of Haematology*, 13, 790.

Natvig, H. & Vellar, O. D. (1967). Studies on haemoglobin values in Norway. *Acta Medica Scandinavica*, 182, (2), 193.

Natvig, H., Vella, O. D., & Andersen, J. (1967). Studies on haemoglobin values in Norway. *Acta Medica Scandinavica*, 182, (2) 183.

Parson, P. L., Withey, J. L. & Kilpatrick, G. S. (1965). The prevalence of anaemia in the elderly. *Practitioner*, 195, 656.

Petrakis, N. L., Wiesenfeld, S. L., Sams, B. J., Collen, M. F., Cutler, J. L. & Siegelaub, A. B. (1970). Prevalence of Sickle-Cell trait and glucose-6-phosphate dehydrogenase deficiency. *The New England Journal of Medicine*, 282, 767.

Rees, E. G., Moore, R. M. A., & Wycherley, P. A. (1969). Unsuspected anaemia; the case for population screening. *Journal of the Royal College of General Practitioners*, 17, 155.

Rose, M. S. (1971). Epitaph for the MCHC. *British Medical Journal*, 4, 169.

Simpson, J. & Gourley, C. A. (1971). Anaemia in women factory workers. *Health Bulletin*, (Edinburgh), XXIX, 197.

Scott, D. E. & Pritchard, J. A. (1967). Iron deficiency in healthy college women. *Journal of the American Medical Association*, 199, (12), 147-150.

Wintrobe, M. M. (1967). *Clinical Haematology*. London: Henry Kimpton.

Wycherley, P. A. (1973). Personal communication.

23 *Carcinoma of the Breast* B. E. P. Wookey

'Screening should always be done in a calculated fashion, on a selected population.'

A. Levene, 1973.

Carcinoma of the breast is the commonest malignant disease in women in Britain, and the incidence is slowly increasing. Despite improvements in surgical techniques and a greater knowledge of the hormonal influences in the disease, the overall cure rate has scarcely improved over the past 30 years.

With this background there has been a renewal of interest during the past decade in methods for detecting the condition in the very early stages, and in particular before it is noticed by the patient, by which time more than 50 per cent of growths have already spread beyond the confines of the breast. Survival rates for breast cancer are greatly influenced by the histology of the tumour as well as the clinical staging, and to be successful early detection methods would certainly need to pick up the more malignant tumours before they are palpable on clinical examination.

A number of investigations are being carried out in Europe and the United States to assess different methods of early detection and the subsequent effects on survival rates for the study groups. Since 10 years seems to be the earliest date following treatment at which survival rates can be satisfactorily assessed, definite information on the subject is inevitably slow to be produced, and the present position remains unclear.

METHODS OF EARLY DETECTION

1 Palpation by the Clinician

This is the simplest and most obvious method of detection. It is difficult to detect lumps much smaller than three centimetres, particularly in women whose breasts normally or premenstrually have a nodular texture, and not infrequently several examinations may be necessary in doubtful cases. A high degree of concentration is required by the examiner, and this may not be easy when examining a lot of patients in one session. To be even moderately effective, examinations probably need to be repeated at least yearly, which is quite impracticable in general practice except under experimental conditions, or when screening is confined to a small selected group of women.

In our own practice (Wookey, 1971) women attending a Well-Woman clinic, primarily concerned with cervical cytology, at five yearly intervals have all had breast examinations. Over the first six years of the clinic a total of 1,690 examinations were made. Only one case of breast cancer was detected at the clinic, but during this period four other women developed the disease, all of whom had attended the clinic at least once, the shortest interval being 10 months after attendance. Others have also recorded disappointing results (Stark and Way, 1970), but in the United States, Gilbertson in Minneapolis has shown that by regular yearly palpation it is possible to improve the overall five-year survival rate in a group of women to 83 per cent. Even in this survey about one third of the cancers presented between the yearly examinations, and these patients had worse survival rates than those detected at the examinations, presumably because they had more rapidly growing tumours (Gilbertson, 1966).

2 Self-Palpation

Because of the limitations of routine periodic palpation by the doctor, patients may be instructed to examine their own breasts at regular intervals. Most women can be taught to do this with the aid of a simple instruction pamphlet, and some manage to develop a regular routine following menstruation or at some fixed date each month. Risks of inducing a cancer-phobia seem to have been exaggerated, but it is doubtful if many women persevere for long. At our Well-Woman Clinic every woman is now instructed in self-palpation, but so far none has returned to report a lump as a result.

Self-palpation instruction is simple and seems at present to be worthwhile when women are attending their doctor for cervical smears, family planning or post-natal examinations. Pamphlets about it might also be provided in the waiting room.

3 Thermography

Thermography involves measurement of the temperature of

infra-red radiation emitted by the body. Breast carcinomas tend to be hotter than surrounding tissue, and apparatus is available which can detect temperature differences of less than 0·1°C. Thermography has been in use experimentally for over 10 years, but is still being developed, and at present it has not been shown that it improves survival rates when used with palpation alone. The principal drawbacks are that centrally located tumours can easily be missed, and it is unreliable in younger women, especially those on an oral contraceptive. It has the advantage of not exposing the patient to radiation hazards. Thermography has also been used in conjunction with mammography and it seems that to some extent the two methods are complementary to each other (Stark and Way, 1970; Davey and Pentney, 1973).

4 Mammography

Mammography is the technique of taking soft tissue x-rays of the breast. It has been in use for a number of years but initially it was found to be difficult to obtain satisfactory contrast on the films, and the proportion of false-negative and false-positive results was too high for the method to attract widespread interest.

Recent developments have greatly improved the technique, and such machines as the Senograph, a low voltage, constant potential x-ray apparatus with a molybdenum anode, now give good results. This machine is easily handled and enables breasts to be x-rayed from a greater variety of angles than conventional apparatus. Normally lateral and cranio-caudal views are taken of both breasts. Interpretation of the films requires a good deal of skill and experience and, as with thermography, the method is unsuitable in younger women owing to the density of breast tissue. Although radiation exposure is low, this might become a hazard with regular mammography over a large number of years.

A number of trials have shown that mammography in conjunction with palpation is more effective in detecting early cases of breast cancer than palpation alone. An important study of the value of mammography has been conducted by Shapiro and his colleagues in New York, where between 1963 and 1966 a randomly-selected group of 31,000 women aged 40-64 were offered yearly palpation and mammography, and compared with a similarly selected and consti-tuted group of 31,000 controls. In their latest report they have been able to show a substantial reduction in lymph node involvement in cancer cases amongst the study group, and a significant drop in the death rate in this group 3½ years after the end of the trial period (Shapiro, Strax and Venet, 1971). However they conclude that though the results are encouraging, a much longer period of follow-up, probably 10 years, will be required before it can be deduced that screening reduces mortality from the disease.

Also in the United States, Gershon-Cohen and his colleagues, carrying out mammography and palpation on 1,120 women over a 10-year period, have shown that in comparison with national figures for breast cancer, the 33 cases detected by them had smaller tumours (most couldn't be detected by palpation), a much smaller proportion had lymph node involvement, and five-year survival figures should be about 80 per cent (Gershon-Cohen et al., 1967). Again, more time is required before these figures can be interpreted as a definite improvement in survival rates.

5 Xero-radiography

This is a development of the Xerographic image-recording process used in photocopying documents etc, and it is possible that it will eventually replace existing mammography techniques. The process is dry and non-chemical and depends on the ability of an electrostatically-charged selenium plate to react to light by 'leaking' the charge from heavily exposed areas, whilst retaining it in dark areas. Fine powder can then be 'blown' across the surface and will adhere to the charged areas whence it can be transferred and fused to a paper or plastic material for inspection.

The most modern Xero-radiographic equipment consists of two automated units, the Conditioner which is concerned with the charging of the plates, and the Automater which is concerned with development and transfer of the image to special paper. Both are about the size of a small table and can easily be moved about. The system can be used with conventional x-ray machines, no dark room is required and the prints, which are permanent on plastic coated paper, can be produced in 90 seconds.

The advantages of Xero-radiography of the breast are that details are more clearly defined than on conventional film and thus easier to interpret, there is a wide exposure latitude which means that operator errors are less critical, and because the plates are very sensitive less radiation exposure is required to produce good prints compared with other types of mammography.

Much of the pioneer work on breast Xero-radiography has been carried out by Wolfe in the United States (Wolfe, 1972). In a comparison with conventional mammography techniques (Wolfe, Dooley and Harkins, 1971), it was shown that the diagnosis of malignancy was significantly more accurate from Xero-radiographs than from conventional mammography films. Further trials of this promising technique are at present in progress.

6 Blood Tests

Research work has been progressing to discover a recognisable factor in the blood of patients with cancer, or those in whom there is a high risk of cancer. A carcinoembryonic antigen has been found in the plasma of patients with some tumours, including breast cancer, but unfortunately it is also present in some other diseases. It has also been shown that the lymphocytes of patients with cancer are sensitized to protein derived from the central nervous system and from human tumours, and that this test is positive in the very early stages of malignancy. Once again, problems have arisen because the test is also positive in some neurological conditions.

Investigations are also being carried out to detect chemical (mainly hormonal) changes in the urine of women with breast cancer or those at high risk, and although neither this work nor that described on the blood have progressed beyond the research stage, it seems possible that a practical screening test of this type will eventually emerge.

Discussion

All the reports on the uses of the more sophisticated equipment described have emanated from research projects or from highly specialized centres, and the practical problems of extending such facilities throughout the National Health Service in Britain are enormous. Even if clinical trials eventually justify such a course, there is likely to be strong competition in terms of finance and resources from other branches of medicine.

The obvious person to carry out routine screening is the family doctor, because of his close knowledge of, and contact with his patient, and because she is much more likely to respond to screening appeals from him than from others. It would however be quite impracticable for him to screen all his female patients over, say 35 or 40, once per year or anything like it. Even doing so every five years for cervical cytology requires considerable time and resources if a high screening rate is to be attained.

Furthermore it would obviously be impossible to install mammography equipment, or even the simpler Xero-radiography apparatus, in the doctor's premises. The cost would be prohibitive and the equipment underutilized except possibly in very large health centres. If screening were to be confined to clinics operated directly by the AHA (e.g. at the local hospital) it is likely that the same patchy response from the public would result as has occurred in many Local Health Authority cervical cytology clinics, and the expense involved would be hard to justify.

There are obviously considerable problems to be overcome, and screening for breast cancer for the whole population seems highly unlikely in the foreseeable future. What does seem more likely, if the results of current clinical trials prove sufficiently encouraging, is a limited screening programme aimed at groups of women with a higher than average risk of developing the disease. Identifying such women remains a problem, and eventually blood or urine tests may be able to pick out susceptible individuals, but even with present knowledge a case could be made for screening those over 40 in the following categories:

1 Nulliparous women, or those whose first child was born after age 30.

2 Women with a history of previous breast biopsy for benign or malignant conditions, including of course those who have undergone mastectomy for carcinoma in the other breast.

3 Those with a family history of breast cancer.

It ought to be possible to compile a list of such women in many practices without outside help, particularly if screening of one sort or another is already being undertaken; but if not the District Community Physician and his staff would be well placed to help in this sort of work. Such lists, with records of attendances etc., might well be computerized at Area or Regional level.

Women in the groups listed might then be offered yearly breast examination by their doctor, combined when appropriate with other screening procedures. This would be followed by Xero-radiographic (or mammography) examinations at the X-ray department of the District General Hospital, with reports being sent to the family doctor. It seems clear that this equipment would have to be based at the District General Hospital and under the control of the consultant radiologist, but provided free and open access was available for screening, and transport problems were overcome, this should not create difficulties. In rural areas there seems no reason why the Xero-radiographic apparatus could not be transported with ease to any peripheral unit which housed suitable X-ray equipment. The unified Health Service after 1974 should make co-operative screening programmes of this nature much easier to carry out, with perhaps a Health Care Planning Team co-ordinating the whole programme within the District.

In addition to routine screening, the mammography equipment would also be available as a diagnostic facility in normal clinical practice, and this would help to justify the high installation costs. A number of surveys have shown that in experienced hands, the technique is extremely accurate in distinguishing benign from malignant breast disease in women with palpable breast lumps, and thus it should be possible to reduce the number of breast biopsies carried out at present. Naturally, if biopsy is omitted or deferred, very careful follow-up is essential.

The relationship between breast feeding and subsequent breast cancer has attracted interest for some years, and reports have differed as to the protection afforded by breast feeding. It does seem, however, that a number of successful periods of lactation in early adult life may reduce the likelihood of breast cancer later on, and indeed it would hardly be surprising if breasts which had carried out their normal physiological function were less prone to disease than those which had not.

Unfortunately breast feeding is probably only one of a number of environmental factors which influence the development of breast cancer, and until more is known of the aetiology of the disease the incidence is unlikely to be significantly reduced. Nevertheless, in view of the many other advantages of breast feeding, general practitioners and their nursing staff might well exert more influence on their patients than at present in efforts to persuade them to breast feed their babies.

Conclusion

It will be clear that breast cancer screening is, to say the least, a controversial subject at the present time (1974). Public pressure at a political level is mounting for some form of national screening service on the lines of the cervical cytology service, but however much one may sympathise with the sentiments behind such moves, the long-term value of the various methods described for the early detection of the disease remains unproven. There is cause for optimism that regular mammography carried out on high-risk groups may bring about the first significant reduction in mortality rates for many years, but the results are not yet conclusive enough to justify the cost and effort of a national screening service. Further into the future, detection of early cases, or better still, the identification of those at risk, by blood or urine tests seems a real possibility.

REFERENCES

Davey, J. & Pentney, H. (1973). Preliminary findings from a women's screening unit. *The Practitioner*, 210, 541.
Gershon-Cohen, J., Ingleby, H., Berger, S. M., Forman, M. and Curcio, B. M. (1967). Mammographic screening for breast cancer. *Radiology*, 88, 663.
Gilbertson, V. A. (1966). Survival of asymptomatic breast cancer patients. *Surgery, Gynaecology and Obstetrics*, 122, 81.
Levene, A. (1973). Contribution to a cancer screening symposium. *British Clinical Journal*, 1, no. 1.
Shapiro, S., Strax, P. and Venet L. (1971). Periodic breast cancer screening in reducing mortality from breast cancer. *Journal of American Medical Association 215*, 11, 1777.

Stark, A. M. & Way, S. (1970). Screening for breast cancer. *Lancet,* 2, 407.
Wolfe, J. N., Dooley, R. & Harkins, L. (1971). Xero-radiography of the breast: a comparative study with conventional film mammographv. *Cancer,* 28, 1569.
Wolfe, J. N. (1972). Xero-radiography of the breast. Springfield, Illinois: Charles C. Thomas.
Wookey, B. E. P. (1971). A well-woman clinic in general practice. *British Medical Journal,* 1, 396.

24 Mental Illness
E. Wilkes

'It is sometimes suggested that screening for mental health is not a practical proposition. Nevertheless the magnitude of the mental health problem is such that techniques should be investigated. The present survey and results show a technique that appears to offer a valid mental health screening procedure.'

R.J. Donaldson, R.J. Kerry and J.E. Orme, 1969.

'Screening for psychiatric disorder must remain at the experimental phase and is not ready for inclusion in the medical services.'

M.R. Eastwood, 1971.

Although we think of mental health screening as something applicable to the community survey or as a help in the management of individual patients, it is not necessarily restricted to these roles. For example, an American survey of the medical personnel who had direct care of patients as compared with colleagues who did not have such direct care, and with a control group of equivalent socio-economic status, showed that the caring doctors had a higher incidence of drug-taking, of marital problems and of psychiatric consultations than the other two groups (Vaillant, Sobowale and McArthur, 1972). One might alter the old phrase to 'physician, screen thyself'.

However, in this chapter it is proposed to discuss only the factors which give urgency to mental health screening procedures, to survey briefly the literature, and to select from it what seems both valuable and practicable for the present conditions of British general practice.

None of the problems involved in the diagnosis and management of mental illness are unique. Indeed all of them are, to a variable degree, tractable and transient; yet the problems differ so much in degree from those encountered in other areas of medical practice that they nearly become differences in kind.

239

Most practitioners have graduated from medical schools in which psychological aspects of illness were discussed frequently and sensibly, but not as a central concern—that was the acute episode typified by the emergency appendicitis or the myocardial infarct. Yet the practitioner sees only five or six new cases of acute appendicitis or myocardial infarct each year (Fry, 1973) and these will loom less large in his day's work than his hospital experience has led him to expect. The incidence of minor psychiatric disorder on the other hand may mean that for the bulk of his work the doctor has neither training nor motivation.

Mental illnesses apparently accost him on a massive scale. Dohrenwend and Dohrenwend (1969) have reviewed the literature but the actual figures vary predictably with the population and even more with the observer. Taylor and Chave (1964) found that in every thousand patients 1·9 were admitted to a psychiatric hospital, 4·4 were referred to a psychiatric outpatient departemnt, 81 had treatment from the family doctor, and a further 330 had neurotic symptoms. Michael's survey (1960) indicated that in a London general practice 815 out of every thousand at risk had symptoms. In the same year Kessel (1960) found a psychiatric morbidity prevalence over one year of 50 per 1,000 patients, to which should be added morbidity with a conspicuous psychiatric component in another 90, as well as physical complaints without any confirmed organic basis in another 380 patients. A more recent survey found a psychiatric prevalence of psychosis in 5·9 per 1,000, of psychoneurosis in 88·8 per 1,000, and of psychophysiological problems in 45·7 per 1,000 (Shepherd et al., 1966). Middle-aged women were the biggest group and only 10 per cent of those with psychiatric symptoms were referred to a psychiatrist. Eastwood (1970) thought that 8 per cent of men and 24·5 per cent of women had psychiatric disorders and that the practitioner missed the diagnosis in one fifth of the men and in a quarter of the women. Those diagnosed by the practitioner had longer histories, more severe illnesses and a higher consultation rate.

This failure to assess psychiatric disorder accurately can be as damaging as with any other untreated acute illness. Barraclough, Nelson and Sainsbury (1968) in an analysis of 25 suicides found that nearly all of them had seen a general practitioner within a few weeks of suicide, that retrospective interviews with the family and scrutiny of their medical records revealed signs of depression in 80 per cent, but in only a few had the diagnosis been made and not one had received antidepressive therapy.

Yet the general practitioners clearly are not sitting idly. They are writing out annually over 250 million prescriptions—5·6 per patient at a cost of some £8,500 per doctor per year (Fry, 1973). 2·8 per cent of the population have been on psychotropic drugs for over a year (Woodcock, 1970) and the annual increase of the prescribing rate in the years 1965 to 1970 of the most popular tranquillisers was one to four million. Over the same period tricyclic antidepressive prescriptions increased by 320 per cent (Parish, 1971). The number of patients dependent on barbiturates—often socially valuable and responsible middle-aged women who resist any reduction or change of regime—is estimated at three million.

Implicit in these figures is a tremendous palliation of suffering and nervous disability; and there must be also the unwilling perpetuation of errors of clinical judgement. The coloured bottle of watery medicine was extremely valuable for most of the minor, self-limiting stress symptoms in the old-fashioned days of general practice. That 'the bottle' has been replaced by potent drugs gives the doctor due cause for nostalgia but little room for corrective manoeuvre. He is by instinct no pusher of powerful drugs. Indeed his treatment of advanced and painful malignant disease is, like that of his hospital colleagues, given often timidly and ineffectively, too little and too late. Why then the enormous deployment of psychotropic drugs?

One factor is the exaggerated and unrealistic expectation of badly briefed patients who cannot easily accept the difficulties and discomforts of the human predicament and who require that the pains of life be soothed away, whether due to a bereavement or a driving test, by the doctor's pill. This is a socially acceptable attitude—indeed it is the norm—but there are signs that in the next decade this may change. Now that intentional drug overdose is the commonest single cause for emergency medical admissions to hospital (Smith, 1972), few practitioners are complacent about the role they are playing. Most of the drug overdose cases are young people and practitioners may gradually become more cautious in their prescriptions as the facts are brought home to them. Many of the older and respectable drug-takers will stay on their preparations till they die, despite their and their doctors' unease; for, as with obesity, prevention is the only effective treatment. But as patients become more knowledgeable, they too will hesitate about starting something that cannot easily be finished.

Another important factor in the prescribing of psychotropic drugs is the attitude of the doctor to those patients who present either with nervous symptoms or with physical symptoms probably of nervous origin. Most doctors have not yet graduated to practice through a vocational training scheme and may not even have heard of Balint (Balint 1964, Balint et al., 1970). With many brilliant and devoted exceptions therefore, when faced with patients who are not physically ill, the doctor may treat his own impatience and bewilderment by writing a prescription. This may help. It may even work very well indeed. At the least, it serves as the doctor's admission ticket to his next consultation since it is so much quicker and easier than a calm, time-consuming discussion of the problem—a discussion for which the doctor may be badly equipped.

At the same time there is an increasing depersonalisation of primary medical care. With the amount of psychiatric disability in the community a personal doctor would be a really valuable support; but the doctor is himself by no means exempt from the prevailing social pressures. The general practitioner now, like his patients, requires more leisure than twenty years ago. His appointments system may even out the work-load but it can also be manipulated to discourage consultations with the more diffident but disturbed patient. As the single-handed doctor is gradually replaced by the group practice, the pooling of skills becomes on occasion less obvious than the sharing of off-duty. In some Health Centres the doctors still work in professional isolation so that the only things centralised are the heating, the secretarial work and the duty rota. At their worst such practices are as anonymous as any out-patient department, lacking only their clinical reliability.

The deputising services are now used by some three quarters of practitioners in the big cities. These effectively deal with 50 per cent of the doctor's night calls, five per cent of his home visits, but less than one per cent of his doctor-patient contacts. This seems an efficient and acceptable service (Williams, Dixon and Knowelden, 1973) but cannot buttress a doctor-patient relationship eroded already by other changes.

Home visiting, for example, is rapidly decreasing. The unjustifiable frequency of home visiting forty years ago was geared more to the retention of income than clinical need and dates from a time when the doctor had little to offer but himself. With an increased capacity for cure has come an increased disengagement. We realise, of course, that the home visit was not always a waste of time. The dirty kitchen with its pile of empty whisky bottles by the back door can be a vital sign unattainable in any streamlined office consultation. Yet in one thousand USA physicians questioned, 25 per cent did no home visits at all and 60 per cent did only between one and five per week (Gross, 1966).

If we work on a rota and do no visits we can still know our patients; but the increasing mobility of modern society means that, from a Canadian example (Wolfe and Badgley, 1972), one in three patients will probably need to establish rapport with a new doctor, because the old doctor will have moved on, every five years; but if the doctor does stay for 15 years, over half his patients will by then have removed (Beamen and Duwors, 1966). This occurs when 70 per cent of the practice population are consulting the doctor once a year or not at all (Wolfe and Badgley, 1972). Although it is said that after two years 85 per cent and after seven years 97 per cent of patients will have seen their doctor (Kessel and Shepherd, 1965), these figures are probably high for small town or country practices.

We can then summarise the background difficulties thus: a medical school education that may be ill-adapted to general practice, unrealistic demands by the patient, a diminished personal contact between doctor and patient, all combined with a large body of psychiatric illness, needing diagnosis and management.

In this environment, the commonest problem in general practice is the minor anxiety state. This can present in many different ways and often gives a much less florid picture than those available for demonstration in the psychiatric out-patient departments. They often occur in constitutionally susceptible people who have battled on for years with their problems but with a greater than average effort, and whose episodes can be remittent and self-limiting (Kerry, Orme and Wilkes, 1970), but are often chronic and of poor prognosis (Cooper, Fry and Kalton, 1969). Loneliness, boredom and affluence encourage symptoms. Young mothers and middle-aged women are the largest groups. Bad temper and irritability, tension and tears, the need for support without nearby friends or relatives to supply it, difficult young children or children who no longer need their mother, marital problems and a positive family history for minor mental illnesses, these are all too familiar to the experienced practitioner. As a consequence there is a danger of too easy and indiscriminate an acceptance by the doctor of these everyday complaints that attend upon him. Many must be able to recall the lady whose difficulties responded well for years to a therapeutic listen and a repeat prescription, and whose fatal illness was diagnosed late because the new symptoms were hidden among the old. This is inevitable since even neurotics die in the end.

What is much less defensible is the error perpetrated by good but harrassed doctors who diagnose neurotic symptoms without any adequate exclusion of organic disease. This situation is exemplified by the following true and unremarkable history.

A lady in her early fifties with no previous neurotic disorder went to see her doctor because she was feeling so very tired. The diagnosis of menopausal neurosis was made, and repeated several weeks later when she returned to say that she was feeling yet weaker and more tired. At this time a pinkish vaginal loss worse after coitus had been present for some months, but a brisk post-menopausal haemorrhage was needed to attain the eventual diagnosis of a disseminated carcinoma of cervix and to end all further talk of neuroticism.

Such a case highlights the dilemma of the general practitioner who lives in a world dominated at times by headache or fatigue, of breathlessness at rest but not on exertion, of bowel disturbance and chest pains, a huge haystack in which lies the needle of important, early, treatable disease. If any effective mental health screening is available, clearly it must be the general practitioner's tool since his need is greatest and it is his challenging responsibility neither to refer unnecessary trivia nor to block expert help from reaching patients in real need.

Screening will consist in practice of three elements: the diagnostic interview, which should be a basic skill; the medical, family and social history dependent on the interview plus the good records often deplorably absent in practice; and the specially designed questionnaire. The questionnaire is mainly a symptom check-list and can only be as reliable as the answers it is given. This reliability is increased by correlation with demographic and other relevant data, and is obviously suitable for computer analysis. One study of this type used the Minnesota Multiphasic Personality Inventory (MMPI) plus demographic data, a relative's history and other psychological test scores (Sletten, Altmann and Ulett, 1971). Merely from this automated check-list cases could be picked out who were more likely to be violent and so the clinician was alerted as to which patients were three times more likely to run away. The authors forecast that 'it will not be long before clinicians will demand computerized suggestions to help them care for their patients as they now demand laboratory reports'.

The Mayo Clinic in another paper on an automated personality inventory also based on the MMPI reported good acceptability by patients and increasing enthusiasm over the years by their physicians for this facility (Pearson et al., 1964). A comparison of over 10,000 patients by this means showed abnormal profiles in 42·7 per cent of medical and in 74 per cent of psychiatric cases. Large-scale handling of data is demonstrated by their intention to analyse 50,000 profiles in this way. More sophisticated studies claim good results from a computer programme applying the logical decision-tree to psychiatric diagnosis (Fleiss et al., 1972).

The MMPI is the most widely respected of the personality inventory scales. It is however a 566-question profile that despite its acceptability to American patients is not, by its sheer size, acceptable as a routine screening test. When combined with interview and demographic data, however, the MMPI gives good diagnostic indications and is of value in the further assessment of patients who have been found to have psychiatric problems by simpler means.

There are many shorter and simpler questionnaires and self-rating scales. Many items recur, and originate from work done years ago. These different tests all have their enthusiastic advocates and their number is hinted at by the title of a paper 'What! Another Rating Scale? The Psychiatric Evaluation Form' in which is described a procedure for measuring psychopathic traits and impairment in role functioning (Endicott and Spitzer, 1972b). Another paper seeks to compare, in measuring the relationship between depression and anxiety, the help received from the Beck Depression Inventory, the Zung Self-Rating Depression Scale, the Costello-Comfrey Scale for Depression and Anxiety, the Zuckerman Multiple Affect Adjective check-list, and the MMPI (Mendels, Weinstein and Cochrane, 1972). Correlation was still found difficult and at this stage one is tempted to agree with Cooper (1970) who thought that 'it may well prove to be unrealistic to expect comparatively crude questionnaire procedures to achieve clear-cut differentiation between personality traits and symptoms of illness'.

On the other hand, there are questionnaires that may not be suitable for general practice but still have a genuine though limited value. Current and Past Psychopathology Scales (CAPPS—Endicott and Spitzer, 1972a) give a complex but reliable guide to the severity of an illness and its prognosis by covering past and present functioning. The In-Patient Multidimensional Psychiatric Scale (IMPS—Lorr and Klett, 1967) correlated well with the clinical diagnosis reached after interview and differentiated usefully between mania and paranoid schizophrenia (Kerry and Orme 1972). The Cornell Medical Index or CMI, (Brodmann, Erdmann, Lorge, Wolff and Broadbent, 1949) succeeds in separating the normal from the neurotic patient (Culpen, Davies and Oppenheim, 1960) but it is a self-administered four-page document containing 195 questions and 18 sections, of which the last six deal with emotional disorders. Again too lengthy for our purposes, 20 items selected from it in a psychiatric survey led Eastwood (1971) to the somewhat pessimistic pronouncement that heads this chapter.

The Hamilton Rating Scale in depression (Salkind, 1969) is considered concise and sensitive, but by comparison with the Beck Depression Inventory (Beck, Ward and Mendelson, 1961) it is not self-rating, it does not have a 'cutting score', and it is more time-consuming.

The Eysenck Personality Index measures the degree of extroversion and of neuroticism in a patient (Eysenck and Eysenck, 1964, Eysenck 1959). The extroversion rating seems fairly consistent but the neuroticism rates vary more with the course of the illness.

The EPI distinguishes well between the normal and the neurotic patient, adds to accuracy of prognosis (Kerr, Schapira, Roth and Garside, 1970) and despite a rather poor correlation with the CMI (Verghese, 1970) is short, straight-forward and nearly a practical possibility for the general practitioner.

In the event, however, only two tests are thought suitable for routine use by the general practitioner—the Orme questionnaire (Orme, 1965) and the modified Beck Depression Index (Beck and Beck, 1972). These are simple, unembarrassing, quick to administer and score, and alone deserve a more detailed description.

The Orme Questionnaire is reproduced in Appendix A to this chapter. It consists of 13 questions plus seven dummy questions that are not scored. It should take less than five minutes to complete.

Each question is typed on a separate card and is handed to the patient, one card at a time. A box is provided with three compartments labelled Yes, No and Don't Know. The patient goes quickly through the questions, putting the cards into the compartments as is correct for him. On the back of each card is the scoring code so that the final score is quickly reached. Don't Know scores 1, but since the dummy questions are inserted just to interfere with the patient's appreciation of the test, they are never scored. Scorable answers score 0 in the right compartment but 2 in the wrong compartment. The theoretical maximum score is thus 26.

From the testing of nearly 500 patients in public health clinics we know that only two per cent of normal patients will score 18 or more, while 67 per cent of psychiatric patients reach that score (Donaldson, Kerry and Orme, 1969). In a survey in a general practice with most of the patients well known to their doctors the test attained an accuracy of over 90 per cent in its positive findings and the abnormal scores also correlated well with their MMPI profiles (Evans, Wilkes and Dalrymple-Smith, 1969).

The positive findings are non-specific as to psychiatric diagnosis. Negative findings can of course be false—intelligent but unco-operative neurotics, hysterics and schizophrenics can all give scores within the normal range. We can reasonably say, however, that patients scoring 18 or more are likely to be vulnerable or neurotic personalities and, given a high standard of clinical judgement and the reasonable exclusion of concomitant organic disease, the Orme Questionnaire is a helpful guide to the likelihood of psychiatric disorder. It has revealed up to five per cent of abnormal scorers in the community. Further study of these by interview and MMPI has shown that anxiety, depression and social difficulties of various kinds are the main problems to be uncovered, though about a fifth of the abnormal scorers have paranoid or schizoid features.

Neuroticism seems to be the factor most easily diagnosed through the symptom check-list questionnaire. It may well be, therefore, that Rawnsley's modification of the Cornell Medical Index or the Middlesex Hospital Questionnaire are in no way diagnostically inferior. But the speed and simplicity of the Orme Questionnaire also underline the limitations of the test and enhance its suitability as a general practice screening technique.

The Beck Depression Inventory (BDI) aims at an equivalent function in picking up cases of depression. This is so frequent a general practice responsibility that Kline (1967) thought that depression was the commonest psychiatric illness treated outside of institutions. Salkind (1969) found that of 80 consecutive consultations in general practice 48 per cent of the patients were in a depressed state. Rawnsley (1968) thought that most cases of depression were treated solely by the general practitioner. The last two authors both thought that the BDI helped in diagnosis and also in assessing the severity of cases and both thought the BDI suitable for use in general practice. They had used the BDI in its original form (Beck, Ward and Mendelson, 1961). Since then the modified version has reduced the 21 items of the original version to 13, while retaining a correlation of 0·96 with the full BDI (Beck and Beck, 1972). The full version took ten minutes to score, but the shorter version should take a good deal less than this. It is reproduced in Appendix B, together with the recommended scoring.

There is, however, a little doubt as to whether the scoring is not too sensitive. Beck and Beck class 5-7 as a mild and 8-15 as moderate cases of depression: but our society is a difficult and changing society, and to feel bewildered by it, helpless before its more vicious and degenerate features, and to lack at times hope and energy and optimism may well be signs of sanity rather than of emotional disturbance. In this situation 10-15 may be taken as perhaps a reasonable score for moderate depression. There is no argument about scores of 16 or more signifying severe depression.

Even in cases of severe depression, however, physical complaints such as almost unendurable pain may dominate the clinical picture. These somatic symptoms will settle as the depression responds to treatment (Beck, 1972), but the BDI can help in differential diagnosis at perhaps an earlier stage. In a series of manic depressive patients one third produced physical symptoms as their main complaint but the BDI differentiated well between depression and anxiety when compared with the depression scale of the MMPI (Beck and Beck, 1972).

It is not claimed that the BDI is clinically superior to, say, the British Hospital Progress Test designed by Victor Cantor: but in its abridged form the Beck Depression Inventory is as easy to use as the Orme Questionnaire, and in these two well-validated and easy techniques we seem to have practical methods for indicating to the doctor the degree of non-specific neuroticism or vulnerability, of anxiety or of depression, that faces him across the desk. These episodes are often self-limiting (Rawnsley, 1968) and they are the very stuff of general practice.

These techniques could also be of tremendous screening value in restricting psychotropic drugs to those who really do need them. This factor could push Mental Health Screening with unexpected speed more into the foreground of routine medical care.

These screening techniques are just methods of weighting a clinical history, yet they must be exploited sensitively and not rigidly. Our professional conservatism is so great that we are less likely to use them clumsily than not to use them at all. One can only say that the need is clear and the techniques are ready and waiting.

Screening techniques in the field of mental health can never be a substitute for the thirty or forty minute interview. This can usher in a close and mutually respecting relationship between doctor and patient while surveying a whole life's background and difficulties. These techniques merely guide the doctor towards those patients who should have his full attention for a duration of time that may be routine in hospital practice but is a rare and lengthy luxury in the hurly-burly of general practice outside the gates.

APPENDIX A. Orme Questionnaire

1.	Do you often want to be with people who will 'cheer you up'?	Yes (scores 2)
2.	When you go to bed do you lie awake a long time before falling asleep?	Yes (scores 2)
3.	Have you ever walked in your sleep?	Buffer (scores 0)
4.	Do you feel adjusted to life?	No (scores 2)
5.	Do you cope fairly well with emergencies?	No (scores 2)
6.	Have you ever fainted or 'blacked out'?	Buffer (scores 0)
7.	Do failures make you work harder?	No (scores 2)
8.	Have you ever done things and later on found you don't know you have been doing them?	Buffer (scores 0)
9.	Are you inclined to worry without any reason for doing so?	Yes (scores 2)
10.	Do you feel you are no good and will never make a success of life?	Yes (scores 2)

11.	Can you usually fall asleep at any time of the day?	Buffer (scores 0)
12.	Are you upset if people make fun of you?	Yes (scores 2)
13.	Do you get downhearted if people don't appreciate you enough?	Yes (score 2)
14.	Are there events in your life which you should be able to remember but can't?	Buffer (scores 0)
15.	Do you have periods of feeling irritable when you don't want to see anyone?	Yes (scores 2)
16.	Can you relax and take it easy when you have time to do so?	No (scores 2)
17.	Are you quick in making decisions?	Buffer (scores 0)
18.	Do you sometimes wake in the night and through worrying have difficulty in going back to sleep?	Yes (scores 2)
19.	Do you make friends easily?	Buffer (scores 0)
20.	Have you ever had a sudden sense of dread and danger for no reason?	Yes (scores 2)

SCORING CODE suggested for back of cards

X - buffer and never scored
N2 - 2 when in 'No' compartment only
Y2 - 2 when in 'Yes' compartment only
N.B. - All 'Don't Knows' except buffer items score 1
Scores of 18 or more are considered abnormal

APPENDIX B. Beck Depression Inventory, short form.

Instructions: This is a questionnaire. On the questionnaire are groups of statements. Please read the entire group of statements in each category. Then pick out the one statement in that group which best described the way you feel today, that is, *right now!* Circle the number beside the statement you have chosen. If several statements in the group seem to apply equally well, circle each one.

Be sure to read all the statements in each group before making your choice.

A. (Sadness)
3 I am so sad or unhappy that I can't stand it.
2 I am blue or sad all the time and I can't snap out of it.
1 I feel sad or blue.
0 I do not feel sad.

B. (Pessimism)
3 I feel that the future is hopeless and that things cannot improve.
2 I feel I have nothing to look forward to.
1 I feel discouraged about the future.
0 I am not particularly pessimistic or discouraged about the future.

C. (Sense of failure)
3   I feel I am a complete failure as a person (parent, husband, wife).
2   As I look back on my life, all I can see is a lot of failures.
1. I feel I have failed more than the average person.
0   I do not feel like a failure.

D. (Dissatisfaction)
3   I am dissatisfied with everything.
2   I don't get satisfaction out of anything anymore.
1   I don't enjoy things the way I used to.
0   I am not particularly dissatisfied.

E. (Guilt)
3   I feel as though I am very bad or worthless.
2   I feel quite guilty.
1   I feel bad or unworthy a good part of the time.
0   I don't feel particularly guilty.

F. (Self-dislike)
3   I hate myself.
2   I am disgusted with myself.
1   I am disappointed in myself.
0   I don't feel disappointed in myself.

G. (Self-harm)
3   I would kill myself if I had the chance.
2   I have definite plans about committing suicide.
1   I feel I would be better off dead.
0   I don't have any thoughts of harming myself.

H. (Social withdrawal)
3   I have lost all of my interest in other people and don't care about them at all.
2   I have lost most of my interest in other people and have little feeling for them.
1   I am less interested in other people than I used to be.
0   I have not lost interest in other people.

I. (Indecisiveness)
3   I can't make any decisions at all anymore.
2   I have great difficulty in making decisions.
1   I try to put off making decisions.
0   I make decisions about as well as ever.

J. (Self-image change)
3   I feel that I am ugly or repulsive-looking.
2   I feel that there are permanent changes in my appearance and they make me look unattractive.
1   I am worried that I am looking old or unattractive.
0   I don't feel that I look any worse than I used to.

K. (Work difficulty)
3   I can't do any work at all.
2   I have to push myself very hard to do anything.
1   It takes extra effort to get started at doing something.
0   I can work about as well as before.

L. (Fatigueability)
3   I get too tired to do anything.
2   I get tired from doing anything.
1   I get tired more easily than I used to.
0   I don't get any more tired than usual.

M. (Anorexia)
3   I have no appetite at all anymore.
2   My appetite is much worse now.
1   My appetite is not as good as it used to be.
0   My appetite is no worse than usual.

ESTIMATED DEGREE OF DEPRESSION ACCORDING TO BDI SCORE

Range of Scores	Degree of Depression
0–4	None or minimal
5–7	Mild
8–15	Moderate
16+	Severe

Note comments re scoring scale on page 247

REFERENCES

Balint, M. (1964). *The Doctor, the Patient and his Illness,* 2nd ed. London: Pittman.

Balint, M., Hunt, J., Joyce, D., Marinker, M. & Woodcock, J. (1970). *Treatment or Diagnosis.* A study of repeat prescriptions in general practice. London: Tavistock Publications. J.B. Lippincot Co.

Barraclough, B. M., Nelson, B. & Sainsbury, P. (1968). The diagnostic classification and psychiatric treatment of 25 suicides. *Proceedings of the Fourth International Conference for Suicide Prevention.* Los Angeles: Delmar Publishing Co. Inc.

Beamen, J. & Duwors, R. E. (1966). Dynamics of residential population change in six prairie cities. *Canadian Medical Association Journal,* 94, 955.

Beck, A. T., Ward, C. H. & Mendelson, M. (1961). An Inventory for measuring depression. *Archives of General Psychiatry,* 4, 561.

Beck, A. T. & Beck, R. W. (1972). Screening depressed patients in family practice: a rapid technic. *Postgraduate Medical Journal,* 52, 81.

Beck, A. T. (1972). *Depression: Causes and Treatment.* Philadelphia: University of Philadelphia Press.

Brodmann, K., Erdmann, A. J. Jr., Lorge, I., Wolff, H. G. & Broadbent, T. H. (1949). The Cornell Medical Index—an adjunct to medical interview. *Journal of the American Medical Association,* 140, 530.

Cooper, B., Fry, J. & Kalton, G. W. (1969). A longitudinal study of psychiatric morbidity in a general practice population. *British Journal of Preventive and Social Medicine,* 23, 210.

Cooper, J. (1970). The Leyton Obsession Inventory. *Psychological Medicine,* 1, 48.

Culpen, R. H., Davies, B. M. & Oppenheim, A. N. (1960). Incidence of psychiatric illness among hospital out-patients: an application of the Cornell Medical Index. *British Medical Journal,* 1, 855.

Department of Health & Social Security Symposium (1973). The medical use of psychotropic drugs. *Journal of the Royal College of General Practitioners,* 23, Supplt.2.

Dohrenwend, B. P. & Dohrenwend, B. S. (1969). *Social Status and Psychological Disorder.* A causal inquiry. New York: Wiley.

Donaldson, R. J., Kerry, R. J. & Orme, J. E. (1969). A community mental health screening procedure. *Acta Psychiatrica Scandinavica,* 45, 198.

Eastwood, M. R. (1970). The physical status of psychiatric emergencies. *British Journal of Psychiatry,* 116, 545.

Eastwood, M. R. (1971). Screening for psychiatric disorder. *Psychological Medicine,* 1, 197.

Endicott, J. & Spitzer, R. L. (1972a). Current and past psychopathology scales. *Archives of General Psychiatry,* 27, 678.

Endicott, J. & Spitzer, R. L. (1972b). What! Another rating scale? The Psychiatric Evaluation form. *Journal of Nervous and Mental Diseases,* 154, 88.

Evans, S. M., Wilkes, E. & Dalrymple-Smith, D. (1969). Presymptomatic diagnosis. *Journal of the Royal College of General Practitioners,* 17, 237.

Eysenck, H. J. (1959). The differentiation between normal and various neurotic groups on the Maudsley Personality Inventory. *British Journal of Psychology,* 50, 176.

Eysenck, H. J. & Eysenck, S. B. G. (1964). *Manual of the Eysenck Personality Inventory.* University of London Press.

Fleiss, J. L., Spitzer, R. L., Cohen, J. & Endicott, J. (1972). Three computer diagnosis methods compared. *Archives of General Psychiatry,* 27, 643.

Fry, J. (1973). Present state and future needs of general practice. Report from General Practice No.16. 3rd ed. *Journal of the Royal College of General Practitioners,* 23, Supplt. 1.

Gross, M. L. (1966). *The Doctors.* New York: Random House.

Kerr, T. A., Schapira, K., Roth, M. & Garside, R. T. (1970). The relationship between the Maudsley Personality Inventory and the course of affective disorders. *British Journal of Psychiatry,* 116, 11.

Kerry, R. J., Orme, J. E. & Wilkes, E. (1970). Personality testing: a new diagnostic aid. *The Practitioner,* 205, 217.

Kerry, R. J. & Orme, J. E. (1972). Psychiatric diagnosis and the In-Patient Multidimensional Psychiatric Scale. *British Journal of Psychiatry,* 121, 541.

Kessel, N. & Shepherd, M. (1965). The health and attitudes of people who seldom consult their doctor. *Medical Care,* 3, 6.

Kessel, W. L. N. (1960). Psychiatric morbidity in a London general practice. *British Journal of Preventive and Social Medicine,* 14, 16.

Kline, N. S. (1967). Psychopharmacologic drugs. *Postgraduate Medical Journal,* 42, 268.

Lorr, M. & Klett, C. J. (1967). *In-Patient Multidimensional Psychiatric Scale.* Palo Alto: California Consulting Psychologists Press.

Mendels, J., Weinstein, N. & Cochrane, C. (1972). The relationship between depression and anxiety. *Archives of General Psychiatry,* 27, 649.

Michael, S. T. (1960). Social attitudes, socio-economic status and psychiatric symptoms. *Acta Psychologica et Neurologica Scandinavica,* 35, 509.

Orme, J. E. (1965). The relationship of obsessional traits to general emotional instability. *British Journal of Psychology,* 38, 269.

Parish, P. A. (1971). The prescribing of psychotrophic drugs in general practice. *Journal of the Royal College of General Practitioners,* 21, Supplt. No. 4.

Pearson, J. S., Swanson, W. M., Rome, H. D., Mataya, P. & Brannick, T. L. (1964). Automated Personality Inventory. *Mayo Clinic Proceedings,* 39, 823.

Rawnsley, K. (1968). *The Early Diagnosis of Depression.* Early Diagnosis Paper No.4., London: Office of Health Economics.

Salkind, M. R. (1969). Beck Depression Inventory in general practice. *Journal of the Royal College of General Practitioners,* 18, 267.

Shepherd, M., Cooper, B., Brown, A. C. & Kalton, G. W. (1966). *Psychiatric Illness in General Practice.* London: OUP.

Sletten, I. W., Altmann, H. & Ulett, G. A. (1971). Routine diagnosis by computer. *American Journal of Psychiatry,* 9, 67.

Smith, A. J. (1972). Self poisoning with drugs—a worsening situation. *British Medical Journal,* 4, 157.

Spiro, H. R., Siassi, I. & Crocetti, G. M. (1972). What gets surveyed in a psychiatric survey? *Journal of Nervous and Mental Diseases,* 154, 105.

Taylor, Lord, & Chave, S. P. W. (1964). *Mental Health and Environment.* London: Longman.

Vaillant, G. E., Sobowale, N. C. & McArthur, C. (1972). Some psychologic vulnerabilities of physicians. *New England Journal of Medicine,* 287, 372.

Verghese, A. (1970). Relationship between the Eysenck Personality Inventory N Score, the Cornell Medical Index M-R Score and the psychogalvanic reflex. *British Journal of Psychiatry,* 116, 27.

Williams, B. T., Dixon, R. & Knowelden, J. (1973). BMA Deputizing Service in Sheffield 1970. *British Medical Journal,* 1, 593.

Wolfe, S. & Badgley, R. F. (1972). *The Family Doctor.* Milbank Memorial Fund. Vol. 1, No. 2.

Woodcock, J. (1970). Long-term consumers of psychotropic drugs, in Balint M. *et al.*

IV Screening Techniques

25 Questionnaires

J.R. Murray

'Them that asks no questions isn't told a lie.'

Kipling.

The success or failure of screening surveys depends very largely on the quality of the questionnaire. Once the aims and objects of the survey have been clearly defined, work can begin on the form that the questionnaire will take. It will help enormously if the problems that are likely to occur at the stage of analysis of the results are considered from the outset. A questionnaire designed with analysis in mind will be neater, easier to use and save a great deal of work at a later date.

Validity and reliability

Questions must be phrased so that the answers give precisely the information needed. There should be no ambiguity; the respondent should understand exactly what the question means. All patients answering a given question ought to interpret it in the same way. This may seem obvious but it is surprising the number of surveys that are published with results that lack validity because the questions have been badly constructed, leaving the results open to various interpretations. Reliability of answers must also be considered. If the same question is asked at a later date, given no change in the patient's circumstances as related to the question, the answer should be the same.

The use of technical jargon will confuse patients. However, even widely accepted terms may be misinterpreted on occasions. We all know of the patient who thinks that having his bowels open is vomiting and the other who thinks it is the same as passing urine.

Questions that are too wide in their scope will produce answers that are difficult to summarise and classify. Other questions may be so narrow as to give precise but limited information.

It is important to ask questions that will receive honest answers. Some questions are hardly worth asking at all—'How many cigarettes do you smoke a day?' 'How much alcohol do you drink each day?', 'How frequently do you make love to your wife?' There are too many personal implications behind the questions for them to be answered truthfully. The patient is more likely to give what he thinks ought to be the answer.

What is the meaning of the answer to a question such as 'Do you think you would benefit by having a wheelchair?' Supposing the patient answers 'Yes', does this mean that he genuinely does believe that the quality of his life would be greatly improved by having a wheelchair, or does he mean 'not really, but anything going free I'll take'? Perhaps he feels that the questioner is trying to help him and he says 'Yes' so that he doesn't cause disappointment. He may even mean 'If I have a wheelchair, someone will have to push me around and I could do with some extra attention.' Conversely, 'No' can mean 'I don't believe the quality of my life would be enhanced by one', 'I have already cost the Welfare State a fortune in medical care and I don't want to be greedy', 'Someone will have to push me around and I don't want to be a burden', or 'I'm damned if I'll let you put me in a wheelchair'. The question asks for an answer that lacks reliability and validity. Moreover it also illustrates another mistake in the construction of questions. By its wording the question implies that a wheelchair will be provided if the answer is 'Yes'. It may well be that the patient's condition would deteriorate if a wheelchair were given, even though he would like one. It could also be that it is financially impossible to provide enough wheelchairs for those needing them.

Intimate questions are likely to be answered untruthfully unless tactfully phrased, or asked by someone who has the patient's full confidence. Leading questions are a mistake, but the leading sexual question is a disaster. 'What problems do you have with your sex life?' For a start, the patient is likely to be upset by the insinuation that he must have sexual problems. Secondly, he or she is unlikely to want the details of his or her sex life committed firmly to paper.

The question 'Do you have any problems with the curse?' illustrates two other points. If answered merely by the affirmative, it means nothing unless further details are requested. Moreover, the use of loaded words such as 'curse' can invalidate the answer. Although it is commendably colloquial, its use does imply that the questioner expects the respondent to have problems and the patient may feel obliged to answer 'Yes' so that the questioner doesn't regard her as being 'odd' or 'unclean'. If the next question asks her to list details of the problems she has with her periods, she may then be in the position of having to exaggerate minor symptoms or even to invent some.

Combined or double questions should also be avoided as the meaning of the answer isn't always clear. For example, what does the answer 'Yes' mean when applied to the question 'Do you suffer from diarrhoea or vomiting?' This question also shows the problems involved in using words that are not clearly defined. Diarrhoea means different things to different people, as we all know only too well.

Although it is terribly frustrating to find at the analysis stage that too few questions have been asked, there are risks attached to asking too many. Boredom can easily occur to both interviewer and patient.

> 'I have answered three questions and that is enough,'
> Said his father 'Don't give yourself airs!
> Do you think I can listen all day to such stuff?
> Be off, or I'll kick you downstairs!'
>
> Lewis Carroll.

Types of Questions

Questions can be closed or open. With the closed question the respondent has no need to write anything. The answer is given by ticking, circling or underlining one of a printed list of possibilities. This is particularly useful for self-administered questionnaires (see below). It is important that the questions are readily understood and that they really do ask for a specific answer. The patient should be well briefed and the words used clearly defined. These questions are relatively crude and require careful pilot work; however, coding is simple and can be built into the questionnaire.

e.g. Q. Have you in the past suffered from any of the following? (Please ring the number in the appropriate column)

	Yes	No	Don't Know
Scarlet fever	1	2	3
Rheumatic fever	1	2	3
Mumps	1	2	3

Other examples of closed questions:

Q.   Please place a tick in the box next to the statement that
     most applies to you.
     (Please tick only ONE box).
     Self Hate

I don't feel disappointed in myself	☐	1
I am disappointed in myself	☐	2
I don't like myself	☐	3
I am disgusted with myself	☐	4
I hate myself	☐	5

The above question (from the Beck Depression Inventory) illustrates
a statistical point. An odd number of questions allows the patient to
choose the 'safe', middle answer; if an even number is used, the
patient has to commit himself.

Q.   Please place a tick in the column that you think is most
     appropriate when applied to the following characteristics
     of drug A.

	Very important	Some importance	No importance
Single daily dose			
Capsule form			
No gastric irritation			

Q.   The patient is asked to imagine a line representing pain as
     shown below. He or she is then asked to place a cross on
     the line at a point that most appropriately represents the
     pain that he is presently suffering

No pain |————————————| The most severe
at all   pain I've ever had.

These last three methods not only record information but also
grade it.

Open questions require the respondent to write relatively lengthy
answers. For instance, drug addicts could be asked the question:-

Q.   'Describe the feeling you have inside you when you are desperate for a "fix".'

A great deal of information can be obtained from these questions but they can be very difficult to code.

Data Collection

Basically there are two ways in which information can be obtained—either by direct questioning or by the individual completing a self-administered questionnaire.

Direct questioning has the advantage that one is able to ask more complicated questions and to use open questions more often. Terms used in the questions can be explained to the patient who has difficulty in understanding them, and probing can occur. However, it is more time consuming and expensive of skilled labour. It is also open to interviewer induced bias. Changes in tone of voice, agreement with the patient, helping the reticent patient may all lead to inaccurate answers. Probing can often cause more problems than it solves. The personality of the interviewer and his particular mood will also influence the replies.

The interviewer must be trained and thoroughly briefed about the aims and objects of the trial and the meaning of the questions. 'Back-up' notes to questions will help. Health visitors, social workers, district and practice nurses, and the GP himself may be involved in the collection of data.

Social problems are best assessed in the home, whereas physical examinations and laboratory investigations are more easily carried out in the surgery. The questions should be interesting for both interviewer and patient, and one topic should flow smoothly into the next. The confidential nature of the survey must be stressed, especially when the GP is not the interviewer. The patient should, of course, be fully informed of the reasons for the survey.

Self-administered questionnaires are less time consuming and relatively inexpensive. Questionnaires can be mailed to each household or distributed to patients as they present at the surgery. They are particularly useful as a means of informing the group to be screened of the programme intended and to find out which patients qualify to be included in the survey and which of these wish to participate. The patient may then attend the surgery for direct questioning.

The last point is illustrated by recent Social Services Department surveys of the physically and mentally handicapped in the local community. An initial questionnaire was delivered to every household in the district using volunteers from local youth organisations. After a few weeks the forms were collected. The questions were mainly of the closed variety and were simple to answer. The layout was attractive and the questions polite and interesting. The questionnaire was designed to explain the reasons for the survey and to find the handicapped people in the area. Those patients/clients qualifying for inclusion in the main part of the survey were then visited by sociology students from the local university and a detailed personal or direct questionnaire completed. The direct questionnaire collected the most important information.

Self administered questionnaires are inevitably cruder than personal, direct ones and rely more heavily on closed question techniques. An attractive layout, interesting questions that are designed to help the respondent feel that the survey has his interests at heart, an initial explanation of the survey stressing the confidential nature, all help to increase the rate of return. It is particularly important to avoid technical terms. However, do not insult the better educated whilst trying to make sure everyone understands the questions. Answers should be made easy and consistent, e.g. ticks for every answer. Keep open questions to a minimum. The answers to open questions can be limited by the use of boxes and lines that restrict the amount of space available for the reply. The intelligent use of different type forms, insets and headings will help the patient to understand the exact point of each question and aid the reply. The patient must be briefed adequately in the opening paragraph and all instructions should be crystal clear.

The main disadvantage of the mailed questionnaire is the poor return rates. A 40 per cent—60 per cent return rate is to be expected.

Whichever type of questionnaire is chosen, a great deal of pilot work will be necessary if it is to be competently constructed.

Specific Surveys

The actual questions to be asked will obviously vary with the survey. Previous chapters will have given ideas. Questionnaires used by previous researchers of the topic to be screened may have been published, and the librarians of the Royal Colleges, the BMA, Royal Society of Medicine and local post graduate centres may be able to obtain photostat copies. These will give valuable background ideas for your own scheme.

When the questionnaire has been drawn up, invite colleagues to criticise it and then try it out on a pilot sample of the population to be screened. The inadequacies of the format will rapidly become evident.

A4 paper is a convenient size for records. It gives ample room for questions and answers and would conform with the Department's projected recording system. Moreover, folded into four, it fits neatly into the existing record envelopes.

Processing the Answers

This is a simple procedure with precoded and most closed questions. The answers are readily represented numerically and can then be recorded on IBM punch-cards and filed in appropriate stacks, or read electronically, converted to punch-tape and fed into a computer (*See* Chapter 6).

For small surveys, edge-punched cards are very useful. These have holes around the edges related to specific answers. Using a pair of clippers, a wedge is cut between the edge of the card and the hole. The card can be designed so that it is the original questionnaire. The cards are separated into appropriate stacks merely by inserting a needle into the requisite hole and letting the punched cards drop out. This is a cheap method that doesn't require sophisticated equipment.

Open questions are more difficult to process. The data has to be converted to numerical form by strict classification. This will inevitably involve rejecting information. It is therefore very important to define carefully the aims and objects of the survey, and to remember them at this stage.

The answers to each separate question are collected together and tabulated. By examining the list carefully a number of categories are devised. More than twelve categories become unwieldy, especially when using edge-punch cards. The categories are then coded and tried on another sample of results to check whether they need further amendment.

Code books or sheets are then drawn up for the use of the coders (e.g. E book code sheets produced by the Royal College of General Practitioners). If a secretary is employed as coder, it is important to brief her well so that she is capable of checking for inconsistencies. The more stages and people involved in recording information, the more frequently will errors occur. Try to keep the handling stages to a minimum.

Statistical analysis of the results is best performed by the expert. Most hospital groups have statisticians, and local universities will have departments of mathematics. Frequently they can be persuaded to help in the survey results and analysis. This stage involves techniques not really lending themselves to management by the enthusiastic amateur, who can easily misrepresent information painfully collected. It is best to call in the help of the statistician at an early stage in planning the questionnaire.

'All things began in order, so shall they end.'

Sir Thomas Browne.

The main reason for screening is to provide a prophylactic medical service to the community. The patient should be made aware of the reasons behind the survey and how the survey can be to his direct advantage if he participates in it. There will be many general practitioners who will want to discover latent illness in their patients, and will not be interested in publishing the results. However, it is very important to be able to analyse results obtained, even if papers are not going to be written. Unless the GP can see his results clearly tabulated, the success or otherwise of the survey will not be apparent. A useless exercise may continue to take up valuable time with no real benefit to anyone. Conversely, a startling piece of epidemiological information may be overlooked.

What may seem to be data processing for its own sake may turn out to be a real service to mankind.

REFERENCES

Some of the ideas and principles discussed in this chapter are to be found in the books by Payne, Cannel, and Oppenheim listed in the Bibliography on pp. 329-330.

26 *Automated Blood Tests*   *B.T.B. Manners*

'All our knowledge brings us nearer to our ignorance . . .
Where is the wisdom we have lost in knowledge,
Where is the knowledge we have lost in information'
Chorus I, *The Rock*. T.S. Eliot.

The wide acceptance of chemical screening tests will present the doctor with a great mass of numerated data. However, the technological revolution in automated chemistry is not paralleled by our understanding either of the data or of the natural history of the disease studied, whether treated or untreated. Further, biochemical data alone have limited diagnostic and prognostic value.

The ability of continuous flow analysis (e.g. 'Autoanalyser') methods to estimate 20 substances in a single sample of blood permits screening for diseases which are associated with biochemical abnormalities. This ability to perform biochemical screening tests is not in question; the problem lies in deciding for which disease to screen, and whether recognition of the disease in the symptomless individual will bring mutual benefit to the doctor and his new patient (Carmalt, 1973).

Quality control of results provided by chemical analyses is important, because laboratory errors can affect the clinical value of results. Errors outside laboratory control include faults in collection, (prolonged use of tourniquet, squirting blood through the needle), preservation and labelling of samples, and the failure to state what drugs have been taken by the individual (which may render the results ridiculous).

Normality

A common trap is to deduce that because certain ill persons have a particular biochemical abnormality, it follows that the presence of the same abnormality in a symptomless individual necessarily means disease. In practice few analyses are pathognomonic for a particular disease. Limitations in the usefulness of a test lie in its specificity, sensitivity, analytic accuracy and the extent of deviation from normal.

The normal range of any analysis is usually dependent on age, sex, recent food and drink, time of day or even of month. Current practice defines the normal range of a substance as the mean value, for the stated population, plus or minus two standard deviations. In a normally distributed population, this includes 95 per cent of individuals. Hence by definition five per cent will be outside the normal range. If sufficient independent measurements are estimated (e.g. 20 tests) every individual may be expected to show one 'abnormality'. Hence biochemical abnormality is a statistical concept, and requires clinical judgement before it is equated with disease; the latter is a clinical concept, implying an adverse effect on the host.

Diseases suitable for detection by biochemical screening

General. Before using a screening test, the possible diagnosis suggested by the use of the test must be considered, also the prevalence of the disease in the studied population, and which further diagnostic methods will establish the diagnosis.

Mass screening involving a whole age group is used for common disorders. For unusual diseases it is wisest only to screen those who are already at high risk because of factors in the personal or family history; this is first line screening by history.

Diabetes and ischaemic heart disease (IHD) are common diseases in western society and are associated respectively with hyperglycaemia and with hyperlipidemia. Although the positive relationship between diabetes and hyperglycaemia is accepted, the degree of hyperglycaemia necessary for diagnosis is arguable. The relationship between IHD and hyperlipidemia is inconstant; the value of treating hyperlipidemia to reduce IHD remains to be proved; paradoxically the detection of hyperlipidemia is widely advocated. Both these diseases are closely linked with the manner of western civilization— lack of exercise at work and leisure, mental stress, cigarette smoking, alcohol, refined sucrose, and saturated animal fat. Obesity and hypertension point the way to both diabetes and ischaemic heart disease.

Diabetes. Epidemiological surveys show increasing diabetes in affluent countries, but comparatively little in primitive unmechanized societies. It has long been recognized that diabetes is a disorder of civilization whilst famine reduces its incidence. Contributory factors include a higher proportion of elderly people in the community, more obesity and lack of muscular exercise. It is likely that Rousseau's 'noble savage' had a low prevalence of diabetes and IHD to compensate for his lack of sophistication!

The problem of the upper limit of normal for blood sugar was discussed in the Bedford diabetic survey of 1962 (Butterfield, 1964). The concept that diabetes is defined by a capillary blood glucose level of 120 mg per cent taken two hours after a 50 g glucose load was questioned, since this level would result in nine per cent of the adult population being labelled diabetic. However if a level of 200 mg per cent is regarded as the upper limit of normal, three per cent of the population is diabetic; this is the group which is labelled diabetic by Butterfield. Those with levels between 120 and 200 mg per cent are named 'borderline'; their frequency of retinopathy, proteinuria, neuropathy, IHD and family history of diabetes lies intermediate between high prevalence in the diabetic group and normal values in the nondiabetic group. Many clinicians accept a level of 150 mg per cent as a compromise (Keen, 1968). This matter is discussed further in Chapter 17.

Although it is widely assumed that detection and treatment of the presymptomatic diabetic is beneficial, a note of caution has been sounded by work showing no difference in morbidity between diabetics treated by diet and hypoglycaemic drugs, and the control group treated by diet alone (University Group Diabetes Programme, 1971).

Ischaemic Heart Disease. With regard to IHD there is an epidemic of thrombotic atherosclerotic disease in western civilization, especially amongst young and middle aged men. The case for presymptomatic diagnosis is commanding. Raised serum lipids, especially cholesterol, are epidemiologically predictive of increased risk of IHD in men. When linked with knowledge of age, cigarette smoking, weight and blood pressure, muscular activity and a family history of IHD, it is possible to talk of predicting an actual risk of IHD for the individual (BMJ, 1973).

Saturated animal fat in the diet causes a disproportionately great increase in plasma lipids; its substitution by unsaturated vegetable fat improves the survival rate in secondary prevention of IHD (Bierenbaum et al., 1973). Drugs such as cholestyramine and clofibrate can reduce plasma lipids and may also diminish the risk of IHD. Such reduction seems feasible, especially if accompanied by low sucrose and low saturated fat diet. Primary prevention trials to assess the effect of diet and drugs on hyperlipidemia and IHD are in progress.

Until these results are known, there must be reservation in recommending mass screening for hyperlipidemia. Screening for hyperlipidemia using cholesterol levels alone may miss some cases, and ideally cholesterol levels should be accompanied by estimation of fasting plasma triglycerides and lipoprotein electrophoresis.

Hypothyroidism. Next to diabetes, IHD, and thyrotoxicosis, one of the commonest metabolic disorders is hypothyroidism. Although the prevalence of classical myxoedema is low, there is probably a large undetected pool of hypothyroidism which does not exhibit clinical 'myxoedema' (Evered and Hall, 1972). Nevertheless this grade of hypothyroidism represents thyroid failure with non-diagnostic symptoms of ill health.

The precise recognition of hypothyroidism requires estimation of PBI (now being replaced by serum thyroxine), T_3 resin uptake, and autoimmune profile for detection of thyroid autoantibodies. However, apart from the PBI, these tests are not automated. Serum cholesterol levels have no place in screening for hypothyroidism; the screening test is the PBI. High values of PBI are sometimes due to drug effects, but can occasionally suggest previously unsuspected thyrotoxicosis.

Liver disease. Screening tests for liver dysfunction are also popular. Because of the difficulties of effectively treating alcoholic liver disease or chronic active hepatitis (other than abstinence from alcohol), enthusiasm for seeking these diagnoses by screening should be tempered by caution.

Specific problems (Normal ranges often vary between laboratories.)

Liver function tests. Automated tests include bilirubin, SGOT, SGPT (relatively specific for liver disease), and alkaline phosphatase; non-automated tests of liver function include prothrombin time, protein electrophoretic strip and autoimmune profile. The last indicates smooth muscle antibody and antinuclear factor in chronic active hepatitis, and mitochondrial antibodies in primary biliary cirrhosis. The normal value of bilirubin is <1·2 mg per cent; SGOT < 30 i.u. per cent and alkaline phosphatase < 15 KA per cent.

Raised bilirubin usually indicates hepatic cellular disease or obstruction; rare alternatives are haemolytic anaemia (diagnosed by blood film, reticulocyte count) or failure to conjugate bilirubin (Gilbert's disease). Although neither specific for liver disease nor sensitive for quiescent cirrhoisis, SGOT and SGPT are helpful in demonstrating hepatic cellular damage. Obstructive liver disease (cholestasis) in a healthy population is usually due to gall stones, and the alkaline phosphatase shows a proportionately greater rise than the SGOT. A raised alkaline phosphatase may also occur in diffuse bone disease (Paget's disease, osteomalacia, hyperparathyroidism); if doubt arises, 5-nucleotidase is elevated in obstructive biliary disease but not in bone disease. Cholestasis is sometimes due to the contraceptive pill.

Mass screening by liver function tests can be unrewarding—usually detecting normal (slightly raised SGOT) convalescence from recent infective hepatitis, gross degree of alcoholic liver damage, or rarely chronic active hepatitis. Effort would be better directed at those who already have a history of one or more episodes of jaundice, or of weight loss, anorexia and nausea, or of abdominal pain, or those suspected of alcoholism.

Diabetes. Normal capillary blood sugar (usually 10 mg per cent higher than venous blood): 40-180 mg per cent at random. The natural history of diabetes unfolds over many years, there being a finite time during which metabolic abnormalities are demonstrable but the individual has either no symptoms or has nonspecific ill health.

Definitions of Diabetes.

1 The *latent* diabetic (Fitzgerald and Keen, 1964) shows hyperglycaemia when under temporary stress such as pregnancy, steroid therapy, rapid weight gain, myocardial infarction, and severe infection, but reverts to normal when 'stress' is removed.

2 The *asymptomatic* diabetic (subclinical, chemical) is symptomless but has persistently abnormal glucose tolerance test (GTT) with normal fasting glucose.

3 The *symptomatic* diabetic may be:-
  (a) Mild—with vague ill health or vascular disease, an often normal fasting glucose, but elevated glucose two hours after a 50 g glucose load.
  (b) Severe—abnormal GTT with raised fasting glucose, dehydration and hyperlipidemia.

A level of 200 mg per cent two hours after a large meal or a 50 g glucose load is diagnostic of diabetes. High levels one hour after loading may occur in partial gastrectomy cases, but the two hour glucose is normal or low.

Although glycosuria is a useful means of detecting diabetes in young people who are expected to have a normal or low (hence renal glycosuria) renal threshold for glucose, this assumption cannot be made in the elderly, in whom screening should be by blood and not by urine alone. Glucose does not appear in the urine of some diabetics until blood levels exceed 250 mg per cent (Butterfield, Keen and Whichelow, 1967). Blood is collected two hours after a 'hearty' breakfast or a 50 g glucose load.

Calcium Metabolism. Normal calcium: 8·5-10·5 mg per cent. Hypercalcaemia is rare and is most often due either to hyperparathyroidism, carcinoma metastatic to bone, or to florid sarcoidosis. Hyperparathyroidism may be associated with bone disease (fracture and bone pain), renal disease (stones, raised blood urea and creatinine) or abdominal pain. Screening for hyperparathyroidism should be restricted to these groups; it seems unwise to subject an apparently healthy individual to the ardours of establishing this diagnosis.

High risk groups for developing hypocalcaemia (without hypoproteinaemia) are those who have had a partial gastrectomy (malabsorption syndrome causing osteomalacia) or partial thyroidectomy (due to parathyroid hypofunction), or those who have symptoms of osteomalacia (bone pain, deformities, muscular cramps and weakness).

Iron Metabolism. Normal iron: 80-160 μg per cent. Although serum iron levels have been used in many screening programmes to aid the diagnosis of anaemia, the value of the test is debatable. Lowered iron levels are indicative of iron deficiency if total iron binding capacity (TIBC) shows less than 16 per cent saturation. In many chronic conditions, fall in serum iron is paralleled by fall in TIBC (e.g. rheumatoid arthritis) and hyposaturation does not occur. There seems little reason for estimating iron in mass screening programmes unless the haemoglobin is low. If the haemoglobin is low, and particularly if there is hypochromia and microcytosis, there is some value in estimating serum iron/TIBC.

Groups with a high risk of iron deficiency anaemia include multiparous women, or those with menorrhagia, 'aspirin eaters', partial gastrectomy patients, those with recurrent diarrhoea, and those with a history of hiatus hernia or peptic ulceration.

Proteins. Normal protein: total 6-8 g per cent; albumin > 4·0 g per cent. Estimation of total plasma protein is of little value. Separate albumin and globulin levels provide more information. Albumin is reduced in malnutrition, malabsorption, severe liver disease and nephrosis. Hypoglobulinaemia associated with recurrent severe infection is rare; hyperglobulinaemia is more common but is a nonspecific abnormality caused by many chronic inflammatory and neoplastic conditions, and has little more significance than a raised ESR. The most valuable protein test is electrophoresis (not automated); here the sharp gamma band of myeloma can be differentiated from the broad gamma band of cirrhosis, collagen disease (including rheumatoid arthritis) and chronic infections. This test is recommended for those with a high ESR, possible liver, gut or bone disease and those with backache aged over 50 years.

Urea and Creatinine. Normal: urea 15-40 mg per cent; creatinine < 1·5 mg per cent. The object of these tests is to detect early renal failure because reversible factors may be treated; e.g. renal infection, ureteric obstruction (prostatism), hypertension, or analgesic nephropathy.

These are crude tests, since severe impairment of renal function occurs before they rise. Further, there is a normal gradual increase in both measurements with increasing age. If these tests are normal, significant renal disease may still exist and be suspected on microscopy and culture of urine, blood pressure recording, urine concentration tests, and creatinine clearance. If urea and creatinine levels are raised, confirmatory evidence of renal disease can usually be found. These two tests are a measure of glomerular filtration rate and not of urine concentrating ability. In chronic pyelonephritis the latter falls first.

Urea levels may be misleadingly elevated by high dietary protein or by excessive tissue breakdown, while creatinine is less affected. In ambulant individuals, with normal diet, the advantage of creatinine is diminished.

Urea estimations are probably justified in a mass screening programme. High risk groups are those with hypertension (including previous toxaemia of pregnancy), recurrent urinary infection (especially acute pyelonephritis, prostatism), backache, headache, anorexia and nausea, or 'aspirin eaters'.

Lipid Metabolism. Normal: cholesterol 140-300 mg per cent; triglycerides < 150 mg (fasting) per cent. Hyperlipidemia is characterised by elevation of fasting cholesterol and triglyceride levels with a characteristic electrophoretic lipoprotein strip. The commonest varieties are Type II (raised cholesterol and a β band on the strip) and Type IV (raised triglycerides and a preβ band on strip). The condition is sometimes familial, sometimes due to diet (high sucrose, high saturated animal fat, high alcohol intake) or associated with disease such as diabetes, hypothyroidism, biliary obstruction, or nephrosis.

Screening for hyperlipidemia in young and middle aged men may now be accepted as justifiable. Since determination of triglycerides and lipoprotein strips are not automated, the relatively nonspecific and nonsensitive automated measurement of cholesterol will temporarily suffice in mass screening: full testing should be reserved for high risk groups—obese, hypertensive, smoking, diabetic, males—especially if there is a family history of IHD.

Uric Acid Metabolism. Normal: uric acid—males <7 mg per cent; females < 6 mg per cent. Because of the high prevalence of gout, uric acid is often estimated in screening programmes. However the upper limit of normal is not well defined, differing values applying to postmenopausal or premenopausal women, and to men. Also, uric acid levels increase in parallel with rises in blood urea due to renal failure; hence a raised uric acid level should be checked against blood urea.

Although it is generally true that patients with clinically typical gout have raised serum uric acid levels, in practice many exacerbations are associated with normal levels. Also hyperuricaemia is sometimes found in non-gouty individuals, and here the value of primary prevention by the use of allopurinol has yet to be accurately defined.

There is a tenuous link between hyperuricaemia on the one hand, and on the other, IHD and hypertension. Hence although it is debatable whether uric acid levels should be included in mass screening, the test is recommended for those with a history of arthritis or renal disease, or hypertensive young or middle aged males.

Hypothyroidism. Normal: PBI 4-8 μg per cent. PBI levels can be measured automatically. There are few causes of falsely low levels in healthy individuals, and a low PBI is highly suggestive of hypothyroidism. More accurate tests of thyroid function are available as kit methods (serum thyroxine, T_3 resin uptake).

Because of the likelihood of a large number of hypothyroid individuals with a long duration of nonspecific ill health in the community, and because effective treatment by thyroxine is readily available, the use of PBI in future screening programmes should be strongly considered. High risk groups are those with a goitre, a history of partial thyroidectomy, or with a family history of thyroid disease.

Conclusion

The need for biochemical screening relating to certain metabolic disorders is discussed. The tests suggested for mass screening are glucose for diagnosis of diabetes, urea for renal failure, and cholesterol for ischaemic heart disease. Estimations of uric acid for gout, proteins and enzymes for liver disease, calcium for hyperparathyroidism or osteomalacia, and iron for anaemia should be performed in those already primarily screened by history and hence placed in a 'high risk group'. The eventual role of automated thyroid function tests in detecting hypothyroidism is suggested.

REFERENCES

Bierenbaum, M. L., Fleischman, A. I., Raichelson, R. I., Hayton, D. & Watson, P. B. (1973). Ten year experience of modified fat diets on younger men with coronary heart disease. *Lancet* 1, 1404.

British Medical Journal, (1973). The odds on getting a coronary. 1, 290.

Butterfield, W. J. H. (1964). Summary of results in the Bedford Diabetes Survey. *Proceedings of Royal Society of Medicine,* 57, 196.

Butterfield, W. J. H., Keen, H. & Whichelow, M. J. (1967). Renal glucose threshold variations with age. *British Medical Journal,* 2, 505.

Carmalt, M. (1973). The general practitioner and the laboratory: chemical screening. *Modern Medicine,* 18, 575-581.

Evered, D. & Hall, R. (1972). Hypothyroidism. *British Medical Journal,* 1, 290.

Fitzgerald, M. G. & Keen, H. (1964). Diagnostic classification of diabetes. *British Medical Journal,* 1, 1568.

Keen, H. (1968). Diabetes Mellitus. In *Presymptomatic Detection and Early Diagnosis.* Edited by C. L. E. H. Sharp, and H. Keen, London: Pitman.

University Group Diabetes Programme (1971). *Diabetes,* 19, Supplement 2.

27 The Electrocardiogram M.H.F. Coigley

Electrocardiography has been considered outside the scope of general practice until recently. Indeed it is still considered so by very many physicians who do not appreciate or have not experienced the conditions and capabilities of modern general practice. These include both hospital doctors and general practitioners.

However, general practice has a long tradition of electrocardiography—the longest. Augustus Waller (1887) recorded the first human electrocardiogram (Guthrie, 1945). He was a general practitioner in Kensington near where the Royal College of General Practitioners now stands, and by using an anterior and posterior chest lead attached to a capillary electrometer, he crudely recorded the electrical impulses within the heart. Later, following Einthoven's invention of the string galvanometer, Sir James Mackenzie in general practice in Burnley, Lancashire until the age of 54 when he came to London, was probably as instrumental as anyone during the first 20 years of this century in making electrocardiography a routine part of the examination of the heart.

Waller, although his apparatus was far too imperfect to produce a worthwhile tracing, was credited by Einthoven with introducing the term electrocardiogram.

Two previous observations are important, as they produced the information on which electrocardiography is based. In 1856 Kölliker and Müller demonstrated that electrical changes took place when the isolated frog's heart contracted, and in 1880 Burdon-Sanderson and Page showed that the excited muscle in the frog's ventricle was electrically negative with respect to the unexcited muscle.

The electrical principle

We now know that in the resting phase, the myocardial cell surface is electrically positive whilst the interior is negative. As the excitatory impulse travels through the cell, the surface becomes electrically negative as well, and there is no potential difference between the interior and the exterior. The cell is then said to be depolarised. Whilst it is in this state, it cannot be excited to contract—it is refractory. Subsequently, the positive ions rearrange themselves along the surface, and a wave of repolarisation passes through the cell. It is this series of events which is mirrored in the electrocardiogram.

The path of the excitatory impulse through the myocardium can be likened to an electrical wave charged positively along its advancing crest followed by a negative trough. In the ventricles the impulse travels outwards from the endocardium to the surface, so that there is a difference of potential between the deeper parts of the myocardium and the surface layers, i.e., between collective masses of depolarised and still polarised cells respectively. This constitutes a dipole and it is this collective difference of potential between depolarised (negative) and polarised (positive) layers of myocardium which is recorded by the electrocardiogram (Ashman, 1948). As the advancing positive front of depolarisation approaches the surface, an electrode placed at this point will record an upstroke or R wave. At the moment that the impulse reaches the surface, the whole thickness of the muscle is depolarised, there is no difference in potential to record, and the R wave rapidly returns to the base line or iso-electric point. The positively charged ions rearrange themselves around the surfaces of the cells, and the process of repolarisation spreads as a similar wave in the wake of the depolarisation wave, giving rise to the T wave. This may be followed by another small positive or U wave. [There is some dispute about this. According to Lepeschkin (1957) the T wave travels in the opposite direction, the subepicardial cells becoming repolarised first, and so positive in relation to the endocardial cells, so the T wave is positive. Others

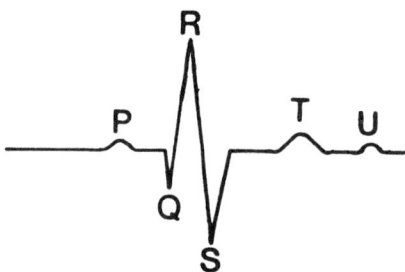

Fig. 7. The changes of potential accompanying a normal heart beat.

such as Paul Wood (*Diseases of the Heart and Circulation,* 1968) have not been able to confirm this.]

The process is always the same, so if an electrode is placed behind the wave of depolarisation (or in the mean axis of the sum of the resultant forces of depolarisation, which is towards the apex of the heart), e.g., at or towards the right shoulder, a negative potential will be recorded as an S wave falling below the baseline, (e.g. lead AVR). In practice, the left ventricle is depolarised before the right so that a unipolar electrode placed over this ventricle, say V5 or V6, will record a positive R wave as the impulse travels towards it, falling to the baseline on complete depolarisation. The wave of excitation passing through the right ventricle has not finished, however, and as it is passing away from the recording electrode, an S wave will follow. An electrode placed over the right ventricle (V1) will show the same configuration, but the R and S waves will reflect the right and left ventricular excitations in that order. As the mass of the left ventricle exceeds that of the right, the R wave will be of greater amplitude over the left ventricle, and the S wave will dominate over the right ventricle.

In practice, two other factors operate. The first is, of course, the initial wave of excitation from the S-A node through the atria to the A-V node, producing the P wave. Secondly, the initial spread of the ventricular impulse is from the left side through the interventricular septum, producing a small negative wave, the Q wave, through any electrode placed over or east of the septum, and an initial R wave through any electrode placed west of the septum, i.e., over the right ventricle. A Q wave is never recorded over the right ventricle in a normal heart.

Any electrode placed over infarcted muscle will record no deflection from this electrically inactive area. Below it, however, across the cavity of the heart will be active muscle with its excitatory wave (having a positive front and negative wake) passing from endocardium to epicardium, i.e., away from the electrode—an initial negative or Q wave will in these circumstances follow the P wave. Likewise, the repolarisation will be recorded as passing away from the electrode, and a negative or inverted T wave will wind up the complex. These two phenomena are the keys to detecting infarction.

Anoxia of the myocardium causes disturbance of the de- and repolarisation process. There is argument about the exact mechanism of this, but the result is an elevation or depression of the S-T segment from the isoelectric line, and it is this shift of the S-T segment which is important in detecting the myocardial ischaemia of coronary artery disease.

The changes of left ventricular hypertrophy and strain are best seen in the left chest leads I and V5-V6, and consist of legthened R waves and inverted T waves.

I have mentioned these particular changes briefly, because they are the most significant when considering routine cardiography in the middle age range of 30-65 yrs., and frequently occur silently and presymptomatically.

The electrocardiogram as a screening technique

The electrocardiogram is now three score and ten years old, and has been a routine investigation in clinical medicine for two to three generations. But the application of routine screening measures to 'cohorts' of patients has only been practised to any extent during the last twenty-five years. The electrocardiogram has a definite place in such screening programmes, but it must be emphasised that tracings must not be looked at in isolation, and the minimum information must include:

1 Age
2 Build, i.e., height, weight and girth
3 Current medication
4 History and any previous ECGs
5 Physical signs

There have been several studies of the routine use of the electro-cardiogram, but as a true screening measure they have mostly been hospital based, and have helped to highlight the fact that the incidence and manifestation of ischaemic heart disease varies with different populations (e.g., the USA has twice the death rate from ischaemic heart disease of Norway, Sweden and Holland, countries which have comparable life styles).

During the first fourteen years of follow up in the Framingham study, 188 ECG-documented infarctions occurred in 5,400 people, and one in eight (12 per cent) of these were silent, i.e., were discovered only by routine electrocardiography. Those with prior ECG abnormalities, hypertension and diabetes were especially prone to unrecognised infarctions. About one in four of these were dead within five years. As Kannel (1973) says, 'The frequent periodic use of the ECG is at present the only feasible method for detecting asymptomatic infarctions.' We might also add left ventricular hyper-trophy, (ECG) manifest myocardial ischaemia, and the probability of impending infarction.

In the Framingham survey, interventricular block and myocardial irritability as evidenced by ventricular ectopic beats in the resting ECG were associated with a three-fold increased risk of sudden death (Gordon & Kannel, 1971).

In general practice various investigators have reported on the use of the electrocardiogram. For instance in 1969 Evans and his colleagues during a wide ranging screening project in a Derbyshire practice carried out a six-lead (leads not specified-? any V leads) ECG on 355 people. People who were obese or hypertensive were given preference, so this was not a true random sample. However, 66·5 per cent were normal, 16·6 per cent were reported as showing possible ischaemic changes, 11·5 per cent as showing possible hypertensive changes and the rest showed minor (unspecified) abnormalities.

In the Hartford Hospital, Connecticut, USA, 4,172 routine ECGs were studied, 1,248 (30 per cent) being taken at a physician's request, and 2,924 (70 per cent) as a pure screening procedure in out-patients (Fieldman 1968). Of these 1,248 request ECGs, 763 (61 per cent) were abnormal with 365 (29 per cent) showing major pathology, and of the 2,924 routine ECGs 1,197 (41 per cent) were abnormal and 380 (13 per cent) showed major pathology. The author concludes 'In the Hartford Hospital Outpatient Department screening has provided a yield of abnormality sufficient for it to be recommended as a routine hospital procedure'.

This may be so, but by definition all patients attending hospitals are more likely to have some pathology, and a higher yield of ECG abnormalities than in general practice may be expected. For instance, in this survey there were many patients from the diabetic clinic.

In general practice, the same criticism may be levelled to some extent at the routine (rather than strict screening) use of the ECG, as it is more likely to be employed among selected groups, the largest being those with chest pain of some kind. Nevertheless, in a survey of 118 tracings taken over twelve months, Evans and his partners (1973) found that 19 or (16 per cent) were taken during a routine general examination. Of the total (118) 47 per cent were abnormal, a similar figure to the 49 per cent quoted by Morgan *et al.* (1970) for a hospital based general practitioner referral service.

The use of electrocardiography as a routine procedure in general practice brings with it certain difficulties. These include:

1 The difficulty in obtaining skilled personnel.
2 The increase in the workload and time involved.
3 The availability of trained readers and their training.

But the advantages are very real and include:

1 The equipment can be brought to the patient instead of vice versa.
2 Immediate availability of the tracing to the attending physician.
3 Immediate availability of patient records.
4 The availability of a captive population, broken down by age and sex in any screening exercise.

These advantages are worth noting. In clinics set up solely for screening such as that of the Institute of Directors where some of these advantages do not operate, the patient may feel, for instance, that it is in his interest to conceal part of his medical history, a symptom such as chest pain or therapy such as digitalis, all factors which may lead to different and erroneous interpretations of an electrocardiogram.

As electrocardiography is a time-consuming procedure involving capital and running expenditure, there is obviously no place for it in general practice comparable with sphygmomanometry, urinalysis, blood analysis, cervical smears etc. Indeed many screening programmes in general practice have omitted electrocardiography (e.g. Taylor, 1970) but others have included it (Evans, Wilkes and Dalrymple-Smith, 1969; Turner, 1968; Pike, 1972). As a method of screening large numbers of asymptomatic people as a routine, say yearly, when attending for another reason, it is hardly practicable at present.

What then is its scope? With the aid of an age and sex register it is certainly possible to screen selected groups of symptomless people. However, great dedication, time and expense would be involved. In the general practice setting, electrocardiography is far more likely to be used widely in screening groups with known or suspected pathology, in particular hypertensives, patients presenting with chest pain or syncope, and diabetes.

Screening selected groups

There is a strong case for screening selected groups by age, sex and of course by occupation. Indeed this has been done for one or two decades with airline pilots, and more recently train and bus drivers. London Transport now carry out periodic ECGs on bus drivers from the age of 50 years, and in 1972 3·7 per cent of 161 symptomless drivers showed definite evidence of myocardial ischaemia (Raffle in a personal communication to Jackson, 1973). However, the age of 40 years would certainly be preferable as the starting point for periodic check ECGs for it is in the ensuing decade that cardiovascular disease takes the greatest toll in male mortality.

Air pilots are subjected to a stricter periodic ECG check, being examined on entry and five yearly until aged 30 years, then two yearly until 40 years of age, then annually for the next decade, followed by six monthly recordings from then on (Jackson, 1973). Is this enough? Anyhow, are more frequent examinations practicable? We shall never know, but would the immediate pre-flight ECG of the captain of the ill-fated Trident LG-ARP 1 have shown any ischaemic change? The necropsy report revealed coronary atheroma with an intimal haemorrhage in one artery (Practitioner, 1973).

Equipment available

Historical. Einthoven's invention of the string galvanometer in 1902 opened the way to everyman's electrocardiography. His principle of making a silver or gold sheathed quartz string (i.e. a light object with very little inertia) deflect when a current was passed through it whilst in a magnetic field was revolutionary. However, the only method of recording this movement was by photographing its shadow, a cumbersome operation necessitating waiting some time for the result. Modern instruments are all based on two main principles: (1) the amplification of small potentials of about 1 millivolt (originally by valves, now by transistors); and (2) the development of direct writing mechanisms. These mechanisms are very heavy compared with the quartz string, so that considerable amplification of the incoming potentials is needed to move them.

Various writing methods have been tried including capillary pens with special ink, capillary jets of ink and heated styli.

The first two methods give good tracings provided the fine glass capillary does not become blocked or damaged. The second is particularly sensitive as the ink is squirted into absorbent paper without the pen actually touching it, so eliminating friction. However these methods are not particularly robust, and their extreme sensitivity can be a disadvantage and unnecessary when interference has to be eliminated. They have been almost entirely superseded by the heated stylus. Usually this consists of a fine loop of platinum wire heated to red heat. Black paper coated with a white oxide in wax is then drawn along in contact with the heated stylus. The white covering is melted by the hot pen, and the black paper shows through, so revealing the tracing.

Power Supply. The power supply of these instruments is either by mains electricity, or batteries, or both. The general practitioner even in this day and age may be faced with the necessity to record an ECG with no mains power available, so that he would be well advised always to purchase a machine that will run on batteries. The most acceptable machines, of which there is a good selection now, are those which have batteries rechargeable by the mains and will run direct from mains power as well. Obviously a truly portable machine must be chosen, but those that are too small tend to give more than their share of trouble. It is also important to note that the most common and annoying form of interference is that produced by the mains current—in Britain producing a fine regular saw-tooth effect at

50 cycles/second—and that this is best eliminated by injecting an opposing current of equal strength and opposite direction. Therefore machines operating on batteries alone may be more liable to unsuppressable mains interference, as an opposing mains pulse is not available.

Electrodes. Three basic types of electrode are in common use. The conventional flat metal one, necessitating using electrode jelly or cream for good contact, is still the commonest. The development of non-corrosive, non-greasy creams has made these more acceptable. However, some makers provide wet pad electrodes with no extra aid, and this can be satisfactory. The latest idea is the nutmeg grater type, of which the author has no personal experience. It is probably true to say that an adequate chest electrode has not yet been produced. Have two or three to hand for various degrees of adiposity and hairiness, and a safety razor as part of your equipment.

Electrode 'jelly'. Water soluble, non-corrosive jelly is now obtainable and should always be used.

Controls. All modern machines have a lead selector which is merely switched to the lead required prior to recording, the connection to the patient being made within the machine. Some machines, however, will only operate at the standard speed of 25 mm/s and at the standard amplitude deflection of 10 mm/millivolt. It is very useful to be able to double the drive speed to 50 mm/s in order to spread out and more easily interpret a tracing with a very rapid heart rate and/or some dysrhythmias, and to halve the amplitude in order to contain the very large deflections sometimes obtained over the left ventricle with chest leads. The small extra expense entailed is well spent.

Cost. The average cost of a modern portable electrocardiograph is about £275 and should be well within the scope of any group practice. The cost of electricity will vary, being negligible if taken from the mains direct or into rechargeable batteries, but being up to £10 per year for replaceable batteries. Recording paper is not cheap. It must be remembered that frequently more' is used than is necessary. A maximum of four complexes is needed for interpretation, with one longer strip to ascertain rhythm. In one investigation the cost of paper over one year (118 readings) was £4·62 or 3·9p per recording (Evans *et al.*, 1973).

Training of doctors and staff

Sources of instruction. We have all been brought up from our earliest student days to know the electrocardiogram as one of the commonest aids to diagnosis, but we may never have got to grips with the basic principles, or the memory may have faded.

To revise there is no doubt that a good lecturer can in two or three hours do more than a book can in twenty or thirty, so the first thing to do if you are coming back to this subject is to attend a course of lectures. At the same time approach your local cardiologist or intensive care unit, and make a regular trip to see the ECGs.

Specialist books are almost all overdetailed, and confusing, but the author can recommend without hesitation *Cardiographic Technique* by Schott and Snelle. After this, the sections on electrocardiography in the larger text books of medicine and cardiology are probably the most useful. We must not, however, forget the publications distributed by some of the pharmaceutical firms. These are short, deal with basic principles and patterns, and can be an invaluable aid which is not submerged in theoretical detail.

The doctor. It is essential to have at least one partner who is conversant with ECG interpretation. If the few earlier remarks are kept in mind, the basic logicality of the subject will be realised, and although at first some time will be spent in orienting each lead in the mind this tends to become nearly automatic quite soon—at least for the tracings of common abnormalities such as simple arrhythmias, ischaemic changes, infarction and ventricular hypertrophy. Deviation of the electrical axis can be important and should be recognised. Likewise, heart blocks of all types can be identified.

The technician. The technician is best chosen from existing practice staff. A practice nurse is ideal, as probably she is known already to most of the patients. She should be instructed in some basic theory, and should also spend one or two sessions in a department of electrocardiography.

Preferably she should take all ECGs except in emergencies. This will lead to standardized technique and what is very important, standardized treatment of the machine which will give better and longer service as a result.

What to record

The leads. So that all electrocardiograms may be read worldwide, there is a standard method of recording by leads. The agreed twelve-lead ECG comprises both bipolar and unipolar leads.

The bipolar or standard leads (Einthoven, 1908). The trace recorded by these leads is the resultant of the changes in electrical potential occurring beneath two electrodes. A current flowing towards the positive electrode will record an upstroke. The leads are:

LEAD I	Right arm (−ve)	Left arm (+ve)
LEAD II	Right arm (−ve)	Left foot (+ve)
LEAD III	Left arm (−ve)	Left foot (+ve)

These standard bipolar leads were to persist in use alone until the mid-1930s.

The unipolar leads. These are the chest or V leads and the unipolar limb leads. The trace recorded by these leads is near enough the exclusive result of the changes in potential occurring beneath one electrode only, the independent or the exploring electrode. The other electrode comprising the leads has zero potential, and is termed the indifferent electrode. This is made up in the chest or V leads by connecting the three limbs to a central terminal, and in the unipolar limb leads by connecting the other two limbs to a single terminal. These terminals are then lead off to the electrocardiogram.

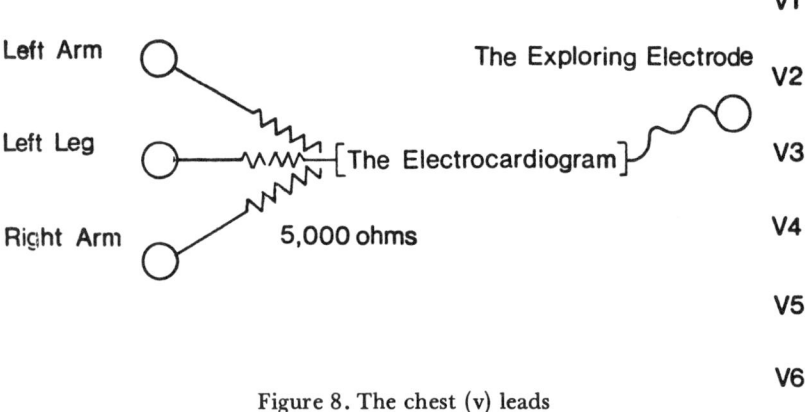

Figure 8. The chest (v) leads

In the chest or V leads the independent electrode is movable or exploring, and in the unipolar limb leads it is fixed.

The Chest or V (for voltage) leads (Fig. 8). Wilson introduced these leads in 1934. They are now in common international use. Two relevant considerations are: (1) that being very near the heart, the exploring electrode will receive greater changes in potential than the limb electrodes; and (2) that small variations in the placement of the exploring electrode will produce greater differences in the trace than similar variations in the limb electrodes, which are at much greater distances from the heart.

The pairing of an indifferent electrode with an exploring electrode on the chest had been practised already, but the technique of making the indifferent electrode uninfluential electrically had not been grasped. For instance, a lead comprising an indifferent electrode on the right arm and exploring electrode on the chest reflects the sum of the potentials under each electrode. These leads have been and are still used by some cardiologists. They are described by the letter C for chest, followed by R, L or F for limb involved, and are termed respectively CR, CL and CF followed by the numerals 1-6, indicating the position of the chest lead just as in the V leads.

Wilson and his colleagues, however, made use of the fact that the algebraic sum of the potentials from the three limbs is zero. They connected these electrodes (through a 5,000 ohm resistance, to minimise differences in skin resistance) to a central terminal to form the indifferent electrode of zero potential, and paired this with the exploring chest electrode.

The agreed sites for the chest electrode are for each lead:

V1 4th intercostal space to right of sternum
V2 4th intercostal space to left of sternum
V3 midway between V2 and V4
V4 5th intercostal space at intersection by midclavicular line
V5 at the same horizontal level as V4 on the left anterior axillary line
V6 at the same horizontal level as V4 on the midaxillary line.

The unipolar limb leads. These are constructed in the same way as the V leads, the indifferent electrode being connected to the three limbs, and another electrode on the limb to be recorded being used as the other connection of the lead. They are therefore designated VR, VL and VF. The potentials recorded, however, are often rather small and they are no longer in routine use.

The augmented unipolar limb leads. (Fig. 9). Goldberger (1942) found that by dropping the wire to the central terminal from the limb being recorded, the potential was increased or augmented by 50 per cent. This is now the standard practice, and the leads are designated AVR, AVL and AVF (A for augmented).

In summary, therefore, the standard twelve lead electrocardiogram comprises the three standard leads I, II and III, and then in practice the augmented unipolar limb leads AVR, AVL and AVF, followed by the chest or V leads V1 to V6 in that order, although historically the augmented limb leads and the V leads come in reverse order.

How many leads? A full twelve-lead ECG may seem an impractical

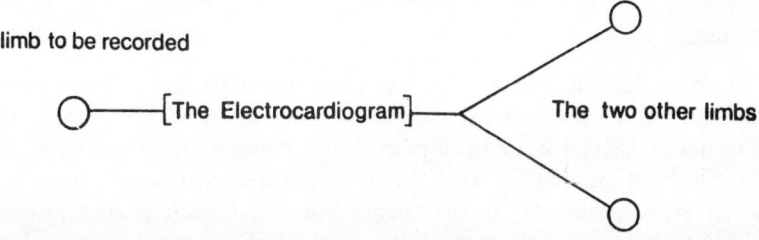

Figure 9. The augmented unipolar limb leads

measure by some. Indeed it has been suggested that for routine mass screening leads I, II and III may suffice. However, factors such as electrical axis and ventricular preponderance may be difficult to elucidate, and it seems difficult to imagine that the unique information gained through the chest leads can be dispensed with. A compromise six-lead ECG might be leads I, AVF, V1, V2, V4 and V6 if time is a vital factor, as these leads would provide information embracing electrical axis, myocardial nutrition and ventricular preponderance or hypertrophy.

The exercise ECG. There is wide controversy over the use of exercise to produce ECG changes in individuals with suspected myocardial ischaemia, and it should not be carried out unless means of resuscitation are to hand. However, there is no doubt that ST changes can be brought to light in some cases, to enhance a clinical diagnosis. In some centres, notably in the USA, the use of the treadmill (variable speed moving belt) with monitoring by pulse rate and ECG is a well established procedure to which anyone with a slight chest pain or 'indigestion' is liable to be subjected.

The Minnesota Code and computer ECGs

Blackburn and his colleagues (1960) suggested the adoption of standardized measurements and other criteria for all ECGs in order to minimise the variability in reporting. He has since published a synopis of these criteria which has become known as the Minnesota Code (Blackburn, 1969). Most epidemiological surveys involving ECG recording now adopt the criteria of the Minnesota Code, and sophisticated electronics can produce a computer printout of the measurement for each tracing, uninfluenced by the human mind and untouched by hand, upon which the clinician may make his judgement. It is not difficult to forsee the day when the general practitioner will feed his ECGs into his own computer terminal, and get the detailed measurements returned in seconds with abnormalities noted for him.

Summary

In this chapter, the author has attempted to lay before you a few practical and theoretical facts which he has at times found particularly difficult to understand. To discuss the place of the ECG in periodical health checks, both asymptomatic and some pathological states, and to quote some sources which may lead one at least to consider whether periodical ECGs may have a place in preventive family medicine. He has also attempted to put the ECG in its historical perspective. He must apologise if to some it has seemed irrelevant or elementary, and to others who may see in it detail and discussion not relevant to general practice. Of necessity he has had to be brief.

It remains to be said that human nature being what it is, many patients feel much better for an ECG (or an X-ray for that matter), but that this unfortunately does not preclude their sudden demise on your front doorstep following a normal tracing. It may, however, if you can honestly and confidently point to some slight abnormality, at its least, have more effect on their reduction of weight and cessation of smoking than your advice alone and with no magic machine.

REFERENCES

Ashman, R. (1948). *The Chest and Heart*. Ed. J. A. Myers & C. N. McKinlay.

Blackburn, H., Keys, A., Simonson, E., Rautaharju, P. & Punsar, S. (1960). The electrocardiogram in population studies: a classification system. *Circulation*, 21, 1160.

Blackburn, H. (1969). Classification of the electrocardiogram for population studies: Minnesota Code. *Journal of Electrocardiography*, 2, 305.

Burdon-Sanderson, J. & Page, F. J. M. (1879-80). On the time relations of the excitatory process in the ventricle of the frog. *Journal of Physiology* (London), 2, 384.

Einthoven, W. (1901). Un nouveau galvonometre. *Archives Neerlandiases des Sciences Exactes et Naturelles*. 2nd series, 6, 625.

Einthoven, W. (1903). Ein neues galvonometer. *Annalem der Physik* (Leipzig). 12, 1059.

Einthoven, W. (1908). Weiteres über das Elektrokardiogram. *Pflügeres Archiv für die gesante Physiologie des menschen und der Tiere*, 122, 517.

Evans, S. M., Wilkes, E. & Dalrymple-Smith, D. (1969). Presymptomatic diagnosis. *Journal of the Royal College of General Practitioners*, 17, 237.

Evans, E. O., Coigley, M. H. F., Lewis, J. V. V. & Woodward, N. A. (1973). Electrocardiography in general practice. *Journal of the Royal College of General Practitioners*, 23, 743.

Fieldman, A. (1968). Evaluation of routine E. C. G. screening of an outpatient population with computer diagnoses. *Journal of the American Medical Association*, 205, 627.

Gordon, T. & Kannel, W. B. (1971). Premature mortality from coronary heart disease: the Framingham study. *Journal of the American Medical Association*, 215, 1617.

Guthrie, D. (1945). *A History of Medicine*. London: Thomas Nelson & Son Ltd.

Jackson, R. (1973). The value of routine electrocardiography. *Practitioner*, 211, 164.

Kannel, W. B. (1973). *The natural history of myocardial infarction—the Framingham study*. Holland: Leyden University Press.

Kölliker, A. & Müller, H. (1856). Nachweis der negativen Schwankung des muskelstroms am näturlich sich contrahirenden muskel. *Verhandlungen der Physikalisch medizinischen Gesellschaft zu Würzberg*, 6, 528.

Morgans, C. M., Gillings, D. B., Pearson, N. G. & Shaw, D. B. (1970). Analysis of an open electrocardiogram referral service for family doctors. *British Medical Journal*, 1, 41.

Pike, L. A. (1972). Screening middle aged man in general practice. *Practitioner*, 209, 690.

Robb, G. P. & Marks, H. H. (1967). Postexercise electrocardiogram in arteriosclerotic heart disease. *Journal of the American Medical Association*, 200, 918.

Rose, K. (1973). Routine electrocardiography for 14 year old football candidates. *Journal of the American Medical Association*,

Schott, A. & Snelle, H. (1963). *Cardiographic Technique*. London: Heinemann.

Taylor, M. P. (1970). Periodic health examinations combined with simple screening tests in general practice. *Journal of the Royal College of General Practitioners*, 19, 146.

Turner, S. (1968). Routine medical examinations—a small series. *Journal of the Royal College of General Practitioners*, 15, 280.

Waller, A. D. (1887). A demonstration on man of electromotive forces accompanying the heart's beat. *Journal of Physiology* (London), 8, 229.

Wood, P. (1968). *Diseases of the Heart and Circulation*. London: Eyre & Spottiswoode.

28 The Chest Film
Ian Gregg

'X-rays do not show diseases; they only throw shadows'.

Screening usually involves the application of various kinds of investigation which are also used in clinical practice for diagnosis or for assessing the degree of severity of an abnormality. Hence, it is often difficult to draw a clear distinction between the use of an investigation for clinical purposes and its use as a screening test. For instance, a general practitioner may refer a patient who has no symptoms nor signs of respiratory disease for a chest radiograph in order to exclude tuberculosis or bronchial carcinoma. At first sight this would seem to be an example of screening, but if the patient had recently lost weight or had felt generally unwell, chest radiography would be a mandatory part of the clinical assessment of such a patient.

Although chest radiography is usually undertaken as an investigation of the respiratory system, it should be remembered that a chest radiograph may also reveal disease or abnormalities in other systems. Information about the cardiovascular system can be gained from the size or shape of the heart shadow and the vascular pattern in the lung fields, while diseases of the skeletal system may be revealed in the ribs or vertebral column. A chest radiograph may also disclose a variety of other disorders such as mediastinal lymph node enlargement, retrosternal goitre, achalasia and hiatus hernia.

25 years ago the value of chest radiography in medical screening was so self-evident as to be beyond dispute. Today, however, as a result of the decline in the incidence of tuberculosis, the situation is very different. In this chapter an attempt will be made to assess the present value of chest radiography in screening, particularly from the standpoint of the general practitioner.

Tuberculosis and mass miniature radiography

Not only was chest radiography the first screening procedure to be introduced on a wide scale into medical practice but its success in achieving the purpose for which it was originally conceived—the presymptomatic detection of pulmonary tuberculosis—has not been equalled by any other form of medical screening which has been introduced subsequently.

The value of any test which is used for screening depends upon a number of factors. Wilson (1966) suggested that, ideally, a screening programme should fulfil ten criteria (Chapter 1, pp.12-13). In retrospect, mass miniature radiography can be seen to have satisfied all his criteria. At the time of its introduction tuberculosis was not only common but of great socio-economic importance: the cost of screening was relatively very small compared with that of treating patients who would not otherwise have been diagnosed until their disease had reached a more advanced stage: chest radiography was a simple test, took little time and was capable of being organised so that large numbers of people could be screened: the yield of cases who were detected was high. Finally, chest radiography proved to be socially acceptable, not only because of its convenience, but also because of the fear of tuberculosis which existed at that time.

The outstanding contribution which the Mass Miniature Radiography Service made towards the control of tuberculosis, coinciding with the development of anti-tuberculous chemotherapy, has led to a situation where the small number of persons who are now found to have tuberculosis no longer justifies the cost of the service.

Bronchial carcinoma

During the same period in which we saw this gratifying decline of tuberculosis an alarming increase occurred in the incidence of bronchial carcinoma. In the majority of patients with this disease the tumour is found to be inoperable at the time of diagnosis and even in patients in whom resection can be carried out, the five-year survival rate is depressingly low. Therefore, it seemed a reasonable proposition that earlier diagnosis might bring about an improvement in this situation.

Unfortunately, the optimism of those who advocated the regular screening by mass chest radiography of persons at special risk (such as heavy smokers in middle age) has proved to be ill-founded. The most important single factor which determines prognosis in bronchial carcinoma is the rate of growth of the tumour, since in general this is related to its local invasiveness and its capacity to metastasise.

Therefore, if a very small tumour is detected in a patient who had a normal chest film six months previously there is a great likelihood of its being highly malignant.

A comparative trial of two large groups of men was carried out by Brett (1966) to assess the value of six-monthly chest films in early diagnosis. One group was examined twice with an interval of three years; in them 51 per cent of the carcinomas which were revealed were resectable. In the other group, which was examined every six months, 65 per cent of the carcinomas revealed were resectable. Somewhat more encouraging results were reported by Nash, Morgan and Tomkins (1968) in a very large survey carried out by the S.E. and S.W. London Mass X-ray Services. Although the length of time between examinations had only a small effect upon the proportion of tumours which were resectable at the time of their discovery, it was found that in men over the age of 55 years this had a highly significant effect upon the survival of those in whom resection could be carried out. When the interval between the discovery film and the previous normal film was not longer than 28 weeks, 76 per cent of men were alive four years after resection. On the other hand, when the interval was between 29 and 52 weeks, only 32 per cent of men were alive four years after resection.

At present one must conclude that X-ray screening for bronchial carcinoma, even if carried out regularly every six months, is not an effective method for improving its prognosis by early detection. It may even prove to be disadvantageous in the prevention of the disease: the author has encountered patients who attend a mass radiography unit every six months and have developed a false sense of security from the knowledge that on each occasion their chest films are reported to be normal and in consequence they continue to smoke heavily with equanimity.

Chronic bronchitis

Chronic obstructive bronchitis is a major public health problem in this country, being one of the most important causes of disability in middle age. Once the disease has become established only conservative treatment is possible, its object being to prevent further progress of the disease. Clearly, it is important to identify chronic bronchitis at as early a stage as possible when preventive measures might arrest its further progress. The only method whereby presymptomatic, structural damage of the bronchi can be detected is by pulmonary function tests. Their use in screening is discussed in Chapter 29.

Chest radiography is of no value as a screening test of early bronchitis. Even in patients who have already become severely disabled by an advanced stage of chronic bronchitis, a chest film often reveals no abnormality. In those patients in whom chronic bronchitis is accompanied by emphysema, the latter has to be widespread and of severe degree before it gives rise to radiological changes (Simon, 1964; Reid and Millard, 1964).

The chief value of chest radiography in chronic bronchitis is to exclude other diseases with which it may be confused or with which it may co-exist. Since smoking is an aetiological factor in both chronic bronchitis and bronchial carcinoma, chest radiography should be carried out regularly to exclude the latter disease. However, the discovery of a carcinoma in patients with chronic bronchitis is chiefly of importance as a guide to their prognosis, since their pulmonary function is seldom good enough to permit resection. Patients with chronic bronchitis should also be X-rayed to exclude tuberculosis (the prevalence of which has been reduced less among elderly persons than in the young) and such conditions as sarcoidosis and fibrosing alveolitis.

Occupational lung disease

For many years before the advent of the Mass Miniature Radiography Service, routine radiography had been used to detect the early stages of pneumoconiosis in coal miners. There is no doubt of the value of screening in this and other occupations which carry special hazards, particularly those which expose workers to asbestos. In the case of miners and large firms, such screening is carried out through the Industrial Medical Service. However, general practitioners should be alert to the possibility that some workers, particularly in small firms, are not screened regularly. Asbestos is used widely by builders, handymen and installers of domestic heating systems: although the risks of asbestosis in such persons are probably not as great as was once feared, they should be referred for chest radiography at regular intervals.

Another group of workers for whom no special provisions for screening exist are farm-workers. In areas where there is a high rainfall, hay becomes contaminated by thermophyllic Actinomyces and the inhalation of their spores gives rise to 'farmer's lung'. Extrinsic allergic fibrosing alveolitis is a similar disease which occurs in persons who keep budgerigars or pigeons and who are liable to inhale dust which has been contaminated by their droppings.

Selective screening

Although chest radiography can no longer be justified as a general screening procedure—that is, the investigation of as many persons as possible regardless of whether or not they have any symptoms suggestive of respiratory disease—its value in selective screening is beyond dispute. The yield of patients found to have active pulmonary tuberculosis or primary lung cancer is much higher among those who have been referred by their general practitioners than it is among persons who have attended a Mass X-ray Unit on their own initiative or have had a chest radiograph as part of a routine medical examination.

The general practitioner should use his knowledge of his patients to identify those who are at special risk. Apart from factors such as smoking and occupation which predispose to lung disease, there are others which should be kept in mind. Diabetics, alcoholics and persons of Irish descent all have an unusually high susceptibility to tuberculosis. Although the screening of immigrants on entry to this country has reduced the likelihood of their arriving with active tuberculosis, they appear to be more susceptible to tuberculous infection if they encounter it after their arrival, particularly if they live under conditions of poverty and overcrowding. The screening of contacts of patients known to have tuberculosis is usually undertaken by Chest Clinics, but sometimes a general practitioner's knowledge of the family enables him to trace contacts who might otherwise have been overlooked.

Teachers and other persons who are in contact with children should have a chest radiograph before they start work in view of the need to safeguard children against tuberculous infection. Doctors and the staff of hospitals or other institutions who are liable to come into contact with tuberculous patients should have an annual chest radiograph.

The risks of radiation from a chest radiograph are negligible, even when repeated at six-monthly intervals, except in women who are pregnant. Whereas formerly it was considered essential that all pregnant women should have a routine chest film, the decline in the incidence of tuberculosis has made this no longer desirable except under special circumstances, as in immigrants, diabetics and those with a previous or family history of tuberculosis.

Occasionally it happens that a person without any symptoms has a chest film which discloses unsuspected disease, such as tuberculosis or carcinoma or, more rarely, pulmonary metastases, a benign tumour (for instance, a hamartoma or thymoma), a pericardial cyst, sarcoidosis or hilar lymph node enlargement. Apart from these radiological abnormalities, which obviously require further investigation, chest radiographs commonly reveal a wide variety of other abnormalities which are seldom of any clinical significance. These include calcified tuberculous foci, fibrotic scars, thickening of the pleura and osteoarthritic changes in the vertebrae.

It should be realised that the reporting of chest radiographs is not as straightforward as some clinicians suppose. Except when a chest radiograph is entirely normal, the radiologist has to decide whether it is important to notify the clinician that there are minor abnormalities. A report of a chest radiograph being normal may only mean that it shows no significant abnormality which requires action to be taken by the clinician.

The radiologist can receive a good deal of help over reporting from information supplied to him by the general practitioner—for instance, the existence of any symptoms or localising signs. It is also of value to inform the radiologist of any history of previous lung disease and of any abnormalities which have been reported on previous chest radiographs. This information may be of crucial importance in helping the radiologist to decide whether an abnormality is old-standing or has arisen recently. Nash (1973) has pointed out how valuable a base-line radiograph may be for comparison with those taken at a later date.

REFERENCES

Brett, G. Z. (1966). The presymptomatic diagnosis of lung cancer. *Proceedings of the Royal Society of Medicine*, 59, 1208.

Nash, F. A., Morgan, J. M. & Tomkins, J. G. (1968). South London cancer study. *British Medical Journal*, 2, 715.

Nash, F. A. (1973). Autologic monitoring exemplified by chest radiography. *Practitioner*, 211, 150.

Reid, L. & Millard, F. J. C. (1964). Correlation between radiological diagnosis and structural lung changes in emphysema. *Clinical Radiology*, 15, 307.

Simon, G. (1964). Radiology and emphysema. *Clinical Radiology*, 15, 293.

Wilson, J. M. G. (1966). Some principles of early diagnosis and detection. In *Surveillance and Early Diagnosis in General Practice*, Ed. G. Teeling-Smith. London: Office of Health Economics.

29 Lung Function Tests

Ian Gregg

'A self-respecting general practitioner should not only possess a sphygmomano-meter but also a peak flow meter or Vitalograph'.

The purpose of this chapter is to discuss the value of pulmonary function tests which can be used by the general practitioner for screening. The most convenient way to deal with the subject is to review the various types of disorder which may affect pulmonary function, then to describe those tests which are suitable for use in general practice and, finally, to discuss their value as screening tests for the detection of respiratory disease.

Disorders of pulmonary function

Pulmonary function is less complex than that of, say, the liver or kidney. The fundamental purpose of respiration is to exchange oxygen and carbon dioxide between the body and the external air and to achieve this three requirements must be fulfilled. First, there must be a large surface area of a very thin membrane across which both gases can easily diffuse into and out of the blood; secondly, there must be an adequate blood supply to this membrane: thirdly, the air which is brought into contact with the membrane must be continually replaced.

It follows that there are three basic ways in which respiration can be disturbed. These are termed disorders of diffusion, perfusion and ventilation. However, it must be emphasised that in many diseases of the respiratory system more than one type of disorder may be present.

Disorders of diffusion. In this type of disorder there is an interference of diffusion, either because the alveolar-capillary membrane becomes less permeable as a result of inflammation or fibrosis (as in sarcoidosis and alveolitis), or because the alveoli are filled with exudate or transudate (as in pneumonia and pulmonary oedema), or because the total surface area of the alveolar-capillary membrane is greatly reduced (as in emphysema).

Disorders of diffusion are readily detected and measured by tests which can be performed in any hospital department of pulmonary physiology but there is no test which is suitable for use in general practice. However, in some cases the pathological processes which give rise to impairment of diffusion may also cause what is termed a restrictive disorder of ventilation. The latter can be detected by simple instruments which will be discussed below.

Disorders of perfusion. The most common cause of this type of disorder is interference of the blood supply to the alveolar-capillary membrane when the pulmonary arteries are obstructed by one or more large emboli or multiple small emboli.

Disorders of ventilation. Delivery of air to the alveolar-capillary membrane depends upon the provision of channels which conduct air from the mouth and distribute it uniformly to the alveoli, and also upon a 'bellows' mechanism which causes air to flow into and out of the lungs. Therefore, there are two ways in which ventilation can be disturbed. Disorders which interfere with the conduction of air are termed 'obstructive' and those which impair the bellows function of the lungs are termed 'restrictive'.

Obstructive disorders of ventilation are the most common of all lung diseases. Airways obstruction is the cardinal disorder in both asthma and chronic obstructive bronchitis. By definition, airways obstruction in the former is reversible, whereas in the latter it is mainly due to structural damage of the airways which is irreversible.

The maintenance of normal respiration depends upon there being a proper balance between ventilation and perfusion. In chronic obstructive bronchitis some alveoli receive no air but remain adequately perfused: this situation gives rise to what is essentially a right to left shunt. Imbalance between ventilation and perfusion is the most common cause of cyanosis in chronic lung disease.

Airways obstruction can easily be detected and measured by simple instruments which are eminently suitable for use in general practice. By means of these tests, which will be described below, it is also possible to determine whether airways obstruction is reversible or irreversible.

Restrictive disorders of ventilation are found in a wide variety of pulmonary diseases. For instance, scoliosis, fibrosis of the pleura and gross obesity all restrict the expansion of the thorax. In certain diseases, such as sarcoidosis, alveolitis and pneumoconiosis, the lungs are abnormally rigid due to inflammatory changes or fibrosis and these similarly restrict the expansion of the thorax. Interference of the nerve supply to the respiratory muscles (as in poliomyelitis and phrenic nerve palsy) also causes a restrictive disorder.

Tests of ventilation function

Disorders of ventilation are the only form of abnormal pulmonary function which can be detected by instruments that are suitable for use in general practice. Two such instruments, the Vitalograph and the Wright peak flow meter are already widely used by general practitioners. Their use is as relevant to the identification and treatment of asthma and chronic obstructive bronchitis as is the sphygomomanometer to the diagnosis and management of hypertension. Both tests measure a single, forced expiration: whichever is used, it is of the utmost importance that the subject who is being tested understands what he is required to do and is persuaded to make a maximal effort.

The Vitalograph. This is essentially a dry spirometer which prov-

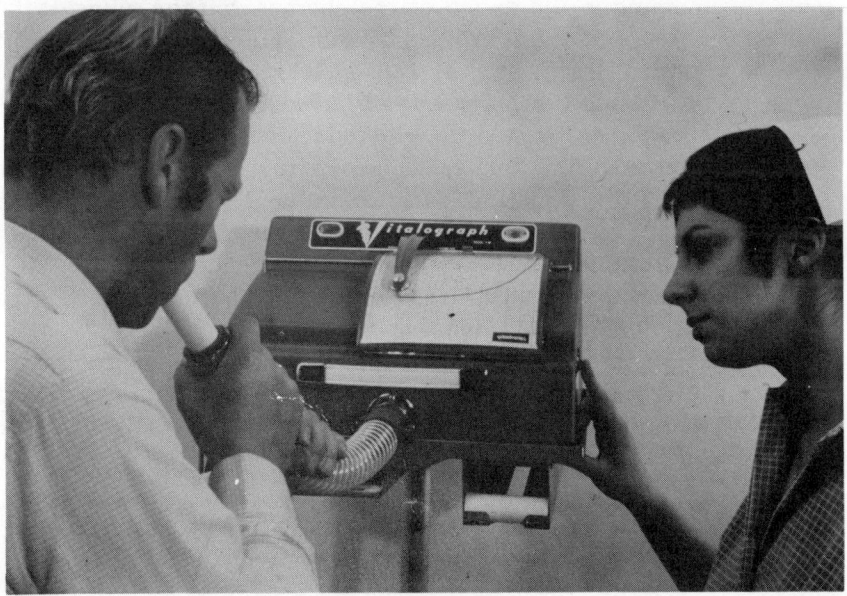

Figure 10. The Vitalograph in use, showing the trace of the subject's forced expiration which has been drawn on the chart. To measure FEV_1 and FVC at BTPS the calibration scale on the *righthand* margin of the chart must be used, i.e. the border nearest the stylus in this view.

ides a recording of the whole of a subject's forced expiration. The expired air inflates an internal rubber bag which causes a stylus to write on the recording chart (Fig. 10). The latter is carried on a frame which begins to move laterally at a fixed speed as soon as the expired air enters the bag. From the tracing it is simple to measure the volume of air expelled in the first second of the forced expiration (FEV_1) and the total amount of air expelled up to the point when the subject cannot expire any further (the forced vital capacity or FVC). In normal subjects the FVC should be attained within 4 seconds and the ratio FEV_1/FVC should not be less than 70 per cent.

It is important to note that the Vitalograph chart has two vertical scales for the measurement of volume. That on the left hand side is calibrated to show the volume of expired air at room temperature, whereas the right hand scale is calibrated to show the volume of expired air at body temperature ($37^\circ C$); in both cases barometric pressure is taken to be 760 mm Hg and allowance is made for the saturation of air by water vapour. The scales are denoted respectively by the initials ATPS, (abbreviation for Ambient Temperature, normal barometric Pressure, Saturated) and BTPS (abbreviation for Body Temperature, normal barometric Pressure, Saturated). A regrettable shortcoming in the design of the chart is that the ruling of the grid is based upon the ATPS calibration. Since normal values of FEV_1 are expressed as volumes of air at BTPS, it is essential to use the right hand scale for measuring observed values of FEV_1 if it is intended to compare them with predicted normal values.

The Wright Peak flow meter. This was originally introduced as a test of ventilatory function for use in epidemiological surveys. During the last ten years it has come to be used increasingly widely by clinicians in hospitals, chest clinics and general practice. It is unexcelled as a rapidly performed test which can be carried out as a part of the clinical examination of patient.

The subject makes a forced expiration into the meter which causes an internal vane to rotate and with it a needle on the dial of the instrument (Fig. 11). From this an immediate reading can be made of peak expiratory flow (PEF).

The relative merits of the Vitalograph and the Wright peak flow meter

Both the Vitalograph and the Wright peak flow meter are highly accurate instruments. As an index of airways obstruction there is little to choose between FEV_1 and PEF, and there is a good correlation between these two measurements (Ritchie, 1962).

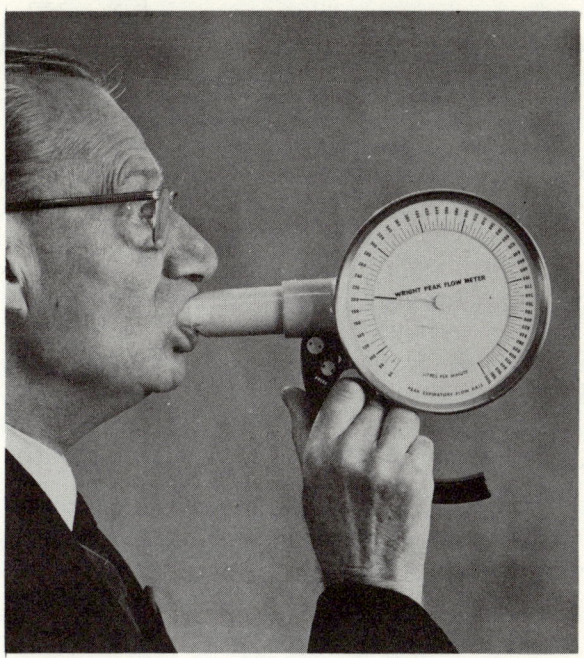

Figure 11. The Wright peak flow meter in use. In this example a PEF of 205 litres/min has been attained.

However, the peak flow meter provides only a measure of airways obstruction, whereas the Vitalograph can enable the clinician to identify restrictive ventilatory disorders also, since it gives the additional measurement of FVC. Thus, a low value of PEF may be due either to airways obstruction or to restrictive disease, whereas a low FEV_1 together with a low FVC (provided that the FEV_1/FVC ratio is more than 70 per cent) is indicative of a restrictive disorder.

The Vitalograph provides a written tracing which can be kept as a permanent record. However, this advantage of the Vitalograph is not so great as is sometimes supposed, since the interpretation of spirograms may require considerable experience. Similarly, the fact that it is possible to derive other indices of ventilatory function in addition to FEV_1 and FVC is of less value to the general practitioner than to the specialist.

Any general practitioner who has to decide whether to buy a Vitalograph or a peak flow meter is well advised to consider the uses, apart from screening, which he will be able to make of whichever instrument he finally purchases. The peak flow meter, being portable and requiring no source of electric supply, is the more convenient of the two instruments to use during consultations. Whereas values of

PEF can be obtained immediately by reading them on the dial of the meter, it takes a short time to measure FEV_1 and FVC on the Vitalograph chart.

In terms of cost the Wright peak flow meter is the more attractive proposition for general practitioners. In a partnership of three doctors each could have a Wright peak flow meter in his consulting room for the same cost as one Vitalograph shared between them.

In October, 1973 a much cheaper version of the peak flow meter was introduced. Preliminary trials of this instrument, which is called a peak flow gauge, have indicated that it gives values of PEF very close to those obtained with the Wright peak flow meter.

The ideal equipment for general practice should be for every doctor to have a Wright peak flow meter or a peak flow gauge for his personal use and to have access to a Vitalograph which is shared by the partners and which can be used for special diagnostic problems.

The use of the vitalograph and peak flow meter as screening tests of symptomless airways obstruction

Although shortness of breath in patients with advanced chronic

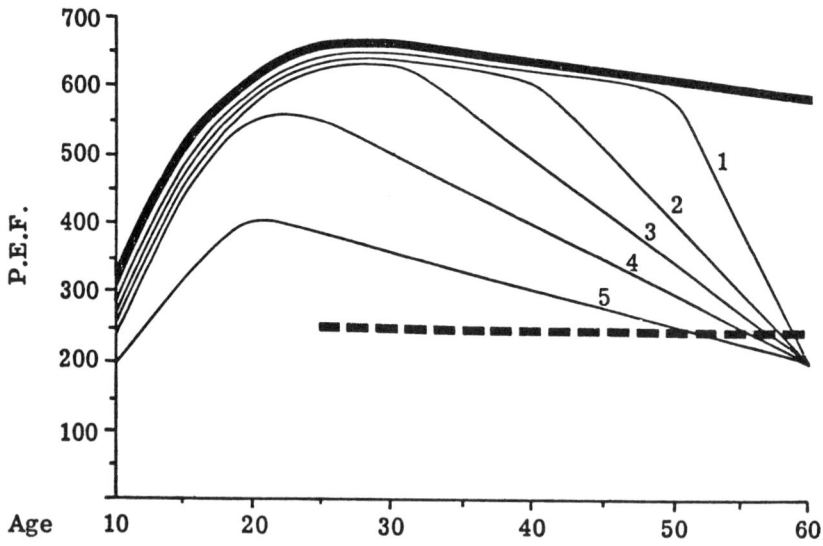

Figure 12. Theoretical ways in which progressive impairment of ventilatory function can develop, all leading to disability at about sixty years of age. The heavy, continuous line represents ventilatory function (PEF) in the normal subject. The interrupted line denotes the level of PEF (about 250 litres/min) at which patients usually first become aware of shortness of breath on moderate exertion. Prospective studies suggest that the most common manners in which progressive impairment occurs are those represented by lines 2, 3 and 4.

bronchitis arises from complex causes, the primary abnormality is irreversible airways obstruction. It is clear that long before a state of disability has been reached, there must have been steadily progressive deterioration of ventilatory function which has occurred over many years. Figure 12 depicts diagrammatically several different ways in which PEF may become reduced with increasing age, leading eventually to disability when it is about 250 litres/minute.

Because of the large reserve ventilatory capacity of the lungs and also because many persons nowadays have sedentary jobs, a considerable degree of airways obstruction may be present without the subject being aware of shortness of breath. It is the contention of those who advocate the use of the Vitalograph or the peak flow meter for screening that such persons can be detected before their function has become seriously impaired. The implicit corollary of this is that the doctor, having thus identified persons with early chronic obstructive bronchitis, can institute measures which will arrest further deterioration or at least prevent its occurring as rapidly as it would otherwise have done.

Although the motives of proponents of screening tests for early chronic obstructive bronchitis are wholly admirable, the considerable practical difficulties which are involved are not sufficiently appreciated: these will be discussed at some length in the sections below.

'Normal values'. It is essential to realise that there is no 'absolute' range of normal values of FEV_1 and PEF, unlike the situation which obtains in the case of, say, blood sugar and blood urea (these being very largely independent of the age or other characteristics of the subjects in whom they are estimated).

Both FEV_1 and PEF are influenced by the age and body build of the subject who is being tested. The only convenient index of body build is height, although this correlates rather poorly with both the dimensions of the thorax and the power of the respiratory muscles which act upon it. Tests which employ forced expiration, such as FEV_1 and PEF, are highly dependent upon these muscular forces. Hence, it is often found that tall, thin subjects have lower values than stocky muscular subjects and, for the same reason, men have a higher range of FEV_1 and PEF than women of the same age and height, whose chests are smaller and whose respiratory muscles are less powerful.

Some guide to the values of FEV_1 and PEF which a subject should achieve can be obtained from prediction tables or nomograms. From these a predicted normal value can be found for men and women of any given age and height, against which the observed value of the subject who is tested can be compared. It is widely accepted that only values which fall outside two standard deviations below the predicted normal value should be regarded as being abnormal. The standard deviation (SD) is a measure of the 'scatter' around the mean regression and in the case of FEV_1 and PEF a large part of this scatter is due to the differences of body build and musculature of individuals of the same age and height.

From prediction tables or nomograms a predicted value of FEV_1 or PEF can be found for any subject of given age and height. By subtracting from this two standard deviations, a value is obtained which respresents the lower limit of normal (LLN) of FEV_1 or PEF. Only those observed values which are less than the LLN can be regarded as being definitely abnormal.

It is a truism, but one which has not received sufficient emphasis, that a screening test can only be as good as its normal values. Ideally, the latter should permit a clear distinction to be made between normality and abnormality. If the range of normal values is very wide, then clearly the test will be valueless for detecting subjects who are, in fact, abnormal but whose observed value still falls within the normal range.

Normal values of FEV_1 and PEF have been derived from various studies of large numbers of supposedly normal subjects. In almost every case, however, smokers were not excluded from the normal series provided that they denied having chronic or persistent expectoration. Since there is considerable evidence that some smokers and ex-smokers, even though they have no symptoms of mucus hypersecretion, nevertheless have lower values of FEV_1 or PEF than persons who have never smoked, the inclusion of smokers in a normal series has two important consequences. First, the mean value of FEV_1 or PEF of the whole series is lowered and, secondly, the scatter of values around the mean, i.e. the standard deviation, is increased. Both these effects reduce the discriminatory value of the predicted normal values.

Normal values of FEV_1. The most widely used normal values for FEV_1 are those which were recommended by Cotes (1968); these are, for males, the series of Kory et al. (1961) and, for females, the series of Ferris et al. (1964). The makers of the Vitalograph have recently published a manual for users of the instrument which includes nomograms for predicting FEV_1 in subjects of both sexes. These were derived from the findings of a small series of healthy factory workers and pensioners in West Germany. It will be seen in Table 19 that the standard deviations in both males and females are larger than those found by Kory et al. (1961) and Ferris et al. (1965) respectively. If the nomograms of the Vitalograph Manual (1973) are used to obtain predicted values, the 'normal' range becomes progressively less discriminatory with advancing age. Thus, in a man or

Table 19. Normal Values of FEV$_1$

MALES

Age	Height (ins)	(cm)	Kory et al. (1961) SD = 0·52L			Vitalograph Manual (1973)* SD = 0·77L		
			Predicted (litres)	LLN (litres)	$\frac{LLN}{Pred.}$ %	Predicted (litres)	LLN (litres)	$\frac{LLN}{Pred.}$ %
20	72	183	4·60	3·56	78%	5·20	3·66	70%
45	69	175	3·50	2·46	70%	3·85	2·31	60%
60	66	168	2·90	1·86	64%	2·95	1·41	48%

FEMALES

Age	Height (ins)	(cm)	Ferris et al. (1965) SD = 0·40L			Vitalograph Manual (1973)* SD = 0·56L		
			Predicted (litres)	LLN (litres)	$\frac{LLN}{Pred.}$ %	Predicted (litres)	LLN (litres)	$\frac{LLN}{Pred.}$ %
20	66	168	3·13	2·33	74%	3·40	2·28	67%
45	63	160	2·40	1·60	67%	2·50	1·38	55%
60	60	152	1·85	1·05	57%	1·90	0·78	41%

*Based upon the data of P.L. Kamburoff, H.J. Woiowitz and R.H. Woitowitz (unpublished).

Although the predicted values of FEV$_1$ given in the Vitalograph manual are in every case higher than the corresponding values of Kory et al. and Ferris et al., the standard deviations for both sexes are much higher. Consequently, the LLN (which is obtained by subtracting 2 standard deviations from the predicted value) is lower, a trend which increases markedly with advancing age. An observed value of FEV$_1$ can be regarded as being abnormal only if the percentage of observed/predicted is less than that of LLN/predicted. It will be seen that the normal values of the Vitalograph's manual are much less discriminating than those of Kory et al., and of Ferris et al.

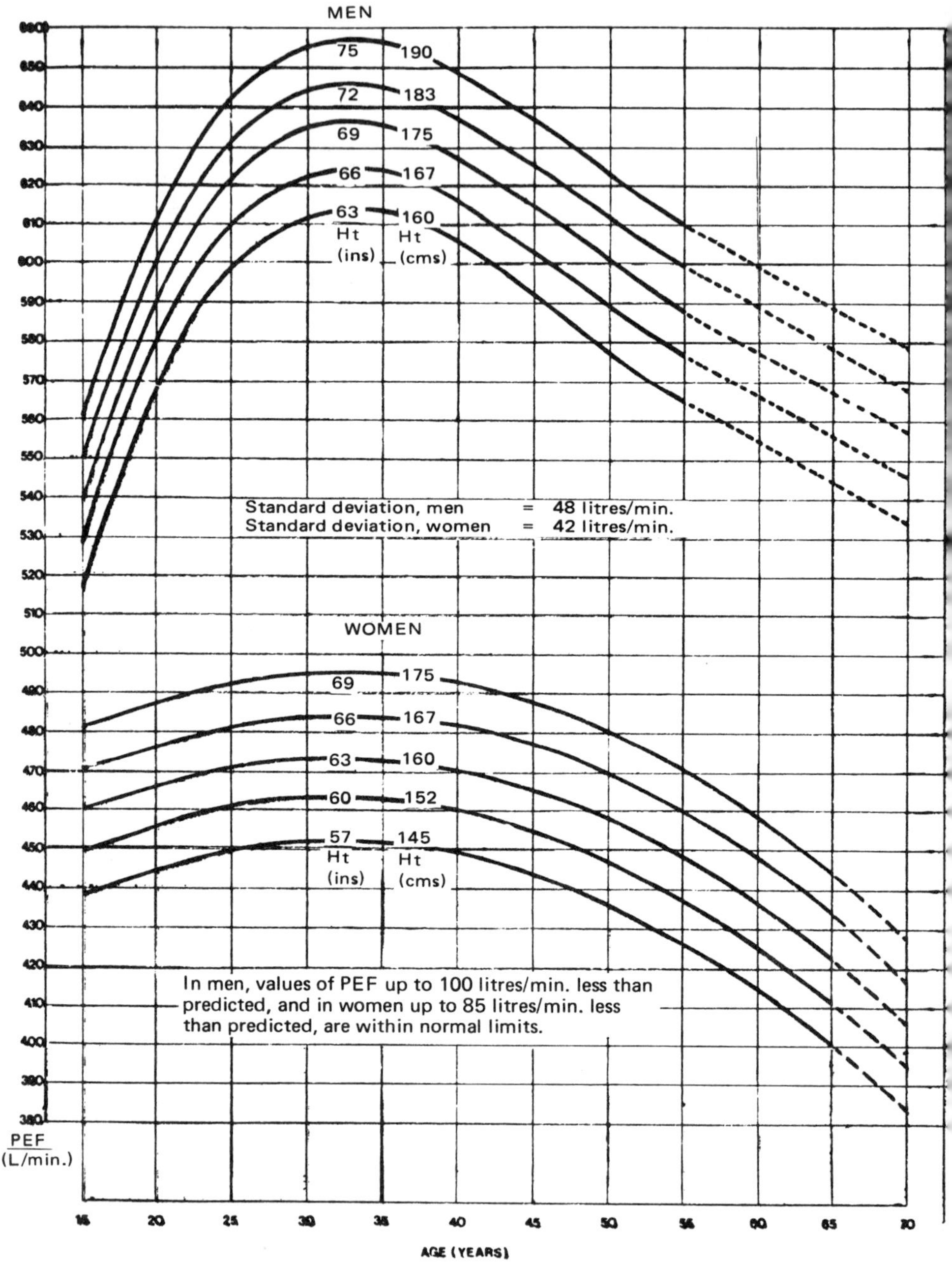

Figure 13. Normal Values of PEF (Gregg and Nunn, 1973).

woman aged 45 years, an observed FEV_1 can only be regarded as abnormal if it is less than 60% of the predicted value (Table 19, p.301).

Normal values of PEF. Cotes (1968) recommended the use of the normal values which were found by Leiner *et al.* (1963) in males and by Pelzer and Thomson (1964) in females. Both these series included smokers and in calculating the regression of PEF it was assumed that PEF falls in a linear fashion from the age of 20 years.

Recently Gregg and Nunn (1973) published their findings of PEF in males and females over the age of 15 years, all of whom satisfied stringent criteria of normality. It will be seen in Figure 13 that the shape of the regression of PEF on age is curvilinear in both sexes: the large difference between the sexes, which emerges at puberty, is due to the more powerful muscular forces of the male. Because of the comparatively small standard deviations in both sexes, an observed PEF which is less than 80 per cent of predicted lies outside the normal range, irrespective of the subject's age or sex (Table 20, p.304).

A simple guide to the use of the normal values of Gregg and Nunn is that in men PEF should be within 100L/min and in women within 90L/min of predicted values.

Compared with the normal series of Leiner *et al.* (for males) and of Pelzer and Thomson (for females), not only are the standard deviations found by Gregg and Nunn smaller, but the predicted values themselves are higher. As a result there is a considerable difference in the LLN depending upon which normal values are used (Table 20).

The following examples will make this clear:

1 A man, aged 45 years and 69 inches tall, whose PEF is less than 520 litres/min is abnormal if the predicted values of Gregg and Nunn are used. Using those of Leiner *et al.* his PEF would be abnormal only if it were less than 450 litres/min.

2 A woman, aged 45 years and 63 inches tall, should have a PEF of at least 380 litres/min according to the predicted values of Gregg and Nunn, whereas if those of Pelzer and Thomson are used her PEF would be abnormal only if it were less than 255 litres/min.

Normal values of FEV_1 and PEF in children. In children aged 5 to 18 years normal values of FEV_1 and PEF can be obtained from a nomogram based on the findings of Godfrey *et al.* (1970).

The limitations of normal values. Because of the wide range of normal values, even in series which have a comparatively small standard deviation, some subjects who are, in fact, abnormal will have values of FEV_1 or PEF which are above the LLN. For instance, a man at the age of 20 years might have an FEV_1 or PEF which is around two SDs *above* the predicted value: considerable deteriora-

Table 20. Normal Values of PEF

MALES

Age	Height (ins)	Height (cm)	Gregg and Nunn (1973) SD = 48 litres/min			Leiner et al. (1963) SD = 60 litres/min		
			Predicted (L/min)	LLN (L/min)	$\frac{LLN}{Pred.}$ %	Predicted (L/min)	LLN (L/min)	$\frac{LLN}{Pred.}$ %
20	72	183	600	504	84%	665	545	82%
45	69	175	615	519	84%	570	450	79%
60	66	168	565	469	83%	510	390	77%

FEMALES

Age	Height (ins)	Height (cm)	Gregg and Nunn (1973) SD = 42 litres/min			Pelzer and Thomson (1964) SD = 67 litres/min		
			Predicted (L/min)	LLN (L/min)	$\frac{LLN}{Pred.}$ %	Predicted (L/min)	LLN (L/min)	$\frac{LLN}{Pred.}$ %
20	66	168	475	391	82%	475	341	72%
45	63	160	465	381	82%	390	256	66%
60	60	152	425	341	80%	325	191	59%

Except in young adults, aged between 20 and 30 years, the normal values of Gregg and Nunn are higher than those of Leiner et al. (males) and Pelzer and Thomson (females). Because the standard deviations in the latter two series are considerably greater, their LLN is lower. Using the normal values of Gregg and Nunn, an observed PEF which is less than 80 per cent of the LLN is abnormal, irrespective of age, height and sex.

tion could occur over the course of 25 years, yet at the age of 45 years he might have an FEV_1 or PEF only just less than two SDs *below* predicted (but still within the normal range). Therefore, some 'rule of thumb' adjustment must be made in evaluating the results of tests of ventilatory function. If the subject is muscular and well-built a value of FEV_1 or PEF which is 90 per cent of predicted value could be abnormal; whereas if the subject is thin and less muscular a value close to the LLN could merely be due to his body build.

The difficulties of interpretation of such borderline values of ventilatory function tests are illustrated in the following example:

3 A powerfully built, stocky labourer aged 34 years and 68 inches tall, smoked 30-40 cigarettes a day but denied expectoration. His FEV_1 was 2·75 litres and his FVC was 3·7 litres (FEV_1/FVC = 74 per cent). Using the normal values of Kory *et al.* his FEV_1 was 71 per cent of predicted and was only just less than the LLN (2·8 litres). Since a man of his body build should have had an FEV_1 higher than the predicted value, it seemed probable that his borderline value denoted the presence of airways obstruction. This was confirmed by his PEF of 480 litres/min which was 76 per cent of predicted (using the normal values of Gregg and Nunn) and considerably less than the LLN (539 litres/min).

Reversible airways obstruction. Airways obstruction occurring in patients with typical asthma gives rise to symptoms which the patient himself can recognise, such as tightness of the chest or wheezing. However, some patients with asthma do not have typical, paroxsymal episodes but have peristent airways obstruction. If they are smokers and if it is found that they have an abnormally low FEV_1 or PEF, it is only too easy to conclude that they have an early stage of chronic obstructive bronchitis. While some part of the airways obstruction in such persons may be irreversible, there may also be a large reversible component which, having once been identified, can then be treated. Therefore, measurement of FEV_1 or PEF should be repeated 5 minutes after the inhalation of isoprenaline from a pressurised aerosol to determine whether improvement occurs in response to the bronchodilator.

The limitations of screening tests for chronic obstructive bronchitis

As yet, there is no ideal screening test for symptomless airways obstruction. Such a test would have to fulfil the following criteria—it should not be influenced by the muscular effort made by the subject who is tested, it should give absolute values which are independent of the subject's body build, and it should be able to discriminate clearly between normal subjects and those with only a minor degree of abnormality. Recently, claims have been made that measurement of the 'closing volume' of the lungs satisfies most of these criteria (Buist and Ross, 1973). Already the measurement of closing volume has been used for screening in one centre in the United States and it has been asserted that the test is capable of revealing abnormalities in smokers who have a normal FEV_1 (Buist et al., (1973). Further experience of the use of this test will be required before it can be recommended for screening. Although the equipment which is necessary for performing the test precludes its use in general practice, it is possible that it could be used in screening programmes which might be undertaken by chest clinics or mass X-ray units to which general practitioners could refer their patients.

The question needs to be asked, however, whether more sensitive and discriminating screening tests would be of any real practical value. At present it is not clear whether the pathological changes which are responsible for abnormality of closing volume are necessarily the same as those which give rise to the development of irreversible airways obstruction (British Medical Journal, 1973).

Selective Screening. A less good case can be made for measuring ventilatory function in every adult who comes to the general practitioner's surgery than can be made for some other screening procedures, such as the measurement of blood pressure and the testing of urine for glycosuria.

Although the screening of large populations may be valuable in epidemiological research, for the clinician it is a pointless exercise unless the identification of an abnormality leads directly to the institution of measures which will arrest further progress of the disease. Therefore, screening for chronic obstructive bronchitis should be selective and should be directed towards those persons who are most at risk of developing the disease. Present knowledge of its pathogenesis suggests that the most important groups to screen are smokers who admit to an intermittent or persistent cough with expectoration ('just the natural smoker's cough'), persons whose occupation exposes them to dust or fumes, persons who are subject to recurrent chest infections and young adults who give a history of having had asthma, bronchitis or pneumonia during their childhood.

While some degree of bronchial damage may well have been incurred before either FEV_1 or PEF becomes unequivocally abnormal, study of Figure 12 shows that considerable impairment of ventilatory function must occur before the onset of disability due to dyspnoea. Therefore, the identification of persons who have a moderate degree of airways obstruction is of value if measures can then be taken to prevent further deterioration. The most important of these is persuasion to give up smoking completely and the prompt treatment of acute episodes of bronchitis with an adequate course of antibiotics.

Conclusions

The Vitalograph and peak flow meter are of value for the selective screening of persons with symptomless airways obstruction. The most discriminatory values of FEV_1 are those of Kory *et al.* (1961) for males, and of Ferris *et al.* (1965) for females (Table 19). In the case of PEF (Table 20) the most discriminatory normal values for males and females are those of Gregg and Nunn (1973).

Comparison of Tables 19 and 20 shows that the percentage of LLN/predicted for PEF is both smaller and more uniform at all ages than that for FEV_1, suggesting that PEF is at least as reliable as FEV_1 for the purpose of screening. Thus, any general practitioner who already possesses a peak flow meter has all that is required to screen his patients for early chronic obstructive bronchitis.

ACKNOWLEDGEMENTS

Grateful acknowledgement is made to Vitalograph Limited, Maids Moreton House, Buckingham, for permission to reproduce Figure 10, and to Clement Clarke International Limited (formerly Airmed Limited), Edinburgh Way, Harlow, Essex, for permission to reproduce Figures 11 and 13.

REFERENCES

British Medical Journal (1973). 'First in, last out' in the lung. Leading Article. 3, 119.

Buist, A. S. & Ross, B. R. (1973). Predicted values for closing volumes using a modified single breath nitrogen test. *American Review of Respiratory Diseases,* 107, 74.

Buist, A. S., Van Fleet, D. L. & Ross, B. R. (1973). A comparison of conventional spirometric tests and the test of closing volume in an emphysema screening centre, *American Review of Respiratory Diseases,* 107, 735.

Cotes, J. E. (1968). *Lung Function. Assessment and Application in Medicine.* 2nd Edition, Oxford: Blackwell.

Ferris, B. G., Anderson, D. O & Zickmantel, R. (1965). Prediction values for screening tests of pulmonary function, *American Review of Respiratory Diseases,* 91, 253.

Godfrey, S., Kamburoff, P. L. & Nairn, J. R. (1970). Spirometry lung volumes and airway resistance in normal children aged 5 to 18 years, *British Journal of Diseases of the Chest,* 64, 15.

Gregg, I. & Nunn, A. J. (1973). Peak expiratory flow in normal subjects, *British Medical Journal,* 3, 282.

Kory, R. C., Callahan, R., Boren, H. G. & Snyder, J. C. (1961). The Veterans Administration army study of pulmonary function: 1. Clinical spirometry in normal men. *American Journal of Medicine,* 30, 243.

Leiner, G. C., Abramowitz, S., Small, J. J., Stenby, B. V. & Lewis, W. A. (1963). Expiratory peak flow rate. Standard values for normal subjects. *American Review of Respiratory Diseases,* 88, 644.

Pelzer, A. M. & Thomson, M. L. (1964). Expiratory peak flow. *British Medical Journal,* 2, 123.

Ritchie, B. (1962). A comparison of forced expiratory volume and peak flow in clinical practice. *Lancet,* 2, 271.

Vitalograph Manual (1973). *The simple measurement of lung ventilation.* Buckingham: Vitalograph Limited.

30 The Audiometer

George Gomez

'How strange a deaf wife to prefer,'
'True, but she's also dumb, good Sir.'

Lessing, 1729-1781.

Of all the diseases seen in the surgery none needs to be sought for more by screening than deafness.

Wilson (1966) described ten postulates as principles of case finding:

1 The condition sought should be an important problem

Our most important deaf patients are children. Unilateral perceptive deafness (usually congenital, or following mumps) is frequently unrecognized and is always incurable. The child's education suffers if he is seated with his deaf ear near his teacher's desk.

Acute otitis media is a common GP disease, never seen in the ENT department in its earliest stages. It usually resolves, but is not infrequently followed by glue ear, not easy to diagnose with an otoscope. The accompanying curable conductive deafness is easily detected and diagnosed with a tuning fork and measured with an audiometer. A perforated tympanic membrane may not heal. Dangerous chronic suppurative otitis media might follow if the perforation is posterior or marginal. A cholesteatoma may develop which erodes bone and may give rise to a brain abscess.

Adolescents and the young middle-aged can also suffer from curable conductive deafness, frequently unilateral at its onset, due to spongy bone formation in the ossicles—otosclerosis. Deafness is also important in the elderly, for increasing age brings presbyacusis to all who live long enough. If not too severe, a hearing aid works miracles both for the socially cut-off, and their unfortunate spouses who have to put up with overloud television programmes.

Noise-induced, incurable perceptive deafness occurs in many occupations ranging from boiler-makers to helicopter engineers, not forgetting members of pop groups playing by their noisy discotheque amplifiers.

The commonest cause of deafness is however wax. This type may come on suddenly in swimmers on holiday.

2 There should be an accepted treatment for patients with recognized disease

Removal of wax is a familiar GP procedure. A non-caustic solvent such as olive oil is best used to soften the wax before syringing the meatus. If there is no history of a perforation a superiorly directed stream of water at body temperature usually works well, though a ruptured tympanic membrane from this cause is seen once or twice a year at most ENT outpatients departments. The elderly patient with a hard plug of wax can often have his deafness cured rapidly by the skilful use of a wax hook under head mirror illumination—as dramatic and satisfying as bursting a wrist ganglion by simple pressure. Wax is normally almost odourless. If it is offensive infection is present, requiring aural toilet, and possibly systemic antibiotics and local hydrargaphen (Ototrane) wicks.

Otitis media and its sequelae are treated with antibiotics in the acute stage and by myringoplasty (patching a perforation with a graft) or tympanoplasty (entire replacement of the tympanic membrane by a graft) when perforations will not heal on their own.

Secretory otitis, or glue ear, with a painless and gradual onset, may need myringotomy when a yellow Evo-stick like discharge can be aspirated. This condition can be diagnosed by the presence of a meniscus visible through the tympanic membrane, when bubbles of air, indicating eustachian patency, may be seen floating in the straw coloured fluid. This disease, common in children, can lead to permanent deafness. Treatment is often the insertion of Shepard's grommets which resemble squashed cotton reels in miniature. They provide aeration of the middle ear, and may remain in position for a year or more, when they are usually extruded naturally, but may sometimes be removed painlessly before the swimming season begins.

Youthful deafness caused by otosclerosis is commonly bilateral but usually one ear is more severely affected, and this one is operated on first by stapedectomy with an 80 per cent success rate.

3 Facilities for diagnosis and treatment should be available

Every family doctor should be able to handle the modern

magnifying otoscope which enlarges the tympanic membrane so that it looks like the side of a glacier. An interest in the deaf cannot be followed up unless the tuning fork tests are understood and accurately performed. In conductive deafness the Rinne test is negative, that is bone conduction is better than air conduction, the opposite of normal. Firm pressure of the foot of the tuning fork on the mastoid with counter pressure by the other hand on the opposite side of the patient's head is essential. The vibrating ends of the fork should be carefully placed exactly opposite the external auditory meatus. In the Weber test when the tuning fork is placed on the vertex, the sound is referred to the deafer ear in conductive deafness, for ambient noise does not reach the ear that is deaf: thus the cochlea of the deaf ear is more sensitive to sound by bone conduction than the normal ear. In perceptive deafness, such as is found in Menière's disease, acoustic neuroma and acoustic trauma, the sound of the tuning fork is heard better in the good ear; for the cochlea of the deaf ear, by definition, does not function.

The Keeler Audio-Tester (Fig. 14) is a fairly inexpensive (£38·00) screening audiometer which measures deafness. Full audiometric assessment requires a silent room in which to perform the test, for

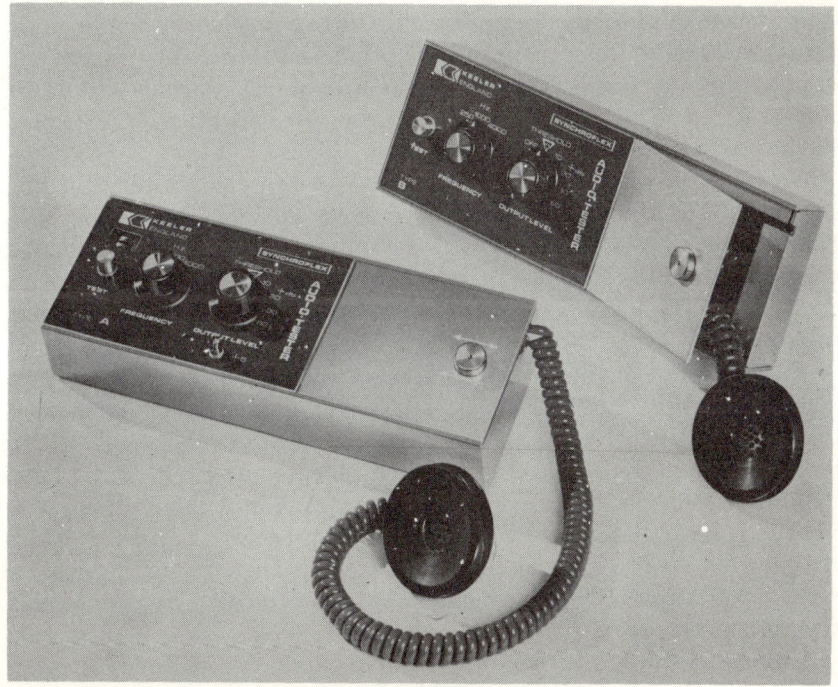

Figure 14. The Keeler Audio-Tester

background noise interferes with auditory acuity. Properly fitting earphones must be used and a full range of frequencies tested, using expensive and complicated apparatus. Such an accurate assessment is not needed for screening purposes if a fail-safe programme is carried out, and all doubtful patients are referred.

The Audio-Tester is a pure tone audiometer which can detect deafness in the normal speech range at frequencies of 250, 1,000, and 4,000 Hz.

The apparatus measures 7 in x 6 in x 3 in (18 cm x 15 cm x 8 cm) and weights 3 lbs (132 gm). It is calibrated to test hearing at threshold (O decibels), and at 10, 15, 20, 25, 30 and 35 db above threshold. There is then a gap to 60-65 db above threshold which enables the patient to hear clearly the sound he is to listen to during the test.

The audiometer, fully transistorised, and powered by a nine volt battery that should last six months, is contained in a metal case. An indicator shows when the battery is run down, and the switch cannot be left on by mistake. The latter need only be touched very lightly: it does not click.

A convenient method of using the instrument with a child is to ask him to hold up his hand, palm towards the doctor. He is told he is a lighthouseman and the doctor is a ship with a magic box sending him signals. When he hears a sound the child must flex his fingers and straighten them out again quickly and decisively. Signals should be sent at irregular intervals. Needless to say the ears must be inspected and any wax removed before beginning the test.

When testing a child there must be a close personal relationship. He should be talked to at first and a guess made of his hearing loss. The audiometer is then used at a louder level than his estimated hearing threshold. Patience may be needed in children with secretory otitis for they may find it difficult to interpret the pure tone audiometer.

The first test made at 1,000 Hz and 60 db. The sound is then reduced to 35, 30, 25, 20, 15, 10, 5 and O db. Threshold level is rarely heard in the relatively noisy conditions prevailing in an ordinary room. This procedure is then repeated at 4,000 Hz and 250 Hz. The other ear is tested in the same way, and the audiogram is recorded. In adults ability to hear such frequencies at 30 db or less is satisfactory. In the case of schoolchildren, persistent hearing loss of over 20 db should be investigated by an otologist before a final diagnosis is made.

There is a fail-safe procedure built in this method, for if the test room is noisy, an audiogram indicating deafness may be recorded when hearing is normal, and the patient is referred. It is most unlikely that a normal audiogram will be recorded when the patient is deaf, however noisy the room in which he is being tested. Care must be taken to fit the ear cup exactly, so that the perforations are opposite the meatus.

Objections to audiometry in the surgery are sometimes raised on the grounds that the procedure cannot be accurately carried out, owing to inexperience of the operator and lack of a silent room. It is sometimes said that if there is any doubt the patient should always be referred for expert opinion. Others say we are far too busy in the NHS open-ended surgery with its conveyor-belt like method, for any GP to concern himself with hearing measurement.

Any intelligent receptionist can be trained to use an audiometer such as that described. Apparent deafness discovered in a relatively noisy test room will be referred and found to be false. A simple hearing test will show up the child who does not want to hear—there are none so deaf as those who will not hear—and his mother can be shown that the child has good hearing. Every child that has had acute otitis media should be tested a month later—few will fail, and those that do should be referred. Poor scholars and those with congenitally deaf siblings should also be tested.

There is some overlap when deafness is being screened with the local authority school examination programmes. A child that has been tested at school and found to be normal should not be asked to come again in the surgery unless for any reason deafness has arisen since the school test.

Reed's pictures are useful when a child's hearing is to be tested. These consist of four pictures in a row, such as of a cup and a duck. The words are whispered by the doctor and the child is asked to point to the appropriate picture. The words are monosyllabic and have similar vowel sounds.

Many doctors would appreciate direct-access audiometry for their deaf patients. Many otologists would agree to this arrangement if they were convinced of the GP's need. They must know, of course, that the deaf patient is not going to be sent for an audiogram with wax occluding his meatus.

4 There should be a recognized latent or early symptomatic stage

This often occurs in otosclerosis, which is of course curable. Secretory otitis begins with insidious deafness, and the sensori-neural deafness of Menière's disease may come on gradually.

The other five of Wilson's postulates all apply to screening for deafness. As described there is a suitable test for the disease, which is acceptable to patients. The natural history of deafness, from its development to declared disease is fairly well understood, and there is an agreed policy of whom to treat as patients. The cost of case finding, including diagnosis and subsequent treatment is reasonable, and is certainly a continuing process.

Sixty-four patients were examined in a south-west London practice during six months. Thirty-six per cent were under 19; 26 per cent were aged 20-49; and 39 per cent were over 50. Their age, sex and disease frequency are shown in Tables 21 and 22. Otitis media in the young, and old tubotympanic disease and presbyacusis in the older age groups were the most common conditions requiring audiometry; two children were seen whose ears had been slapped, resulting in a ruptured eardrum. Unsuspected deafness has been found:

JB, aged eight, was found to be erratic in his work at school. He was excellent in some classes and very poor in others. He was found to be suffering from unilateral deafness, his school performance depending on where he sat in the classroom. He was good when his good ear was directed to the teacher, for he had given up listening with his bad one. His school record improved when his unsuspected deafness was appreciated, so that he could be properly seated in the classroom.

Table 21. Deafness in general practice—64 patients seen in the surgery in six months—age-sex distribution.

Age	Male	Female	Percentage of total
0-20	10	12	36
20-50	8	9	26
Over 50	12	13	39

Table 22. Diseases causing deafness seen in the surgery in six months.

Disease	No of cases
Recent acute otitis media	20
Old tubotympanic disease	13
Presbyacusis	10
Recent trauma to tympanic membrane	3
Acoustic trauma	2
Secretory otitis	3
Mixed deafness	3
Otosclerosis	2
Cholesteatoma	2
Congenital	2
Nerve deafness after measles	2
Nerve deafness after aspirin poisoning	1
Malingering	1

Deaf patients were shunned by the writer for many years. Communication was difficult, and the external auditory meatus was dark, often exquisitely tender, and usually offensive. Only when practice with a head mirror enabled both hands to be used to remove debris was it possible to use a modern magnifying otoscope and a tuning fork to best advantage.

Mr B has been coming to see me for 15 years for his bronchitis. He had always been as deaf as a post, which I thought was incurable. A tuning fork revealed a negative Rinne's test, his conductive deafness being due to otosclerosis. Stapedectomy was performed and his face now lights up when he describes his 'breakthrough'. He had forgotten that floorboards creak and he still has to stop himself from ducking his head when an aeroplane goes over.

Children with earache are frequently seen in the surgery. It is important to make sure that permanent deafness does not ensue:

VH, aged five, had acute earache without discharge for two days. Both tympanic membranes were red, and the right one was bulging. The Rinne's test was negative as expected. There was a history of seven previous attacks. Her mother was deaf in one ear from old tubotympanic disease. Treatment with intramuscular penicillin G 1 mega unit followed by penicillin V for five days, resulted in a dramatic improvement as shown by the audiogram (Fig. 15).

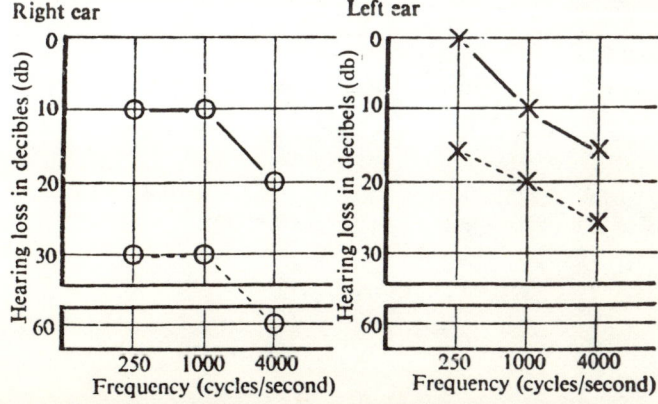

Figure 15. Improvement in auditory acuity after antibiotic treatment of acute otitis media. (Dotted lines before treatment, straight lines after treatment).

Good hearing can be life-saving in today's traffic, as much as in primitive areas where rattle-snakes give audible warning of their presence. It is also vital to the blind, who depend on the echo of their footsteps, and sometimes of their stick, to know if they are about to walk into a lamp-post. They do not like the snow which muffles this echo, for as they say, snow is the blind man's fog.

REFERENCE

Wilson, J. M. G. (1966). Some principles of early diagnosis and detection. In *Surveillance and Early Diagnosis in General Practice.* Edited by G.G. Teeling-Smith. London: Office of Health Economics.

31 Cervical Cytology

Gareth Lloyd

'A final solution of the cancer problem is impossible'.

Smithers, 1956.

The cervical cytotest is the oldest and most widely used of all screening procedures for the detection of malignant disease. Certain guiding principles are important. A positive cervical cytotest does not diagnose cancer, but selects patients who require further investigation. A negative cervical cytotest does not exclude cancer.

Among the Registrar General's figures of deaths due to cancer of women in England and Wales for 1971, 2,315 deaths are attributed to cancer of the cervix. This figure represents 20 per cent of deaths due to malignant disease of the female reproductive organs and five per cent of all deaths in women due to malignant disease (Registrar General, 1971). For women aged below 50, cancer of the cervix is responsible for a quarter of the total deaths due to cancer (Hussain, 1968).

The cervical cytotest is simple, painless, and can be performed quickly. Successful development of the test is the result of the special staining technique described by Papanicolau in 1928 and a cervical scraping method introduced by Ayre in 1947.

The cervical scrape can readily be accomplished in general practice. Since the introduction of a national cervical cytology programme in the United Kingdom in 1964, and up to July 1970, general practitioners have taken 1,330,253 tests, and this represents 30 per cent of tests taken outside hospitals and 18 per cent of all tests taken during this period (Thomson 1971).

In East Lincolnshire, over half of the smears dealt with by the cytology laboratory are taken by general practitioners (Wookey 1971).

Terminology

1 **Pre-invasive carcinoma** (synonyms: Carcinoma in situ; Stage 0 carcinoma; Intra-epithelial carcinoma; Bowen's disease of the cervix). These terms are applied to cellular changes in the cervical endothelium which have histological characteristics of cancer but are present only in the cellular layers above the basement membrane. The term used in the International Classification is Stage 0 carcinoma, and was introduced by Broders (1932). The diagnosis of pre-invasive carcinoma is made on biopsy of the cervix and cannot be made on the basis of a cervical smear alone (Jeffcoate, 1957; Way, 1955).

2 **Pre-symptomatic cancer.** This term is variously used to describe cancer of the cervix which is present but which has not yet caused the patient to perceive symptoms. Such cancer may be pre-invasive or invasive. The cervical cytotest is particularly useful in detecting invasive cancer which is pre-symptomatic, because the results of therapy in these circumstances are very good (Jeffcoate, 1957).

History

The first demonstration of exfoliative cytology can probably be attributed to Leeuwenhoek, who showed a party of visitors to his laboratory in 1710, scrapings from the skin of the arm and from the surface of the tongue. Donné, in 1837, described the cells of sputum, and Barry in 1847 described and illustrated the nuclei of cells. Though Walshe in 1841 referred to his finding fragments of malignant tissue in the sputum of patients with cancer of the lung, it is probable that the diagnosis of cancer by a cytological method was first described by Beale in 1860.

Further reports on the histological finding of cancer cells and on their characteristics appeared during the 19th Century (Virchow, 1858; Biermer, 1855; Troup, 1886). Troup's monograph contains some of the earliest photomicrographs made in pathology. In 1914, MacCarty reported his observations and photographic illustrations of the cancer cell, drawing attention to the prognostic significance of the ratio of nuclear to nucleolar size.

The widespread use of cytological methods of diagnosis of cancer began following the reports of a new technique of staining smears introduced by Papanicolau in 1928. The acridine orange fluorochrome technique, attributable to Papanicolau, results in a more translucent coloration of cells and greater diagnostic accuracy.

An active proponent of the concept of population screening for cervical cancer is T. Ernest Ayre of the Cancer Cytology Foundation of America. Ayre developed the characteristic wooden spatula for obtaining a 'scrape' of the cervix (Ayre, 1962).

Large and small scale population screening programmes have been described, and examples are: The British Columbia Project (Boyes, Fidler and Lock, 1962); The Aberdeen Study (MacGregor and Baird, 1963); The Manchester Survey (Wakefield, 1971) and the Birmingham Programme (Parry, 1971). Stimulus for the establishment, implementation and expansion of the British National Cervical Screening programme has come from many organisations, among whom are the Trade Unions (TUC Congress Resolutions, 1964; 1966) and the BMA (BMJ Supplement, 1964).

The claim of the British Columbia observers that mortality from cancer of the cervix is diminishing as a result of population screening programmes has not yet been adequately supported by the evidence (Fidler *et al.*, 1968, Kinlen and Doll, 1973).

Technique for smear taking

There are two commonly used techniques for collecting cells from the gynaecological tract.

1 Aspiration of the posterior vaginal fornix is the simplest, and was the method used by Papanicolau to obtain cellular material (Papanicolau, 1942). The instrument required consists of a glass or plastic tube slightly bent at one end and attached firmly to a rubber bulb at the other end. The tube is inserted into the vagina as far as the vault. Aspirate is obtained by releasing the compressed bulb whilst moving the end of the tube laterally across the posterior vaginal fornix. A speculum is not necessary to obtain a specimen in this way, and a 'do-it-herself' kit has been described by Davis and Kurz, 1962.

2 The much more widely used technique in the United Kingdom is the cervical scrape, using a wooden spatula described by Ayre (Ayre, 1947). Scraping of the cervix is carried out under direct vision, and for this a speculum and a good source of light are essential. The scrape must be taken from the squamo-columnar junction as well as the ectocervix (Fig. 16).

Specimens obtained by aspirate or scrape should be transferred quickly to a clean glass slide and spread thinly. A fixative is applied, either as a liquid or spray, while the smear is still wet. The name of the patient should be written on the frosted end of the slide.

The vaginal aspirate has the advantage of simplicity, and is more likely to pick up endometrial cells. Examination of aspirate smears is, however, more difficult and time consuming and may reveal very

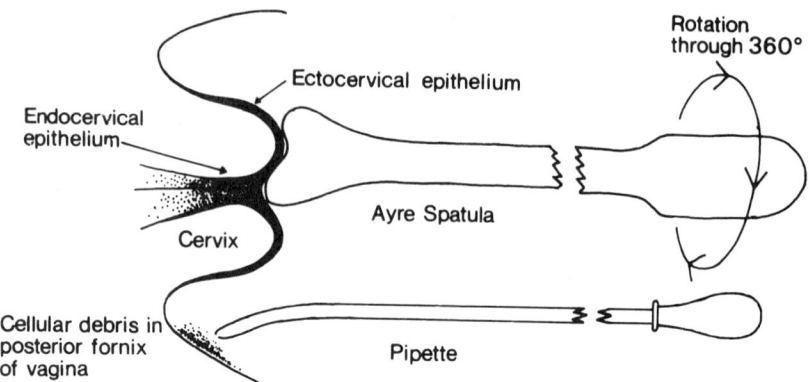

Figure 16. Diagrammatic representation of cervical scrape and aspiration of the posterior fornix of the vagina. The mucus plug at the cervical os should be included with material obtained by means of the Ayre spatula. This mucus plug and the cellular debris in the posterior fornix are disturbed if cytology is preceded by digital examination.

little cervical material. Obtaining an adequate cervical scrape entails a good exposure of the cervix and the services of a trained operator. Nurses can be trained to use a satisfactory technique (Osborne and Leyshon, 1966), though they may still lack the ability to give a judgement on the clinical state of the cervix or of the other pelvic organs. The information provided by such judgement can be very valuable to the cytohistologist.

Rewell (1960), referring to cytological specimens, emphasises that 'success is so dependent on small points of technique beyond the control of the pathologists, and in none is a good preparation so essential to success'.

Whichever technique is used to obtain a smear, sterile equipment should always be used. The general practitioner who is unable to obtain access to a central supply department for instruments, should use a disposable speculum. Perfunctory cleaning and boiling do not destroy monilia or trichomonas organisms, and these are readily transferred from one woman to another. Lubricants tend to spoil the quality of the smear and should therefore be used sparingly. The aspirate of the vagina or the scrape of the cervix should be taken before performing a digital pelvic examination.

During the period of menstruation, cervical scrape or vaginal aspirate should be avoided because of contamination by endometrial debris. The optimum time for a cytotest is during the third week of the menstrual cycle. In all but a few instances, however, the availability of the patient should determine the timing of the cytotest, with the possible exception of the period of menstruation.

In January 1972, the Department of Health and Social Security introduced a modification of the standardised request form which accompanies the cervical smear. Forms are available from Family Practitioner Committees (ECN 877, October 1971). One of the advantages which the form offers the general practitioner is an assurance that a copy is sent ultimately to the patient's own doctor, irrespective of who takes the smear.

Microscopic examination

Examination of the material obtained by vaginal aspirate or cervical scrape is made by a cytologist or trained technician.

The method involves an organised microscopic scanning of the smear. There have been occasional reports of general practitioners undertaking their own scanning of smears (Rivett, 1964). The work of the scanner is made easier when the smear is thinly spread and when the material has come from the correct location. An excessive amount of blood or pus on the smear may interfere with the microscopic appearance.

Electronic scanning instruments have been devised (McMaster, 1965) but have not yet achieved acceptable accuracy.

The cellular changes between the obviously normal cell and the frankly malignant cell range over a wide spectrum. The size of the cell, the size of the nucleus, the density of the nucleus, and the relative amount of cytoplasm are factors which the cytologist has to consider. The ultimate decision is dependent more on the subjective criteria defined by the individual cytologist rather than on standardised objective measurement.

Interpretation of reports

The cytologist will usually report the microscopic findings in some detail. The presence of trichomonas vaginalis or monilia or inflamatory cells may be reported. He may also record his interpretation of the findings, and may state that a smear is normal or abnormal.

Certain features of the report are important and call for emphasis.

1 The cytologist does not make a diagnosis of cancer. The presence of malignant or suspicious looking cells (dyskaryotic or dysplasic cells) may be recorded. Cancer is not determined by the appearance of a cell, but rather by what the cell does. The cells of invasive cancer and carcinoma *in situ* can have similar appearance, and it cannot be determined from a cervical smear or vaginal aspirate if the barrier of the basement membrane is broken.

2 A report which is negative does not exclude cancer. False negative reports are not uncommon. Garrett (1964) found 13 per cent of false negatives in 30 symptomless carcinomas of the cervix. The Manchester Regional Cytology Laboratory found an error rate which meant that 'as many as one in five precancerous lesions remain undetected, among women who had the test only once' (Cytology Newsletter, 1971). This report is based on the re-examination of 7,500 women known to have a 'normal' smear.

3 Infection causes a considerable increase in the number of inflammatory cells deposited on the smear. The normal appearance of non-inflammatory cells may be distorted. In the presence of infection the cytologist may be unable to detect other cellular material, let alone determine their characteristics. Such smears cannot be regarded as normal, and must always be repeated after treatment of the infection.

Use of cervical cytology in general practice

The cervical cytotest has been used in general practice for two main reasons. Some doctors have achieved success with screening programmes, and others have used the test as part of routine gynaecological examination.

Routine gynaecological examination.

For some general practitioners the cervical smear is a part of routine gynaecological examination (Freeling, 1965; Lloyd, 1967). A cervical smear should be taken whenever symptoms suggest disease of the genital tract, and particularly if the cervix appears to be normal on clinical examination. The post-natal examination offers opportunity to take a smear (Scott, 1965).

Abnormalities which may be revealed by a cervical smear include infective or inflammatory conditions as well as neoplastic changes. Trichomonas vaginalis and monilia infection are frequently encountered. Collinson (1968) found ten times as much trichomonas vaginalis as malignant tissue in 354 smears taken in general practice. A cervical smear or vaginal aspirate offers the general practitioner opportunity to confirm a clinical diagnosis of either monilia or trichomonas infection. Cassie and Stevenson (1973) state that cytology is the most reliable method of diagnosis of trichomonas infection.

Screening programmes

Screening can be described as 'The determined investigation of population groups who have "at risk" characteristics of a particular disease.' There is a need to identify the population and the illness, and for an organised programme (Lloyd, 1973).

The general practitioner who maintains an age-sex register of his patients and who has adequate nursing support, is suitably placed to undertake a screening programme for cervical cancer. A number of such programmes have been described. Ashworth (1964) reported a response of 20 per cent to a single invitation to women in the 30-39 age group. More recently, Hodes (1972) reported a 44 per cent response to a first invitation and this was increased by a further 12 per cent after a reminder. Better results have been reported. Scaiffe (1972) obtained an 88 per cent response following repeated invitations to women aged 35-50, and Rose (1972) secured a 91 per cent success among 1,319 'eligible' women in a single group practice. Properly conducted programmes, using the resources available in general practice, including the nurse, can succeed.

The numbers of cancers of the cervix detected in each of these programmes is small and it cannot be established what the outcome would have been for the patients concerned, had the smears not been taken.

Carcinoma *in situ* and invasive cancer

Cervical cytology screening programmes have been endowed on the premise that if they are universally applied, death from cancer of the cervix can be abolished (Green *et al.*, 1970). If this objective is to be achieved, then cancer of the cervix has to be anticipated. The rationale of such anticipation lies in establishing a relationship between carcinoma *in situ* and invasive cancer.

The probability of carcinoma *in situ* becoming invasive has been variously estimated to lie between 100 per cent (MacGregor, 1966), and less than 10 per cent (Green, 1970). Bamforth and Cardell reported in 1962 that of the 653 biopsies of the cervix at Kings College Hospital, London, for the period 1951-1960, squamous cell carcinoma was diagnosed in 125 instances, and in 26 of these areas of carcinoma *in situ* were also encountered. The apparent progression of *in situ* lesions to invasive cancer has been reported by a number of gynaecologists who have observed women who had *in situ* lesions for five to ten years (Sagiroglu, 1963; Copenhauer, 1963; Petersen, 1956; Koss, 1961). Petersen reports the development of invasive cancer in 33 per cent of *in situ* lesions within nine years and four per cent within one year. Koss reported that *in situ* lesions became invasive in 25 per cent, remained stationary in 50 per cent and regressed in 25 per cent. The time interval between the onset of *in situ* lesions and the development of invasive cancer has been calculated to be variously between 4 years (Wilson, 1961) and 20 years (MacGregor, 1966). The general consensus seems to be that the most likely interval is about 11 years.

There is still no absolute evidence that all *in situ* lesions will become invasive, though it can no longer be reasonable to anticipate the outcome. A relationship between pre-invasive and invasive cancer has been sufficiently established to require aggressive treatment of pre-invasive lesions. ·

Women at special risk

Certain women have an increased risk of cancer of the cervix. Non-Jewish women have been found to have a higher incidence (Anderson, 1953; Stern, 1959). Baird (1965) stated that women in social class five had 20 times the incidence of cancer of the cervix compared with the wives of professional men. A very close correlation with socio-economic status is suggested by more recent observers (Wakefield *et al.*, 1973).

Baird suggests that early marriage and multiparity places a woman in a high risk category. Until the age of 40, pre-invasive lesions are more common than invasive cancer; after age 40, the reverse is true (Carter *et al.*, 1965; Petersen, 1956). Wynder (1955) quotes Rozel of Copenhagen as stating that prostitutes have a high incidence of cancer of the cervix. A high incidence of cancer of the cervix in women who maintain poor personal hygiene has also been reported (Lawson, 1957; Rao, Reddy and Reddy, 1959).

An additional risk, compounding that for most of the women already at special risk, is unwillingness to attend cervical cytology test clinics. Only a proportion of women at risk make use of screening facilities for cervical cancer. The ones who do are those in the higher social grades (Stocks, 1955; Lawson, 1957; Boyd and Doll, 1964; Wakefield, 1971). The chance of cancer and of a positive smear is lower among these women (MacGregor and Baird, 1963).

A cytology service offered to the staff of the Manchester Regional Hospital Board and Blood Transfusion Service attracted a response of only 46 per cent, even when patients with good reason for declining the test are excluded. Among the female staff of the Regional Hospital Board, the proportion tested was higher in those aged over 55 (Cytology Newsletter, 1972). Refusal to attend for cervical cytotest has been found to be associated with psychiatric illness, previous hysterectomy, being unmarried, and having had a recent smear test (Hodes, 1972). The fear of cancer, or of operation, and apathy, are suggested by Scaiffe (1972) as significant barriers to the acceptance of cervical smears.

Publicity about cytotests has failed to reach a substantial number of women (Davison and Clements, 1971). Analysis of enquiry among 1,106 women attending Manchester Local Health Authority Clinics for cervical smear tests showed that only 21 per cent cited a poster as their source of information (Cytology Newsletter, 1972).

Conclusion

A satisfactory solution to the vexing dilemma of attaining a high level of screening among the population most at risk does not yet seem to have emerged (Allman *et al.*, 1974). A few well motivated general practitioners have achieved very creditable results. There is, however, no substantial evidence that many general practitioners recognise screening for cervical cancer to be a significant part of their role.

The hopes of many were summarised by Miller in 1967, when he stated 'The epitaph for invasive cancer should now be written'. As yet, this hope is not nearly being realised in general practice.

REFERENCES

Allman, S. T., Chamberlain, J. & Harman, P. (1974). The national cervical cytology recall system: report of a pilot study. *Health Trends*, 6, 39-41.

Anderson, A. F. (1953). Latent cancer of the cervix. *Journal of Obstetrics and Gynaecology of the British Empire*, 60, 353-362.

Ashworth, H. W. (1964). Presymptomatic diagnosis of carcinoma of cervix. *Medical World*, August.

Ayre, J. E. (1947). Selective cytology smear for diagnosis of cancer. *American Journal of Obstetrics and Gynaecology*, 53, 609-617.

Ayre, J. E. (1962). A simple method, that can be used in the doctor's office for detection of cancer of the uterus. *Gynaecologie Practique*, 13, 247.

Baird, D. (1965). The use of continuous suction in gynaecological surgery. *Journal of Obstetrics and Gynaecology of the British Commonwealth*, 72, 259.

Bamforth, J. & Cardell, B. S. (1962). The laboratory diagnosis of carcinoma of the uterine cervix. *Journal of Obstetrics and Gynaecology of the British Commonwealth*, 69, 379.

Barry, M. (1847). *On the nucleus of the Animal and Vegetable 'Cell'*. Edinburgh: Neill and Co.

Beale, L. S. (1860/61). Examination of sputum from a case of cancer of the pharynx and adjacent parts. *Arch. Med.* 2, 44.

Biermer, A. (1855). *Die Lehre Vom Auswurf.* Wurzburg.

Boyd, J. T. & Doll, R. (1964). A study of the aetiology of carcinoma of the cervix uteri. *British Journal of Cancer*, 18, 419.

Boyes, D. A., Fidler, H. K. & Lock, D. R. (1962). The British Columbia project. *British Medical Journal*, 1, 203.

Broders, A. C. (1932). Carcinoma in situ contrasted with benign penetrating epithelium. *Journal of the American Medical Association.* 99, 1670.

B. M. A. (1964). *British Medical Journal*, 2, Supplement, p. 3417.

Carter, B., Wyler, W. K., Kaufmann, L. A., Thomas, W. L., Creadick, R. N., Parker, R. T., Peete, C. H. & Cherry, W. B. (1965). Clinical problems in stage 0 (intraepithelial) cancer of the cervix. *American Journal of Obstetrics and Gynaecology*, 71, 634.

Cassie, R. & Stevenson, A. (1973). Screening for gonorrhoea, trichomoniasis, moniliasis and syphilis in pregnancy. *Journal of Obstetrics and Gynaecology of the British Commonwealth*, **880**, 48.

Collinson, V. F. (1968). A cervical cytology survey in general practice. *Journal of the Royal College of General Practitioners*, **16**, 446.

Copenhaver, E. H. (1963). Obstacles in the control of cancer of the cervix. *Postgraduate Medicine*, **33**, 4.

Cytology, Newsletter, (1971). Vol. 1, No. 3. Issued by the Local Co-ordinating Committee on Cervical Cytology for the Manchester Region.

Cytology, Newsletter, (1972). Vol. 2, No. 1. Issued by the Local Co-ordinating Committee on Cervical Cytology for the Manchester Region.

Davis, H. J. & Kurz, L. (1962). Detection of preinvasive cancer by the irrigation smear technique. *Danish Medical Bulletin*, **9**, 121.

Davison, R. L. & Clements, J. C. (1971). Why don't they attend for a cytotest? A pilot study among a high-risk population. *Medical Officer*, **125**, 329.

Dobell, C. (1960). *Antony Van Leeuwenhoek and his 'Little Animals.'* New York: Dover Publications Inc. 76.

Donné, A. (1837). *Recherches microscopiques sur la nature des mucus et de la matiers des ecoulemens*. Paris.

Fidler, H. K., Boyes, D. A. & Worth, A. J. (1968). Cervical cancer detection in British Columbia. *Journal of Obstetrics and Gynaecology of the British Commonwealth*, **75**, 392.

Freeling, P. (1965). Candidates for exfoliative cytology of the cervix. *Journal of the College of General Practitioners*, **10**, 261.

Garrett, W. J. (1964). Symptomless carcinoma of the cervix. *Journal of Obstetrics and Gynaecology of the British Commonwealth*, **71**, 517.

Green, G. H. (1966). The significance of cervical carcinoma in situ. *American Journal of Obstetrics and Gynaecology*, **94**, 1009.

Green, G. H. & Donovan, J. W. (1970). The natural history of cervical carcinoma in situ. *Journal of Obstetrics and Gynaecology of the British Commonwealth*, **77**, 1.

Hodes, C. (1972). Cervical screening—refusal in general practice. *Journal of the Royal College of General Practitioners*, **22**, 172.

Husain, O. A. N. (1968). *The early diagnosis of cancer of the cervix*. Early Diagnosis Paper No. 3. London: Office of Health Economics.

Jeffcoate, T. N. A. (1957). *Principles of Gynaecology*. London: Butterworth.

Jeffcoate, T. N. A. (1966). Cervical Cytology. Its value and limitations. *British Medical Journal*, **2**, 1091.

Koss, G. L. (1961). Carcinoma in situ. *British Medical Journal*, **2**, 1571.

Kinlen, L. J. & Doll, R. (1973). Trends in mortality from cancer of the uterus in Canada and in England and Wales. *British Journal of Preventive and Social Medicine*, **27**, 146.

Lawson, J. G. (1957). Cancer of the uterine cervix; an enquiry into predisposing factors, with special reference to earlier diagnosis. *Journal of Obstetrics and Gynaecology of the British Empire*, **64**, 488.

Lloyd, G. (1967). Cervical cytology in general practice. *Journal of the Royal College of General Practitioners*, **13**, 63.

Lloyd, G. (1973). The use of investigations in a general practice. *Journal of the Royal College of General Practitioners*, **23**, 326.

McCarty, W. C. (1914). Studies in the etiology of cancer; IV. Notes on the regularity and similarity of cancer cells. *Collected Papers Mayo Clinic*, **6**, 600.

MacGregor, J. E. (1966). A study of clinically and cytologically detected cervical cancers in the city of Aberdeen. *Acta Cytologica* (Baltimore) **10**, 246.

MacGregor, J. E. & Baird, D. (1963). The Aberdeen Project. *British Medical Journal*, **1**, 1631.

McMaster, G. W. (1965). Quantitative scanning of cervical cells. *Journal of Obstetrics and Gynaecology of the British Commonwealth*, **72**, 936.

Miller, T. R. (1967). Translumbar amputation for carcinoma of the vagina. *Obs. Gyn. Survey*, **22**, 167.

Osborn, G. R. & Leyshon, V. N. (1966). Domiciliary testing of cervical smears by home nurses. *Lancet*, **1**, 256.

Papanicolau, G. N. (1942). New procedure for staining vaginal smears. *Science*, **95**, 438.

Parry, W. H. & Wilson, L. A. (1971). Cervical cytology in Nottingham. 1966-70. *Medical Officer*, **125**, 85.

Petersen, O. (1956). Spontaneous cause of cervical precancerous conditions. *American Journal of Obstetrics and Gynaecology*, **72**, 1063.

Rao, P. S., Reddy, R. S. & Reddy, D. J. A. (1959). A study of the aetiological factors in carcinoma of cervix uteri in Guntur. *Journal of the Indian Medical Association*, **32**, 463.

Registrar General (1971). Dicennial Supplement, England and Wales, 1961. Occupational Mortality Tables.

Rewell, R. E. (1960). *Obstetrical and Gynaecological Pathology*. E. & S. Livingstone, Edinburgh and London.

Rivett, G. (1964). Cervical cytology in general practice. *British Medical Journal*, 2, 1531.

Rose Elizabeth, (1972). Cervical cytology survey in a general practice, 1964-1970. *Update* January. 19.

Sagiroglu, N. (1963). Progression and regression studies of pre-cancer (anaplastic or dysplastic) cells, and the halo test. *American Journal of Obstetrics and Gynaecology*, 85, 454.

Scaiffe, B. (1972). Survey of cervical cytology in general practice. *British Medical Journal*, 3, 200.

Scott, J. S. (1965). Care in the puerperium. *Practitioner*, 194, 781.

Smithers, D. W. (1956). Clinical cancer research. *Lancet*, 1, 253.

Stern, E. (1959). Rate, stage, and patient age in cervical cancer. An analysis of age specific discovery rates for atypical hyperplasia in situ cancer, and invasive cancer in a well population. *Cancer*, 12, 933.

Stocks, P. (1955). Cancer of uterine cervix and social conditions. *British Journal of Cancer*, 9, 487.

Thomson, J. G. (1971). Cervical cytology in England and Wales: Some facts. *Health Trends*, 3, 24.

Troup, F. (1886). *Sputum: Its microscopy and diagnostic and prognostic significance*. Edinburgh: Oliver and Boyd.

T. U. C. Congress Resolutions 1964 and 1966.

Virchow, R. (1863). *Cellular pathology as based upon physiological and pathological histology; twenty lectures, February/April 1858*. Translated by Frank Chance, Philadelphia.

Wakefield, J. (1971). The family doctor and cervical cytology. A study of 38,741 women. *Health Trends*, 3, 25.

Wakefield, D. J., Yule, R., Smith A. & Adelstein, A. (1973). Relation of abnormal cytological smears and carcinoma of cervix uteri to husband's occupation. *British Medical Journal*, 2, 142.

Walshe, W. H. (1841). *A practical treatise on the diseases of the lungs and heart*. London: Blanshard and Lea.

Way, S. (1955). *Modern trends in Obstetrics and Gynaecology*. London: Butterworth.

Wilson, J. M. G. (1961). Screening for cervical cancer. *Monthly Bulletin of the Ministry of Health*, (London). 20, 214.

Wookey, B. E. P. (1971). Exfoliative cytology in general practice. *British Medical Journal*, 3, 31.

Wynder, E. L. (1955). Environmental factors in cervical cancer. An approach to its prevention. *British Medical Journal*, 1, 743

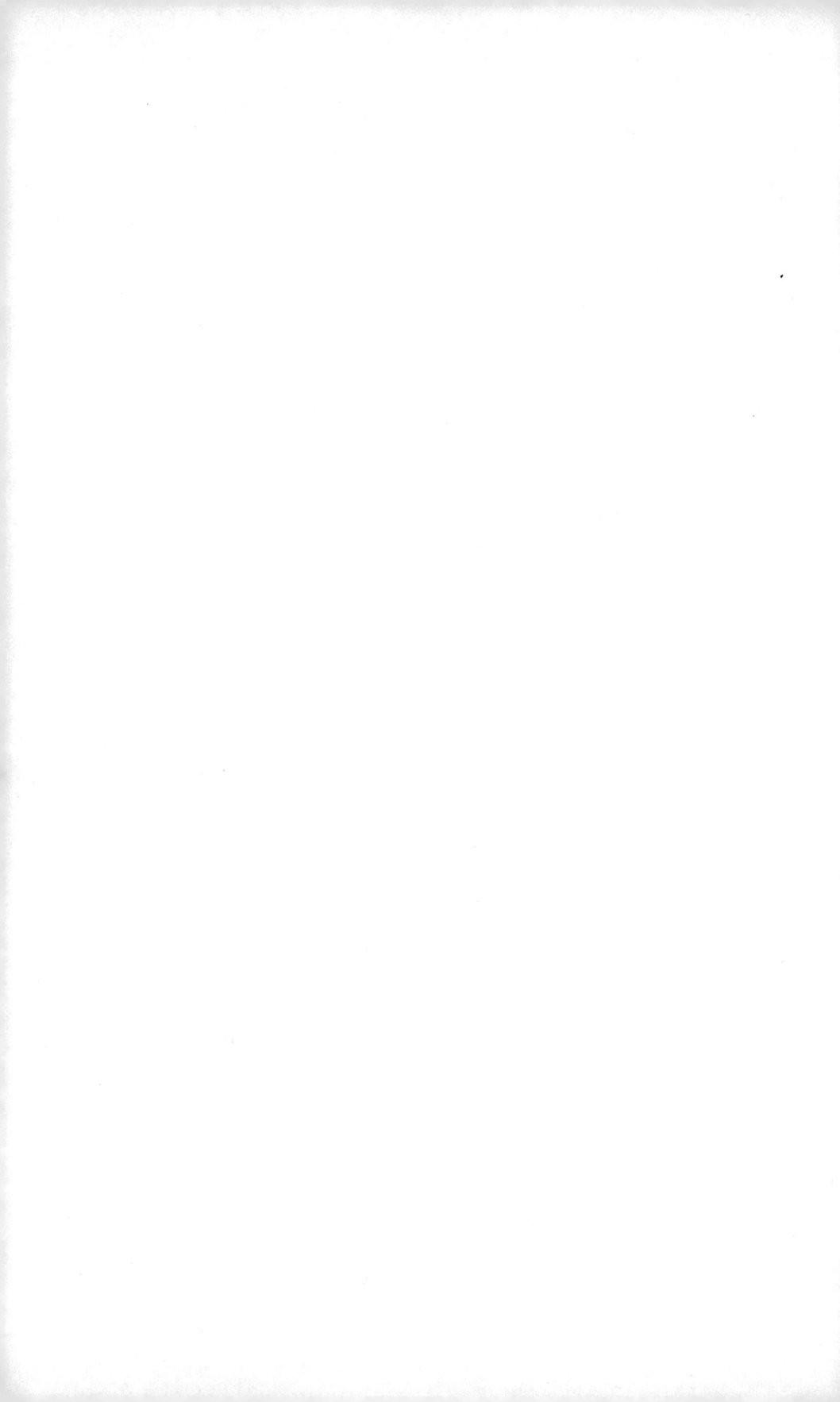

Bibliography

Acheson, E. D. (1968). *Record Linkage in Medicine.* Edinburgh: E. & S. Livingstone.

Asscher, A. W. (1970). *The early Diagnosis of Urinary Tract Infection.* London: Office of Health Economics.

Cannel, C. & Kahne, R. (1957). *The Dynamics of Interviewing.* London: Chapman & Hall.

Cartwright, A. (1967). *Patients and their Doctors: A Study of General Practice.* London: Routledge & Kegan Paul.

Cochrane, A. L. (1972). *Effectiveness and Efficiency: Random Reflections on Health Services.* Nuffield Provincial Hospitals Trust.

Cochrane, A. L. & Fletcher, C. M. (1968). *The Early Diagnosis of Some Diseases of the Lung.* London: Office of Health Economics.

Cotes, J. E. (1968). *Lung Function. Assessment and Application in Medicine,* 2nd Edn. Oxford: Blackwell Scientific.

Craddock, D. (1973). *Obesity and its Management.* 2nd Edn. London: Churchill Livingstone.

Davie, R., Butler, N. & Goldstein H. (1972). *From Birth to Seven,* London: Longmans.

Egan, D. F., Illingworth, R. S., & McKeith, R. C. (1969). *Developmental Screening, 0-5 years. Clinics in Developmental Medicine,* London: Spastics International Medical Publications, in association with William Heinemann Medical Books Limited.

Evans, K. T. & Gravelle, I. H. (1973). *Mammography, Thermography and Ultrasonography in Breast Disease.* London: Butterworth.

Eysenck, H. J. & Eysenck, S. B. G. (1964). *Manual of the Eysenck Personality Inventory.* London University Press.

Ferrer, H. P. (1968). *Screening for Health.* London: Butterworths.

Fry, J. (1966). *Profiles of Disease.* Edinburgh: E. & S. Livingstone.

Gelman, A. C. (1971). *Multiphasic Health Testing Systems: Reviews and Annotations.* Rochville, U.S.A.: U.S. Department of Health, Education, and Welfare.

Goldberg, E. M., Mortimer, A. & Williams, B. T. (1970). *Helping the Aged.* London: Allen & Unwin.

Graham, P. H. (1967). *The Early Diagnosis of Field Defects.* London: Office of Health Economics.

Hodgkin, K. (1973). *Towards Earlier Diagnosis.* 3rd Edn. London: Churchill Livingstone.

Holland, W. W. (1967). *The Early Diagnosis of Raised Arterial Blood Pressure.* London: Office of Health Economics.

Husain, O. A. N. (1968). *The Early Diagnosis of Cancer of the Cervix.* London: Office of Health Economics.

Illingworth, D. G. (1970). *The Health Check in Practice.* Hemel Hempstead: Educare.

Illingworth, R. S. (1972). *Development of the Infant and Young Child, Normal and Abnormal.* 4th Edition. Edinburgh & London: Churchill Livingstone.

Joseph, M. C. & MacKeith, R. C. (1966). *A New Look at Child Care.* London: Pitman Medical.

McLachlan, G., Editor (1971). *Problems and Progress in Medical Care.* Oxford University Press: Nuffield Provincial Hospitals Trust.

McLachlan, G. & Shegog, R. F. A. (1968). *Computers in the Service of Medicine.* Volumes I and II. London: Oxford University Press.

Oppenheim, A. N. (1966). *Questionnaire Design and Attitude Measurements.* Heinemann.

Payne, F. L. (1951). *The Art of Asking Questions.* London: Oxford University Press.

Pearse, I. H. & Crocker, L. (1943). *The Peckham Experiment.* London: Allen & Unwin.

Rawnsley, K. (1968). *The Early Diagnosis of Depression.* London: Office of Health Economics.

Raynor, E. (1971). *Human Development.* London: Allen & Unwin.

Robinson, D. (1971). *The Process of Becoming Ill.* London: Routledge & Kegan Paul.

Sharp, C. L. E. H. & Keen, H. (1968). *Presymptomatic Detection and Early Diagnosis.* London: Pitman Medical.

Smithells, R. W. (1969). *The Early Diagnosis of Congenital Anomalies.* London: Office of Health Economics.

Social Science Research Unit (1969). *A Multiple Screening Clinic, Rotherham 1966: A Social and Economic Assessment.* London: HMSO.

Teeling-Smith, G., Editor (1966). *Surveillance and Early Diagnosis in General Practice.* London: Office of Health Economics,

Vitalograph Manual (1973). *The Simple Measurement of Lung Ventilation.* Vitalograph Limited, Buckingham, England.

Wakefield, J. (1972). *Seeking Wisely to Prevent.* London: HMSO.

Walker, J. B. & Kerridge, D. (1961). *Diabetes in an English Community.* Leicester University Press.

Wilson, J. M. G. & Jungner, G. (1968). *Principles and Practice of Screening for Disease.* Geneva: WHO Public Health Paper No. 34.

Wolfe, J. N. (1972). *Xeroradiography of the Breast.* Springfield Illinois, Charles C. Thomas.

Index

Computer Typesetting by Print Origination, Bootle Merseyside L20 6NS
Printed by Thomson Litho, East Kilbride, Scotland